The Law of Hospital and Health Care Administration

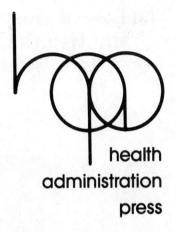

health
administration
press

The Law of Hospital and Health Care Administration

Arthur F. Southwick, M.B.A., J.D.
PROFESSOR OF BUSINESS LAW AND HOSPITAL ADMINISTRATION
THE UNIVERSITY OF MICHIGAN

with contributions on the Anglo-American legal system
and on professional liability by
George J. Siedel III, J.D.
ASSOCIATE PROFESSOR OF BUSINESS LAW
THE UNIVERSITY OF MICHIGAN

health
administration
press

Library of Congress Cataloging in Publication Data

Southwick, Arthur F
     The law of hospital and health care administration.

     Bibliography: p.
     Includes index.
     1. Hospitals--United States--Laws and legislation.
2. Medical care--Law and legislation--United States.
I. Siedel, George J., joint author. II. Title.
[DNLM: 1. Public health administration--United States
--Legislation. 2. Legislation, Hospital--United States.
WX33 AA1 S7L]
KF3825.S65   344'.73'03211   78-4846
ISBN 0-914904-27-2

Preface

This book was prepared in response to a need expressed by graduate students in health administration, School of Public Health, University of Michigan, for text and reference materials relating to the legal aspects of health care. Accordingly, the primary aim was to provide a classroom text for use by students preparing for professional careers in the management of health care institutions.

Such a textbook should also serve as a reference book for further inquiry and research, especially in an area as dynamic as the laws pertaining to health care. For that reason most of the chapters in this book contain extensive citation of current legal authority to support the textual material and as a guide to further study. Because this field has not yet received much attention, professional counsel for health care practitioners and institutions may also find the work helpful. Thus, the book has been written with two purposes in mind: the volume should serve as a base for academic study, while simultaneously fulfilling a role as a reference book for students and for professional legal counsel.

When a course in law is presented to lay students preparing for professional careers as managers of health care institutions, as government officials, or as practitioners of medicine, the purposes of the instruction must be carefully delineated from the outset. These purposes are threefold: to teach students to recognize a legal issue or problem inherent in a given set of facts or circumstance; to present the issues in such a way as to encourage consultation with professional legal counsel; and finally, to convey an understanding and appreciation of counsel's role in advising clients with respect to their legal position. Courses in law for lay students are thus thoroughly justified and indeed mandatory for this reason: an intelligent administrator or manager who is able to recognize a legal issue and to communicate with professional counsel can do much to prevent and minimize legal problems and adversary situations. Students reading and studying law should direct their constant attention to this question: what should counsel and I together do to prevent a legal issue or adversary situation from arising?

Future health care managers and practitioners of the healing arts must also be reminded that their study of this book, though useful, will not equip them to serve as their own legal counsel. As is true of all works on legal matters, this text is intended to provide authoritative information regarding the subject matter covered—but not to supplant professional legal counsel when professional service is needed. Since the facts of a given situation and local law determine the advice given by counsel to a client or the outcome of a given question, individual counsel is indispensable to the health care institution and practicing physician. What the publisher and author hope for is that the work will be a source of information for concerned students, administrators, physicians, and legal advisers to help in identifying legal issues and to provide a general overview of the fundamental principles that guide the possible resolution of those issues.

The most effective method for instruction in law is clearly the study of cases. The facts of any given situation determine both the outcome of litigation and the appropriate administrative policy. Because students studying law for the first time seldom realize this fundamental underpinning of the Anglo-American legal system, they must read cases (and statutes) to appreciate how and why rules of law are developed and to understand the application of rules to solve particular questions. Case instruction also serves to emphasize that rules of law are constantly being changed, expanded, modified; that not all jurisdictions follow the same rules; that courts as well as legislative bodies play an active role in the development of law; and that there is constant interaction between judicial and legislative bodies. In my classroom in Ann Arbor I have students read selected cases in their entirety as a supplement to the text, and we discuss those cases in class.*

A glance at the table of contents will reveal that this book is limited in its scope. Primarily, the subject matter can be identified as "private law"—the law relating to the mutual rights and responsibilities of private individuals and institutions—discussed under five headings:

---

*A list of these cases may be obtained from the author.

Introduction to Law and the Anglo-American Legal System, The Hospital as a Corporation, The Physician-Patient Relationship, The Hospital-Patient Relationship, and The Hospital-Physician Relationship. Most of the material, therefore, relates to the private law of contract, tort, and property. Where it is relevant to private relationships, there is of course extensive discussion of current doctrines relating to constitutional law.

Excluded from this volume is that vast body of developing law known as "public law," the law of governmental regulation of the health care industry. Many students and readers will be understandably disappointed by this omission, realizing that governmental regulation is in many respects of greater current concern to the manager of a hospital or health care institution than is the common law of contract and tort, for example. Nevertheless, I believe that a discussion of the legal aspects of governmental regulation of the health industry is best reserved for a separate book and that the subject should be taught only after the student has studied the private law.

I am indebted to my colleague and friend, Professor George J. Siedel III of the Graduate School of Business Administration, University of Michigan, for his contribution of three chapters: a chapter introducing the Anglo-American Legal System and two chapters discussing the professional liability of a physician to his patients. Professor Siedel has had experience as a practicing attorney and is now committed to the full-time teaching of law to students in other fields. Moreover, he has a real and genuine appreciation for the practice of medicine, since three members of his wife's family are practicing physicians.

This book could not have been written and published without the help and support of three persons who verified all citations of legal authority: Stephen E. Wagner, Stephen A. Cooper, and David B. Miller. At the time of their work they were law students at the University of Michigan and all are now members of the Bar. I am grateful and indebted to each of them. Nevertheless, of course, the ultimate responsibility for the accuracy and the interpretation of case and statutory authority is mine alone.

I am also indebted to Mrs. Rosannah C. Steinhoff, who served as editor of this manuscript. For many years Mrs. Steinhoff was senior editor for the Division of Research, Graduate School of Business Administration, University of Michigan. Now retired from the University she continues to be active in her profession, and it was my distinct pleasure to work with her as she read, challenged, and advised with respect to this work. Although several persons participated in the typing of the manuscript, I wish to thank especially Ms. Judy Kindig, who carefully and in painstaking fashion prepared much of the final copy for the printer.

Portions of the text represent revision, expansion, and updating of some of my earlier writings for law reviews. Acknowledgments for permission to use previously copyrighted material are noted on a separate page.

Finally, my sincere gratitude and thanks are extended to the graduate students in health care administration, numbering more than 200, who used preliminary drafts of this text in my courses. During the three semesters in which the material was presented in manuscript form, their comments and questions were invaluable guides to final revision of the work. They and my other students in this field are the persons who have motivated me to speak and write on a dynamic area of law that is of vital interest and concern to society. Every class hour with these dedicated students has been a delightful experience.

Arthur F. Southwick

Ann Arbor, Michigan
December, 1977

Acknowledgments

The definitions of law, private law, and public law and the description of administrative agencies and the administrative process in Chapter I are from an earlier publication: *The Doctor, the Hospital, and the Patient in England: Rights and Responsibilities* by Arthur F. Southwick, Michigan International Business Studies No. 6 (Ann Arbor: Bureau of Business Research, Graduate School of Business Administration, University of Michigan, 1967), copyright by the University of Michigan. The material is used by permission of the Division of Research, University of Michigan Graduate School of Business Administration.

Chapter VII is revised and expanded from a previous publication: "Legal Aspects of the Emergency Department" by Arthur F. Southwick, in Spencer, James H., *The Hospital Emergency Department*, 1972. Courtesy of Charles C. Thomas, Publisher, Springfield, Illinois.

Chapter XII is revised and expanded from an article contributed by Arthur F. Southwick to Wecht, Cyril H. (ed.), *Legal Medicine Annual 1970*. Courtesy of Appleton-Century Crofts, Publishing Division of Prentice-Hall, Inc. Chapters XII and XIII include materials from two previously published articles by Arthur F. Southwick: "Hospital Medical Staff Privileges," from *DePaul Law Review*, Summer 1969, courtesy of De Paul University College of Law; and "The Hospital as an Institution—Expanding Responsibilities Change Its Relationship with the Staff Physician," from *California Western Law Review*, Spring 1973, courtesy of California Western School of Law.

The Joint Commission on Accreditation of Hospitals has kindly granted permission to quote from the *Accreditation Manual for Hospitals*, 1976 and from the three supplements to the *Manual*.

Contents

PART ONE

Introduction to Law and the Legal System

George J. Siedel III

I

The Anglo-American Legal System

The study of law is essential to the health care professional. With the many social and technological changes of recent years, law has assumed great, some would say exaggerated, importance in the daily affairs of men and women. Nowhere have changes been greater and the legal issues more challenging than in health care. Unfortunately, health care professionals cannot have an attorney constantly at hand when they are confronted with the myriad statutes, administrative regulations, and court decisions that have become so important to health care law. Consequently, they must have a fundamental understanding of the law so that they can at least perceive serious legal problems that do require professional legal counsel.

In this chapter some general concepts essential to any study of law will be examined, with special emphasis on three areas: the sources of the law, the court system, and legal procedure. First, however, a working definition of law will be useful. Defined in its simplest and broadest sense, law is a system of principles and rules devised by organized society for the purpose of controlling human conduct. Society must have certain specified standards of behavior and the means to enforce the standards. In the final analysis the purpose of law is to avoid conflict between individuals and between government and subject. Inevitably conflicts do occur, however, and then legal institutions and doctrines supply the means of resolving the disputes.

Since law is concerned with human behavior it falls short of being an exact science. Much of law is uncertain. Rules of law often fail to guarantee particular results in individual controversies. Lawyers are many times unable to predict with authority the outcome of current conflict. As economic and social conditions change, law must be changed, and these changes frequently produce legal uncertainties.

3

But in a sense uncertainty about the law is a virtue and the law's greatest strength. Its opposite, legal rigidity, produces decay by inhibiting initiative with respect to economic growth and the development of social institutions.

Sources of Law

Law can be classified as either public law or private law, depending upon its subject matter. That body of law which concerns the government or its relations with individuals is classified as public law. In contrast, the term private law refers to the rules and principles which define and regulate rights and duties between individuals. Without doubt these two broad classifications of law have become intermixed in modern societies, and it is not always possible or advisable to assign arbitrarily a given rule of law to one classification or the other. Yet the classifications are accepted as useful in understanding Anglo-American legal doctrine.

The concept of private law embraces much of the law of contracts, property, and tort. The law of contracts is concerned with such matters as the sale of goods, the furnishing of services, the employment of others, and the loan of money. In its broadest sense the law of property regulates the ownership, employment, and disposition of property, including the creation and operation of trusts. Tort law defines and enforces those respective duties and rights which exist between individuals but are independent of contractual agreement between the parties. These three areas of private law vitally influence the conduct of all human enterprise and activity.

In contrast to private law, the purpose of public law is to define, regulate, and enforce rights where any part or agency of government is a party to the subject matter, which includes among other topics labor relations, taxation, antitrust, and municipal corporations. Generally the primary and original sources of public law, substantive and procedural, are written constitutions and statutory enactments by a legislative body, complemented by a third source, administrative law. This fact alone distinguishes public law from private law, since the primary source of private rights and duties is judicial decision, subject to statutory modification and codification. In the following paragraphs, we will examine more closely these four primary sources of public and private law: constitutions, statutes, administrative law, and judicial decisions.

CONSTITUTIONS

The United States Constitution is aptly called the "supreme law of the land," for the Constitution provides a standard against which all other laws are to be judged. In the most basic terms the Constitution is a grant of power from the states to the federal government. All powers not granted to the federal government by the Constitution are reserved in the individual states. The grant of power to the federal government is both express and implied. The Constitution, for example, expressly authorizes Congress to lay and collect taxes, to borrow and coin money, to declare war, to raise and support armies, and to regulate interstate commerce. But Congress may also enact laws which are "necessary and proper" for exercising these powers. To cite one instance relevant to hospital law, the express power of Congress to regulate interstate commerce carries with it the implied power to pass antidiscrimination legislation such as the Civil Rights Act of 1964, an act that will be discussed in greater detail in later chapters.

The Constitution can be divided into two parts. The main body establishes and defines the power of the three branches of the federal government: (1) that of the legislative to make the laws; (2) that of the executive to enforce the laws; and (3) that of the judicial to interpret the laws. As will be seen, this simple breakdown is often imprecise and incorrect, especially in regard to the sources of the law.

Following the main body of the Constitution are twenty-six amendments. The first ten, the Bill of Rights, were ratified shortly after the adoption of the Constitution in order, according to James Madison, to calm the apprehensions of persons who felt that without the specific declaration the federal government might be held to possess these rights. The provisions of the Bill of Rights include the well-known rights to free speech and free exercise of religion, to be secure from unreasonable searches and seizures, to bear arms, to demand a jury trial, to be protected against self-incrimination, and to be accorded due process. Despite the granting of these rights, however, the scope of the first ten amendments is limited: in and of themselves, they only apply to the federal government.

Does this mean that without a provision in the state constitution a state government could take away any or all of the aforementioned rights? The answer, at least before the ratification of the Fourteenth Amendment in 1870, was yes.[1] However, the Fourteenth Amendment in its concluding phrases provides this safeguard: ". . . nor shall any State deprive any person of life, liberty, or property, without due process of law; nor deny to any person within its jurisdiction the equal protection of the laws." The Fourteenth Amendment is

---

[1] *Barron v. Baltimore*, 32 U.S. (7 Pet.) 243 (1833).

especially important for two reasons. First, the Supreme Court has generally defined due process as specifically including the rights set forth in the Bill of Rights. Consequently the states as well as the federal government may not infringe upon these rights. Secondly, and more important to hospital law, what constitutes the "state" or "state action" has been defined very broadly by many courts. Even the operations of a private hospital, for example, might fall under "state action" depending on the interplay of several factors, including the influence of government regulations on hospital policies, the availability of other hospitals in a particular area, the receipt by the hospital of federal or state funding, and the hospital's use of tax exemptions.[2] Whether the activities of a private hospital constitute "state action" is especially important in regard to admission of patients to the hospital and granting hospital staff privileges.[3]

In addition to the Constitution each state has its own constitution which is the supreme law of that state but is subordinate to the federal Constitution. The state and federal constitutions are often similar, although state constitutions are more detailed and cover such matters as the financing of public works and the organization of local governments.

STATUTES

The second source of law, statutory law, is the law enacted by a legislative body, normally the United States Congress, a state legislature, or a local governmental unit such as a city council. In certain branches of hospital law, statutes enacted by each of these bodies will be applicable to a hospital. In regard to discrimination in admitting patients, for example, hospitals must comply with federal statutes such as the Civil Rights Act of 1964 and the Hill-Burton Act, as well as with relevant statutes enacted by states with respect to discrimination, taxation, and licensure, and with local laws. More than half the states and a number of large cities are estimated to have enacted antidiscrimination statutes.

Although, as noted below, statutes have priority as a source of law over conflicting judicial decisions, judges are faced with the task of interpreting statutes; and this is especially difficult if the wording is vague or ambiguous. In interpreting statutes the courts

[2] Siedel, "The Hospital and Abortion," 79 *Case and Comment* 24 (1974).
[3] See, for example, *Simkins v. Moses H. Cone Memorial Hospital*, 323 F. 2d 959 (4th Cir. 1963), *cert. denied*, 376 U.S. 938 (1964); *Eaton v. Grubbs*, 329 F. 2d 710 (1964), *cert. denied*, 359 U.S. 984 (1964); *Sams v. Ohio Valley General Hosp. Ass'n*, 257 F. Supp. 369 (N.D.W. Va. 1966). *Contra: Barrett v. United Hospital*, 376 F. Supp. 791 (S.D.N.Y. 1974), *aff'd.* 506 F. 2d 1395 (2d Cir. 1974).

have developed several rules of construction, and in some states these rules are themselves the subject of a separate statute. Whatever the source of the rules, it is generally agreed that they are designed to help one to ascertain the intention of the legislature. Illustrative of the guidelines a court looks to in determining legislative intent is the following section from the Pennsylvania Statutory Construction Act:

> The object of all interpretation and construction of laws is to ascertain and effectuate the intention of the Legislature. Every law shall be construed, if possible, to give effect to all its provisions.
>
> When the words of a law are clear and free from all ambiguity, the letter of it is not to be disregarded under the pretext of pursuing its spirit.
>
> When the words of a law are not explicit, the intention of the Legislature may be ascertained by considering, among other matters—(1) the occasion and necessity for the law; (2) the circumstances under which it was enacted; (3) the mischief to be remedied; (4) the object to be attained; (5) the former law, if any, including other laws upon the same or similar subject; (6) the consequences of a particular interpretation; (7) the contemporaneous legislative history; and (8) legislative and administrative interpretations of such law.[4]

ADMINISTRATIVE LAW

Administrative law is a third source of law and is that division of public law which relates to administrative government. According to Sir Ivor Jennings, an English scholar, "Administrative law is the law relating to the administration. It determines the organization, powers and duties of administrative authorities."[5] Whenever a question arises concerning the organization and the power of an administrative authority, fundamental principles of constitutional law become relevant. Further, a true understanding of administrative law requires more than a definition of the rules governing the powers and procedural methods of administrative bodies. Administrative law has greater scope and significance than is generally realized and is concerned with more than procedural matters. In fact, this division of public law is the source of much of the substantive law that directly affects the rights and duties of individuals and their relation to governmental authority.

---

[4] 1 Pa. C.S.A. Section 1501 et seq. (1972).
[5] See, generally, Jennings, *The Law and the Constitution* (1959).

The administrative or executive branch of government, in contrast to the legislative and the judicial branches, is often said to include all those departments of government which have the responsibility of carrying the laws into effect. This definition is an oversimplification and hence misleading, because administrative government often does make law and furthermore exercises a considerable amount of judicial or quasi-judicial power. In Anglo-American government, the phrase "administrative government" should be understood as embracing all departments of the executive branch and all governmental agencies created by legislation for specific public purposes.

Examples of administrative agencies or tribunals abound. In the United States they exist at all levels of government: local, state, and federal. Well-known federal agencies are the National Labor Relations Board, the Interstate Commerce Commission, the Federal Communications Commission, the Civil Aeronautics Board, the Federal Trade Commission, and the Food and Drug Administration. At the state level there are workmen's compensation commissions, labor relations boards, boards of medical registration, and numerous other agencies.

The law-making and judicial powers of administrative government result from delegated, or subordinate, legislation. The United States Congress delegates to various administrative bodies the right to initiate statutory law, typically called regulations, or simply rules. The Federal Food and Drug Administration, for example, although an administrative agency, has the power to promulgate rules controlling the manufacture, marketing, and advertising of foods, drugs, and cosmetics. The Internal Revenue Service regulates tax administration. Many other examples could be given.

The amount of delegated legislation has increased tremendously in this century, particularly since World War II. The reasons are clear: economic and social conditions inevitably change as societies become ever more complicated, and legislatures cannot directly provide the mass of rules necessary to govern the society. Part of the legislature's problem is time; but a more significant obstacle is that many elected representatives of the people lack sufficient information and ability to make intelligent provision through detailed rules of law to implement the social policies expressed in primary legislation. Delegating legislative authority makes it possible to put this responsibility in the hands of experts.

All legislation, whether federal or state in origin and application, must be consistent with the federal Constitution. The power to legislate is therefore limited by doctrines of the fundamental law, and the Supreme Court of the United States has the power to declare that

an act of Congress or the act of a state legislature is unconstitutional.[6]
The issue of constitutional law is also raised when Congress delegates
legislative authority to administrative government. Congress may not
abdicate its responsibility by delegating complete authority, even with
respect to a specialized subject matter. Primary legislation must
generally stipulate what regulations an administrative body is
empowered to make. At the level of state government, the legislature's
power to delegate authority is similarly limited. Furthermore the
enforcement of valid regulations typically lodges judicial or quasi-
judicial power in the administrative body, and this again raises a
question of American constitutional law because the federal Constitution vests "judicial power" in the Supreme Court.

JUDICIAL DECISIONS

The last major source of law is the judicial decision. Judicial
decisions are subordinate, of course, to the Constitution and also
to statutes so long as the statute is consistent with the Constitution.
Despite this subordinate role, however, judicial decisions are the
primary source of private law. Private law, especially the law of
contracts and tort, has traditionally had the most influence on hospital
law and is hence of particular interest here.

Historically, judicial decisions came either from the courts at
common law or from equity. The common law—that is, the law
that is common to England—originally developed in England after
the Norman invasion in 1066. Two factors especially influenced its
development in England, where reliance was originally placed on
local courts to administer justice. First, the English court system
became centralized with the development of the royal courts: the
Court of Common Pleas, the Court of King's Bench, and the
Exchequer. An important procedural device utilized by the courts
and developed during the reign of Henry II (1154–1189) was the
writ, an order purchased by the plaintiff which directed the defendant
to appear before the King's Court. Each writ, or form of action,
differed from the others and carried with it the development of
a separate body of substantive law, prompting Maitland to note that,
although the old forms of action are buried and no longer used,
"they still rule us from their graves."[7]

Secondly, the common law courts developed the doctrine of stare
decisis, literally to abide by decided cases. Under this doctrine, courts

---

[6]*Marbury v. Madison*, 5 U.S. (1 Cranch) 137 (1803). (Established the court's power
to declare federal legislation unconstitutional.)
[7]Maitland, *The Forms of Action at Common Law* 2 (1965).

would look to past disputes involving similar facts and determine
the outcome of the current case on the basis of the earlier decision.
The use of earlier cases as precedent has made for stability in the
Anglo-American legal system, since a person embarking on a new
enterprise can surmise the legal consequences of his action from
the judicial decision already rendered in similar circumstances. The
use of earlier decisions to determine the substance of the law
distinguishes the common law from the civil or Roman law system,
which relies principally on a comprehensive code of laws to decide
a case currently under consideration. Civil law is the basis for the
law in Europe, Central and South America, Japan, Quebec, and
Louisiana.

In the United States, stare decisis is a concept that is applied
vertically, but not horizontally, to equal or lower courts in the same
system or to courts from other systems. An Ohio trial court, for
example, would be bound by the decisions of the higher Ohio courts,
that is, the state's appellate courts and supreme court, but would
not be bound by decisions of other Ohio trial courts or by the decisions
of out-of-state courts. Likewise, the federal trial court, the district
court, would be bound by appellate court decision for its own circuit,
but not by the federal appellate decisions of other circuits or by
decisions of other district courts. The one exception applies where
a federal court, in hearing a diversity of citizenship action, must
determine the law by following the decisions of the highest state
court. While not bound to do so, courts in one system will of course
examine judicial solutions in other systems in order to decide a
case of first impression.

While stare decisis provides stability to the Anglo-American judicial
system, the doctrine would also lead to stagnation if courts were
forced to adhere blindly to precedents. Consequently courts are given
some flexibility in modifying the legal rule when the facts vary from
the precedent, or they may even completely overturn their own earlier
decisions. For instance, the Supreme Court of Pennsylvania overruled
its own decisions and held that charitable hospitals in Pennsylvania
are no longer immune from tort liability when their employees are
negligent. Justice Musmanno noted:

> *Stare decisis* channels the law. It erects lighthouses and flys
> [*sic*] the signals of safety. The ships of jurisprudence must
> follow the well-defined channel which, over the years, has
> been proved to be secure and trustworthy. But it would not
> comport with wisdom to insist that, should shoals rise in
> a heretofore safe course and rocks emerge to encumber the

passage, the ship should nonetheless pursue the original course, merely because it presented no hazard in the past. The principle of *stare decisis* does not demand that we follow precedents which shipwreck justice.[8]

The doctrine of stare decisis should not be confused with another important common law doctrine also referred to in its Latin form, res judicata. Res judicata literally means "a thing or matter settled by judgment." Practically this means that, once a legal dispute has been decided by a court and all appeals exhausted, the parties may not later bring suit regarding matters decided already by the court. The complications that can arise in applying this simple rule are illustrated by a medical malpractice case, *Parkell v. Fitzporter.* In that case the plaintiff's left leg was injured in an automobile accident caused by one of the defendant physicians. The driver-physician and the other defendant physician set the leg, but in sewing up the plaintiff's cuts they failed to remove cinders from the street and parts of the plaintiff's clothing, including his garter buckle, which had become lodged in the wounds. As a result, he suffered gangrene infection and permanent injury.

When sued in a malpractice action the physicians raised as a defense the fact that plaintiff had already, while a minor, recovered damages from the driver-physician for his negligence in causing the automobile accident. The court decided, however, that this defense must fail because in the second suit the plaintiff was suing on a distinct cause of action: "These two cases, that is to say, the suit for malpractice in sewing the garter buckle into the wound, and the suit for negligently producing the same wound, are founded on two separate and distinct causes of action."[9] Consequently res judicata, at least according to this decision, will not be a defense if the plaintiff has a separate cause of action, even if the same defendant is named in both cases.

Equity developed as a source of law because of deficiencies in the common law. By the Middle Ages common law procedures had become rigid, and courts could provide no relief to many parties who had just claims. This failure also applied to the relief that might be available, because the common law generally acted only after the fact. Thus the common law court could grant damages to an injured party after an injury but would not order a wrongdoer to cease his illegal behavior before the injury occurred.

As a result of such inadequacies, parties began to seek relief from

---

[8]*Flagiello v. Pennsylvania Hospital,* 417 Pa. 486, 510–11, 208 A. 2d 193, 205 (1965).
[9]301 Mo. 217, 256 S.W. 239, 244 (1923).

the king when the common law could provide no satisfaction. The king, through his chancellor, often aided these parties and eventually established a separate court, the Court of Chancery, to hear the cases. These courts, which attempted to "do equity" and to act in good conscience where the common law courts could not provide relief, developed the law of equity, which differed from the common law in two major respects. First, the courts in equity developed their own remedies—for example, the injunction which enabled the court to provide relief before a wrong occurred. And, secondly, the procedure in the chancery court differed from that in the law courts. Most notably, the parties in the Court of Chancery had no right to a jury trial, and certain rules or maxims were frequently applied, for example, "He who comes into equity must have clean hands."

Gradually, with the development of these rules, equity became almost as inflexible as the common law, prompting Dickens to write in *Bleak House:* "Never can there come fog too thick, never can there come mud and mire too deep, to assort with the groping and floundering condition which [the] High Court of Chancery, most pestilent of hoary sinners, holds . . . in the sight of heaven and earth."

Although the dual system of law and equity was adopted in the United States, both here and in England law and equity eventually came to be administered by the same court. The relevant Michigan statute, for example, provides that the "circuit courts have the power and jurisdiction possessed by courts of record at the common law . . . and possessed by courts and judges in Chancery in England."[10] Despite the merger of law and equity into one court, however, procedural and remedial distinctions remain. For example, the parties in an equitable action are still not entitled to a jury trial, and the equitable maxims are still applied by the courts.

The law derived from judicial decisions is often referred to as the unwritten law because it is not a part of a formal statute or constitution. This term is misleading because court decisions are in fact written, and many are published in bound volumes.[11]

[10] Mich. Comp. Laws Ann., Section 600.601 (1961).
[11] In this book citations are given when cases are mentioned, not only to show where the complete court opinion can be found but also to indicate when and where the case was decided. The citation "374 Mich. 524, 132 N.W. 2d 634 (1965)," for example, shows that the case was a 1965 Michigan case and that the complete opinion may be found in volume 374, page 524, of the Michigan reports, and in volume 132, page 634, of a regional collection of cases, *North Western Reporter*, second series. "309 F. Supp. 548 (D.C. Utah 1970)" indicates that the case was decided in 1970 by the United States District Court in Utah and may be found in the *Federal Supplement.* "504 F. 2d 325 (5th Circuit 1974)" means the case was decided in 1974 by the

The Court System

The primary method of resolving disputes in the United States is through the court system. This will involve one of fifty-two court systems in the United States, since each state and the District of Columbia has its own separate system, in addition to the federal courts. The large number of different courts makes study of the law in the United States extremely complex, especially when courts in different states use divergent approaches in deciding cases. Nevertheless, although law students must often study a "majority" approach and several "minority" approaches to the same legal issue, the complexity also adds a great deal of strength and vitality to the American system because a wide number of resolutions to a particular problem may be tested in individual states before a consensus is reached regarding the best solution.

STATE COURTS

The federal court system and many state court systems utilize a three-tier structure comprising the trial courts, the intermediate courts of appeal, and a supreme court. In the state court system, the lowest tier, the trial courts, is often divided into the court of limited jurisdiction and the court of general jurisdiction. Typically the courts of limited jurisdiction hear criminal trials involving lesser crimes, that is misdemeanors and civil cases where the amount in dispute is limited, normally to less than $10,000. The courts of limited jurisdiction often include a small claims court, where lawyers are not allowed to practice and the usual legal procedure is not followed.

The state courts of general jurisdiction hear the more serious criminal cases involving felonies and civil cases where larger amounts are in question. In some states only the courts of general jurisdiction may grant equitable relief, such as the issuance of an injunction. Because of the tremendous volume of cases, the courts of general jurisdiction are often divided into special courts: a family or domestic relations court, a juvenile court, and a probate court. The probate court is especially important to hospital administrators because, in addition to probating wills and administering estates, this court is often given jurisdiction to hear cases involving such matters as sterilization of an incompetent or the involuntary commitment of a mentally ill person.

U.S. Court of Appeals for the 5th Circuit and may be found in the *Federal Reporter*, second series; and "118 U.S. 356, 6 S. Ct. 1064, 30 L. Ed. 220 (1886)" means the case was decided by the U.S. Supreme Court in 1886 and may be found in three different sets of reports: the *United States Supreme Court Reports*, the *Supreme Court Reporter*, and *Lawyers' Edition*.

At the next tier of many state court systems is the intermediate appellate court. This court has appellate jurisdiction, that is, the power to hear appeals from final judgments of the trial courts. The court also has limited original jurisdiction, with the result that certain cases, for example a mandamus action to force a government official to perform his duty, may be commenced in the appellate court. In exercising their appellate jurisdiction, appellate courts generally are limited to the record from the trial court and to questions of law, not of fact. For this reason there are few cases such as *Garcia v. Nyack Hospital,* where the appellate court decided that the jury verdict was against the weight of the evidence.[12]

The highest tier in the state court system is the state supreme court. This court hears appeals from the intermediate appellate court and possesses original jurisdiction similar to that of the lower appellate court. The supreme court is often charged with other duties, for example adopting rules of procedure and supervising the practice of law in the state. An example of these duties, to be discussed in a later chapter, is the prescription of attorneys' contingency fees in malpractice actions.

FEDERAL COURTS

At the bottom tier in the federal court system the district court, the federal trial court, hears criminal cases involving both felonies and misdemeanors which arise under the federal statutes. The district court hears civil cases involving actions arising either under federal statutes, such as federal civil rights actions, or under the U.S. Constitution. The district court may also hear suits in which a citizen of one state sues a citizen of another state (that is, where there is "diversity of citizenship") if the amount in dispute is over $10,000. In such a case the court will apply the law of one of the states, since there generally is no federal common law.

Appeals from the district courts go to the United States courts of appeals. The United States has eleven circuits, each of which has a court of appeals functioning in the same manner as the state appellate courts.

At the highest rung in the federal court system is the United States Supreme Court. The Supreme Court hears appeals from the United States courts of appeals and from the highest state courts in cases involving federal statutes, treaties, or the U.S. Constitution. One procedure used by the Supreme Court in deciding to hear

---

[12] 49 A.D. 2d 937, 373 N.Y.S. 2d 879 (1975).

a case is to grant a writ of certiorari. This writ is granted very infrequently, for the Supreme Court normally hears a very small proportion of the cases which are appealed to the Court.

ALTERNATIVE METHODS OF RESOLVING DISPUTES

In addition to the court system, two alternative methods of resolving disputes are popular in the United States. First, adjudication of legal rights as defined by any particular area of administrative law is most often accomplished by an administrative agency or tribunal created by statute or constitution; hence many private disputes controlled by administrative law are not resolved by courts at all. For instance, a claim by an injured employee against his private employer for compensation for injury suffered in the course of employment is ordinarily adjudicated in the United States by a state workmen's compensation commission. Undoubtedly far more disputes are settled today by administrative adjudicative bodies than by the ordinary courts. Moreover an administrative agency often has the statutory responsibility and power to initiate enforcement of statutory pronouncements. It may frequently happen that the same agency brings the initial proceeding, hears the case, and decides the dispute. In the United States, for instance, the Federal Trade Commission is empowered by Congress to initiate a proceeding to compel an alleged offender to cease and desist from practicing unfair methods of competition.

Thus an ordinary court, following established and traditional methods of adjudication, may not be involved in administrative justice. Statutes, of course, will prescribe the powers of administrative authorities. The roles of ordinary courts will generally be limited to preventing administrative authorities from exceeding their powers and to granting remedies to individuals who have been injured by wrongful administrative action. Sometimes the statutes will give the right of appeal to a court from a judicial or semijudicial decision of administrative government. Generally the tasks or goals of procedural administrative law should be the same as those of common law in deciding matters of private law: to provide a day in "court," an independent "judge" or body to decide the dispute, and a rationally justified decision. A corollary aim is to transmit to administrative authority the traditional common law procedural concepts so far as is consistent with notions of public welfare.

The other alternative method of resolving disputes is submitting the dispute to arbitration, a method which is often quicker, less complicated, and less costly than commencing an action in court.

Arbitration in connection with the professional liability of physicians will be discussed in a later chapter.

Legal Procedure

The law, either public or private, which creates and defines rights and duties is called substantive law, and most of this book is devoted to the substantive law as it relates to hospitals. Procedural or "adjective" law on the other hand provides the means of enforcing and protecting rights granted by the substantive law. The branch of procedural law to be discussed below is the law relating to the litigation of a case.

The litigation process may be divided into six stages. It should be mentioned at the outset, however, that many cases involving the hospital or physician are settled by negotiation completed before commencement of the litigation process. According to a 1973 report on medical malpractice issued by the Department of Health, Education, and Welfare (HEW):

> On an average working day in 1970, the 26 or so major malpractice insurance companies opened approximately 70 medical malpractice claim files, or about 18,000 files for the year. Not all of these files represented malpractice claims made by or on behalf of patients. In fact, based upon comparable data for files closed in 1970, only 70 percent (or about 12,600) of the files represented claims asserted by patients; the remaining 30 percent were files that in all likelihood will be closed without a claim ever being made. Insurance companies opened these preclaim files solely on the basis of reports by insured doctors and hospitals of adverse medical incidents or threats made by patients.[13]

Of the claims files closed in 1970, the report concluded that 50 percent were closed without a lawsuit, and that 25 percent of the claimants in these cases received compensation.

COMMENCEMENT OF LEGAL ACTION

When claims do go to court, the first stage is commencement of the legal action. A claimant who begins a lawsuit or an "action," becomes the plaintiff and the other party to the action is the defendant. The plaintiff commences his action by filing a complaint in court, which states the nature of his claim and the amount of damages he is seeking. The complaint and all papers subsequently filed in

[13] HEW, *Report of the Secretary's Commission on Malpractice*, at 6 (1973).

court are the pleadings. A copy of the complaint, along with a summons, is then served on the defendant. The summons will advise the defendant that he must answer the complaint or take other action within a limited time—for example, 20 days—and that if the defendant fails to act the plaintiff will be granted judgment by default.

A problem sometimes arises when an action is commenced against a party out of state. As a general rule courts have decided that it is not fair to force a defendant to defend a lawsuit in a state with which he has had no contact. In *Gelineau v. New York University Hospital,* for example, a New Jersey resident contracted hepatitis while being treated in a New York hospital.[14] When the patient brought suit in New Jersey against the hospital the court dismissed the suit because the hospital had no New Jersey facilities or agents and had done no business in New Jersey. The court concluded that if the patient traveled to another state for treatment, he should expect to travel to the state again to bring suit against the hospital.

THE DEFENDANT'S RESPONSE

In the second stage of the litigation process, it is the defendant's turn to pursue several courses of action either independently or concurrently. The defendant will, at the outset, file an answer to the complaint, admitting, denying, or pleading ignorance to each allegation in the complaint. The defendant may also file a complaint against the plaintiff (a countersuit) or against a third party (a third party action) thus bringing a "third party defendant" into the litigation. An example of a third party action would be a suit against a hospital for injuries suffered by a patient when an improperly manufactured bed collapsed. The hospital would sue the retailer and manufacturer of the bed as third party defendants, claiming that they should pay any damages for which the hospital might be held liable.

A countersuit against the plaintiff may be filed in the original court proceeding, as when a hospital which is being sued for malpractice files a countersuit against the patient for unpaid bills, or, in some instances, after the conclusion of the original lawsuit. Such a counterattack is becoming especially popular with physicians who have defended and won malpractice cases, and who then sue the patient and his attorney for malicious prosecution, abuse of process, defamation, or even barratry, which is illegally stirring up or encouraging litigation. These claims are often difficult to prove.

---

[14]375 F. Supp. 661 (D.C.N.J. 1974).

Malicious prosecution, for example, requires proof that the plaintiff instituted suit without probable cause and with malicious motive, that the defendant won the lawsuit, and that he suffered damages as a result of the suit.[15] Despite the difficulties, however, recoveries have ranged up to $21,000 in the countersuits, and physicians are claiming as much as $11 million in suits currently pending.[16] One untoward outcome of these suits might well be a second round of malicious prosecution suits filed against the physicians and attorneys who brought the original malicious prosecution suits.

The defendant in a lawsuit has one other option available at this stage in the proceeding: to ask that the court dismiss the plaintiff's complaint. The defendant may base the motion on a variety of grounds: the court's lack of jurisdiction, a prior judgment on the same matter, or the failure of the opposing party to state a legal claim, assuming that the facts alleged by the plaintiff are true. Although the terminology differs from state to state, the motion to dismiss is usually called a motion for summary judgment or a demurrer. When the motion to dismiss is granted by the court, the judgment is final; thus the losing party can appeal the decision immediately. In many hospital law cases, the trial court will grant a summary judgment, the losing party will appeal, and the appellate court will then decide whether to uphold the trial court decision or to remand the case for further proceedings.

DISCOVERY—THE DEPOSITION

In a few cases there is very little delay between the initial two stages and the decision by the court. In one instance a wife had lost two-thirds of her blood supply because of a ruptured ulcer, but her husband refused to approve blood transfusions because they were Jehovah's Witnesses and bound by the scriptural edict that they not "drink blood." Within a matter of hours the hospital petitioned the district court for permission to administer blood, the district court denied permission, and the case was taken to a court of appeals where an order was signed allowing the transfusion.[17]

More frequently, however, especially in urban areas, there is a 4- or 5-year delay between commencement of the action and trial. During this time, each party engages in the third stage of the litigation process, discovery, which is an attempt to "discover" whether the

[15]Adler, "Malicious Prosecution As Counterbalance to Medical Malpractice Suits," 21 *Clev. St. L.R.*, 51 (1972).
[16]*The National Observer*, February 21, 1976, 4.
[17]*Application of President and Directors of Georgetown College, Inc.*, 331 F. 2d 1000 (D.C. Cir. 1964), *cert. denied*, 377 U.S. 398 (1964).

other party has a strong case, and if so to settle the case as favorably as possible. Discovery is a valuable device that can be used even to ascertain the amount of malpractice insurance coverage or the identity of defendants. In *Cidilko v. Palestine,* for instance, a patient had fallen on the way to the washroom and fractured a hip.[18] The hospital was required to disclose the identity of the nurse who had directed the patient to the washroom instead of giving bedside attention.

Five methods may be used by parties to discover the strength of the other party's case. All are generally limited to matters which are relevant to the subject matter and not privileged. The most common and effective discovery device is the deposition, whereby a party subpoenas a witness who, at a given time and place, will testify under oath before a reporter who transcribes the testimony. The opposing attorney will also be present during the deposition to make appropriate objections and, if he wishes, to cross-examine the witness. Besides being useful as a discovery device, the deposition serves at least two other major purposes. First, it may be read into evidence at the trial itself when the witness is unable to testify. Second, it can be used to impeach the testimony of a witness. For these reasons, especially the latter, persons being deposed should answer the questions exactly as if they were testifying in court. The following excerpts from a malpractice trial illustrate both the use of a deposition during trial and the importance of keeping accurate personal as well as professional records. In this testimony one of the defendant physicians had been called to testify by the plaintiff's attorney. Readers should keep in mind that none of this part of the examination relates to the actual treatment rendered by the physician to his patient:[19]

Q. BY MR. HARNEY: When did you graduate from college?
A. I graduated from Osteopathic College in—
Q. I didn't ask about Osteopathic College.
A. I finished at the University of Utah in 1934. After I finished at the University of Utah—
Q. No. I asked when did you graduate from college? Did you graduate from the University of Utah?
A. I completed all the requirements for my Bachelor's Degree in 1934.
Q. Did you graduate, Doctor, or perhaps you don't know what the word means.

[18] 24 Misc. 2d 19, 207 N.Y.S. 2d 727 (1961).
[19] Sen. Subcomm. on Executive Reorganization, "Medical Malpractice: The Patient vs. the Physician," 91st Cong., 1st Sess. 57–60, 65–66, 69–71, 132–33, 139–42 (1969).

A.   I do know what the word "graduate" means.
Q.   Did you graduate from the University of Utah?
A.   I did not graduate from the University of Utah.
Q.   In your deposition you testified under oath that you
received a degree; isn't that correct?
A.   I have since received a degree from the University of
Utah on the basis of my credits and work I did at the University
of Utah and University of Southern California.
Q.   Now, in your deposition you testified as follows:
    "Q.   Doctor, would you give us your educational
    background, please, beginning with undergraduate
    college? Tell us where you went to school, the ap-
    proximate years, and what degrees you received, and
    so on, right on up the line.
    "A.   University of Utah; I got out of there I think
    it was 1932.
    "Q.   How many years were you there?
    "A.   Four.
    "Q.   Degree?
    "A.   Bachelor of Arts.
    "Q.   Major?
    "A.   Engineering."
A.   That is true.
Q.   You received the degree of Bachelor of Arts in 1932?
A.   As I said, I have since received information from the
University of Utah that I am eligible for my Bachelor of
Arts degree and it would be given to me.
MR. HARNEY: I move to strike that answer. That is all
kinds of hearsay, conclusionary, non-responsive matter.
THE COURT: That will be stricken.
Q.   BY MR. HARNEY: Now, do you have a degree from
the University of Utah or not?
A.   I do not have a degree right now, no.
Q.   When you testified in your deposition, which was taken
on February 27, 1963, that you had a Bachelor of Arts degree
from the University of Utah, that was not a true statement,
was it?
A.   It was true to the extent that I have been notified that
I will get my Bachelor's Degree.
MR. HARNEY: I move to strike that.
THE COURT: It can remain.
MR. HARNEY: I asked if it was a true statement. Obviously
it wasn't. He didn't ever get a degree.
THE COURT: We will let the jury decide that.
Q.   BY MR. HARNEY: You still don't have a degree from
the University of Utah, do you?
A.   All I have is a letter notifying me that I have adequate—
Q.   I say, you don't have a degree?
THE COURT: Answer yes or no, Doctor.
THE WITNESS: No.

Q. BY MR. HARNEY: And you know what a degree is, don't you?
A. I do.
Q. And you knew what a degree was when your deposition was taken?
A. I did.
Q. And you testified that you had a degree in engineering; is that right?
A. Yes, sir.

. . . .

Q. BY MR. HARNEY: Did you spend the entire four years in undergraduate school at the University of Southern California?
A. No, sir. I was working full time and trying to go to school too.
Q. All of the time you spent at the University of Southern California was strictly on the undergraduate level?
A. Yes.
Q. Not medical school?
A. Pre-medical undergraduate.
Q. Not medical school?
A. That's correct.
Q. In your deposition when you testified you were going to medical school there, you were mistaken; is that right?
A. Pre-medical school.
Q. No. In your deposition when you said "going to medical school; I did not graduate" you were mistaken about that, weren't you?
A. You might say I was mistaken.
Q. There is no question about it, is there?
A. I made the correction on my deposition.
Q. No. When you testified under oath as follows:
    "Q. What were you doing at University of Southern
    California?
    "A. Going to medical school. I did not graduate.
    "Q. Why not?
    "A. Uncle Sam called me."
    When you said you were going to medical school
    there, it wasn't true, was it?
A. No. It was pre-medical school.
Q. But when you said you were going to medical school, that was not a true statement?
A. There are a lot of statements in this deposition—I changed them and corrected them to the best of my knowledge.
Q. Now, my only question, sir, is: When you gave that testimony at your deposition, it was not true, was it?
A. It was an error.
Q. Was that due to faulty recollection?

A.   There were a lot of questions that were asked there
that were due to faulty recollection.

. . . .

Q.   Did you take a residency at UCLA in anesthesia?
A.   I did not take a residency where I was appointed as
a—
Q.   No. The question is, Doctor, did you take a residency
at UCLA Medical school? You did or you didn't.
A.   I did not take a full-time residency.
Q.   Did you take a residency, as that word is used in medical
terminology?
A.   No.
Q.   Now, in your deposition you testified as follows:
   "Q.   You said you interned a year?
   "A.   Yes.
   "Q.   From '49 to '50?
   "A.   Yes.
   "Q.   Where was that?
   "A.   In Chicago.
   "Q.   What—
   "A.   Rotating internship. We worked six hospitals.
   Then from '50 to '53 I was in general practice in
   Orlando, Florida. I came to California in May of
   1953. Then I did a preceptorship in anesthesia for
   three years.
   "Q.   Where?
   "A.   Los Angeles.
   "Q.   Under whom?
   "A.   Doctor M. Howard Farber, F-a-r-b-e-r.
   "Q.   Where is he located?
   "A.   I think he is now on Santa Monica Boulevard.
   He was on Vermont. And then I—
   "Q.   That was two years?
   "A.   Yes. Then I went to UCLA and I had a residency
   in anesthesia."
   That wasn't true either, was it?
A.   I made a correction on my deposition at the time.
Q.   But when you gave the testimony under oath, being
questioned by Doctor Dunbar in this deposition, you knew
that you didn't have a residency at UCLA; isn't that correct?
A.   May I explain, your Honor?
THE COURT: You can answer yes or no.
Q.   BY MR. HARNEY: What is there to explain? You knew
it or didn't know it, Doctor.
A.   I had not done a formal residency, no.
Q.   You misused the word "residency" in that deposition,
didn't you?
A.   Misused the word "residency" where you would apply

it as obtaining a certificate upon completion or being a salaried
employee, yes.

. . . .

Q. Did you tell the University of Southern California that
you went to West High School, Salt Lake City, Utah?
MR. HOME: Again I object, your Honor, upon the ground
that it is immaterial.
THE COURT: Overruled.
THE WITNESS: Yes, I attended West High.
THE COURT: You will have to keep your voice up.
THE WITNESS: Yes.
Q. BY MR. HARNEY: Did you tell the University of
Southern California that you graduated from West High
School, Salt Lake City, Utah, in June, 1933?
MR. HOME: Again, I object upon the ground this is
immaterial and not within any issues.
THE COURT: Overruled.
THE WITNESS: I believe that's when I graduated. I don't
remember the exact date.
THE COURT: Nobody can hear you, Doctor.
Q. BY MR. HARNEY: That's when you graduated from
high school?
A. I don't remember when I graduated.
Q. Well, the question is: Did you tell the University of
Southern California that you graduated from West High
School?
A. Yes, I did graduate from West High School.
Q. Salt Lake City, Utah, in June, 1933?
MR. HOME: May I just have a running objection to this
so I don't have to interrupt each time?
THE COURT: Surely.
THE WITNESS: I believe that's when I graduated, yes.
Q. BY MR. HARNEY: When you testified in the deposi-
tion taken in February, 1963, that you graduated from the
University of Utah in 1932 with a Bachelor of Arts degree—
A. I changed that, sir.
Q. Excuse me—and a major in engineering, that was com-
pletely false testimony, wasn't it?
A. I am wrong on my dates, yes.
Q. And you were wrong on the fact that you graduated?
A. I put that there—there was a mistake there, yes.
Q. And you were wrong on the fact that you got a degree?
A. Yes.

. . . .

Q. So in 1933, when you graduated from high school, you
were 27 years of age; is that right?
A. Yes.

Q. And you didn't graduate from the University of Utah
any time in your whole life, did you?
A. I said that this morning.
Q. You didn't attend that institution for any four years
either, did you?
A. Yes, I went—I was there almost four years.
Q. Well, I understand you got out of high school in 1933
and you said in the deposition you went in the Navy from
'34 to '36 and USC from '36 to '41. Now, where did you
get the four years in at the University of Utah?
A. To get the entire picture of this thing, you have to get
all of my scholastic record together.
Q. Well, I am going to do that if I can.
A. I hope you do.
Q. I am sure going to try.
A. I was an orphan—
Q. Doctor, without going into that part of it, I want to
know where you spent the four years at the University of
Utah.
A. Because I had attended two other universities before
I went to the University of Utah. I attended school, college
and high school, where I could attend, where I could get
a job and eat. I had to work and eat, as I lived by myself.
Q. I did too, Doctor, and I certainly admire you and myself,
but the question is: Where did you get the four years in
at the University of Utah?
A. The amount of credits and time that I had possessed
from Northwestern University and University of Nebraska—
Q. When did you attend Northwestern University, now?
A. In 1929. I took courses at—
Q. When you were 13 years of age?
A. Yes, sir.
Q. At Northwestern University?
A. At University of Nebraska.
Q. When you were 13 years of age before you got out
of high school, four years before you got out of high school,
you went—
A. I finished high school, one high school, Central High
School in Omaha, Nebraska, and when I transferred from
Omaha, Nebraska, to Kansas City I had to go back into
high school and take some more credits. I left Kansas City
and went to Chicago. I had to take some more credits. I
went from Chicago to Salt Lake City and my credits were
not in order for the requirements there and I had to go
back and take some more credits at West High School, and
it seemed like wherever I went, each and every one of them
always came up with something, "you are short one credit
here," or "you are short of this" or "you are short of that."
I was determined to go through school. I didn't care if they
said I had to start over in kindergarten, I wanted to go
to school.

Q. All right. Now, where did you spend the four years at the University of Utah? Was that in 1912, '14, '18, '32, '39, or what?

A. It would be around 1932, '33 or '[3] 4.

Q. That would be two years, then?

A. '32, '33, '34.

Q. Two years, not four?

A. Three years.

Q. Three years?

A. Yes.

Q. I thought you didn't get out of high school until '33.

A. I just told you I was short on credits and they said you have to go take this. It seems all the time I was in school no matter where I went, this has to be made up, you have to do this, you have to do that. It is exceedingly difficult while you are working to try and go to school.

Q. I realize that, Doctor, because I worked my way through school. I understand.

Now, do you mean to say that the University of Utah let you in before you had your high school diploma?

A. I had a diploma—as I recall, I had a diploma from high school in Omaha.

OTHER METHODS OF DISCOVERY

A second method of discovery, written interrogatories, is similar to the taking of depositions except that the questions are written. The procedure for using written interrogatories sometimes varies, depending on whether they are directed toward an adverse party or other witnesses.

A party using the third method of discovery—a method especially important to a hospital—may inspect and copy documents and tangible things in the possession of the opposing party, enter and inspect land under the control of the other party, and inspect and copy things produced by a witness served with a subpoena duces tecum, that is, a subpoena requiring the witness to bring with him certain books and documents. Some states have separate rules governing subpoenas for the production of hospital records. Michigan Court Rule 506, for example, provides that a hospital responding to such a subpoena should send to the clerk of court the medical record, or photostatic copies, together with the sworn statement of an authorized hospital official verifying that the record is true and complete. The hospital must also notify the attorneys that it has complied with the subpoena. The medical record will be kept in a sealed container by the clerk and may not be opened without an order from the court. The record will be returned to the hospital forty days after the case has been concluded. The court may order the subpoena to the hospital to be quashed upon good cause shown by the hospital.

A physical or mental examination, the fourth discovery device, may be used when the physical or mental condition of a person is in dispute and good cause is shown for the examination. If the party being examined demands to see a report of the examination, that party waives any privilege he may have regarding the testimony of other persons who have conducted similar examinations, although in some states the privilege may be waived by bringing the lawsuit.[20]

The final discovery method is to request the opposing party to admit certain facts. By using these requests for admission, the parties may save the time and expense involved in unnecessary proof and may substantially limit the factual issues to be decided by the court.

In addition to the above methods of discovery, a pretrial conference will be held a few months before trial so that the judge and the parties may determine what issues are in dispute, discuss settlement, and set a date for trial if settlement is not possible. The pretrial conference also aids discovery because the court will require that parties specify all damage claims in detail, produce all exhibits to be used in the trial, and in some jurisdictions exchange lists of all witnesses to be called at trial. With all these discovery devices available, the calling of an unexpected witness or presentation of other evidence which truly surprises opposing counsel would be extremely rare.

THE TRIAL

The next stage in the litigation process is the trial, but very few cases reach trial. As noted earlier, according to the malpractice report issued by HEW, only 50 percent of the malpractice claims reach the litigation process. Of this 50 percent, 80 percent are settled before trial, and 60 percent of the claimants receive some payment. Of the cases which go to trial, 20 percent are decided in favor of the plaintiff.[21]

A trial begins with the selection of a jury, if either party has requested a jury trial and if the case is one at law, not equity. After jury selection, each attorney makes an opening statement in which he explains what he intends to prove during the trial. The plaintiff then calls his witnesses and presents other evidence, and the defense attorney is given the opportunity to cross-examine each of the witnesses. After the plaintiff has rested his case, the defendant's attorney frequently asks the court to direct a verdict for his client.

---

[20]Cal. Evid. Code, Sec. 996 (West 1965).
[21]HEW, *supra n.* 13, at 10.

Courts will grant the directed verdict if the jury, viewing the facts most favorably to plaintiff, could not reasonably return a verdict in his favor which would be in accord with the law. If the directed verdict is denied, the defendant proceeds with his evidence and witnesses, again subject to cross-examination by the plaintiff.

When all the evidence has been presented, either party may move for a directed verdict. If the judge denies the motions he will instruct the jury as to the law, and the jury will deliberate until reaching a verdict. Many times, after the jury has reached its decision, the losing party asks the court for a "judgment notwithstanding the verdict" and a new trial. The motions will be granted if the judge decides that the verdict is against the weight of the evidence.

The judge and the jury, of course, play key roles in the trial. The judge has the dominant role: he can decide whether evidence is admissible, charge the jury on the law before deliberation begins, and take the case away from the jury by means of a directed verdict or a judgment notwithstanding the verdict. This power narrows the role of the jury to deciding the facts in the case in order to determine ultimately whether the plaintiff has proved his case by a preponderance of the evidence.

To illustrate the interplay between judge and jury in a medical case, assume that a plaintiff shows that an infant choked to death while unattended. The judge must explain to the jury the legal standard of care, that is, new-born infants must not be left unattended for an unreasonable length of time. It is then the jury's responsibility to determine whether the plaintiff met the burden of proving that the deceased infant was in fact left unattended for an unreasonable length of time. However, if the judge concludes that reasonable minds could not differ on the facts, he can take the case from the "trier of fact," the jury, and enter a directed verdict.

Because of the jury's role in deciding the facts, it is of utmost importance that the members of the jury be impartial. If there is evidence that a jury member might have been biased, some courts will overturn the jury decision. In one case, a California hospital was sued by a plaintiff who had undergone surgery there.[22] A jury rendered a verdict for the hospital by a 9–3 vote, a unanimous verdict not being required in California. The plaintiff discovered, however, that one of the jurors was a dentist who had retired two years earlier. During selection of the jury he had been asked about

---

[22] *Clemens v. Regents, University of California,* 20 Cal. App. 3d 356, 97 Cal. Rptr. 589 (1971), noted in 46 *Hospitals, J.A.H.A.* 197 (1972).

his employment and had said he was engaged in ranching and investment planning. He did not volunteer the information that he was a retired dentist. Furthermore, affidavits from the other jurors indicated that he had a general dislike of persons who brought malpractice actions. On the basis of this information, the appellate court overturned the trial court's decision and ordered a new trial.

CONCLUDING STAGES

The next stage in litigation is the appeal. In the appellate court the party who appeals the case, the losing party in the trial court, will usually be referred to as the appellant while the other party will be the appellee. In reading appellate court decisions one must not assume that the first name in the case is the plaintiff because many appellate courts reverse the order of the names when the case is appealed. The case of *Smith v. Jones,* for example, where Smith sued Jones in the trial court, might become *Jones v. Smith* on appeal. The appellate court, as noted above, limits itself to a review of the law applied in the case and normally will not review the facts as determined by the judge or jury. In reviewing the case the appellate court may affirm the trial court decision, modify or reverse the decision, or reverse and remand for a new trial.

The final stage of the litigation process is collection of the judgment. The most common methods of collection are execution and garnishment. A writ of execution entitles the plaintiff to have a local official seize the defendant's property and to have the property sold to satisfy the judgment. A garnishment is an order to a third person who is indebted to the defendant to pay the debt directly to the plaintiff to satisfy the judgment. Often the third party is the employer of the defendant, and he will be ordered to pay a certain percentage of the defendant's wages directly to the plaintiff.

In this chapter, the sources of law, the court system, and legal procedure have been examined. It should be noted, in conclusion, that the procedure used in a criminal trial will differ in several respects from the civil procedure discussed above. A detailed discussion of criminal procedure is beyond the scope of this book, it being the premise, and hope, of the authors that health care professionals will minimize their contact with the criminal justice system.

PART TWO

The Hospital as a Corporation

II

The Organization and Management of a Corporate Hospital

Most hospitals and other institutional providers of health care are corporations, and it is therefore important for all their personnel to understand the fundamental nature of the corporate form of organization.

The Formation and Nature of a Corporation

In the landmark case of *Dartmouth College v. Woodward*, Chief Justice John Marshall of the United States Supreme Court provided the classical definition of a corporation when he wrote that it is "an artificial being, invisible, intangible, and existing only in contemplation of law. Being the mere creature of the law, it possesses only those properties which the charter confers upon it, either expressly or as incidental to its very existence."[1]

Accordingly, a corporation is purely a creation of the legislature and can exist only by virtue of a statute providing for its formation, and the grant of a franchise or charter. Historically in both England and the United States the early corporations were ecclesiastical, educational, charitable, or even governmental in purpose and were usually created by special act of the legislature.

The modern corporation came into prominence in the latter part of the nineteenth century with the passage on a state-by-state basis of general business corporation statutes. In effect, these allow any group of persons, or even a single individual in some states, to incorporate an enterprise for any lawful purpose, as long as statutory

---

[1] 17 U.S. (4 Wheat) 518, 636, 4 L. Ed. 629, 659 (1819).

31

requirements are met. Thus they eliminated the need for special legislative action each time a corporation was created.

The general business corporation acts, as the name suggests, provide for the formation and subsequent operation of the customary and typical form of business corporations organized for profit and embracing a wide range of enterprises, including but not necessarily limited to manufacturing, wholesaling, and retailing. In addition, in many states these acts also permit and control the formation of many private nonprofit corporations, such as hospitals, since quite a number of jurisdictions have no separate corporate statute for nonprofit organizations. About half the states, on the other hand, have a general nonprofit corporation statute containing provisions for this form of enterprise, and more will be said about these acts.

In addition to the general corporation statutes, many states also have separate incorporation statutes governing the creation and operation of particular types of business activity, such as banking and public utilities. There are also special state statutes now which allow professional practitioners of law, medicine, accountancy, and many other licensed occupations to incorporate their practice.

In any event it is important for the manager or executive of a corporation to know the relevant statute under which his employer is incorporated, for this statute will control and govern the conduct of the corporation's affairs. Since a corporation is created by the legislature, the organization has only the powers granted to it by the charter, or expressly specified or implied in the relevant statute.

Implicit also in Chief Justice Marshall's definition is the fact that a corporation is an artificial person or legal entity separate and distinct from the individuals who created the organization or own the corporation. Accordingly, when a constitutional provision or statutory law uses the word "person," it is the general rule that corporations are included within the definition of person as long as the intent of the provision can be fairly said to include artificial beings. For example, the Fifth and Fourteenth Amendments to the federal Constitution provide that no "person" shall be deprived of "life, liberty, or property without due process of law," and the Fourteenth Amendment further reads that no state "shall deny to any person . . . the equal protection of the laws." It has long been held that corporations are embraced within these fundamental doctrines of constitutional law.

On the other hand, a corporation is not a person under state licensure statutes governing the practice of a profession such as medicine, law, or public accounting. A corporation as an artificial person or entity cannot obtain a license to practice a profession because it cannot possess the educational requirements or meet the standards of personal character required for professional licensure. This prohibition on corporate licensure must, of course, be distinguished from those statutes referred to above which sanction licensed individuals to incorporate their practice.

Similarly, a corporation is not a person within the meaning of the Fifth Amendment to the federal Constitution, which protects an individual against self-incrimination, since the purpose and intent of the provision applies only to natural persons.

Although a corporation is generally a person in applications of laws employing that term, it is generally not a "citizen" when that designation is used in written constitutional and statutory provisions. Thus it cannot as an entity vote in an election. More significantly, a corporation is not protected by the Fourteenth Amendment's provision that "no state shall make or enforce any law which shall abridge the privileges or immunities of citizens of the United States." Hence a particular state can require that a corporation incorporated elsewhere pay special taxes, franchise fees, or other fees in return for the privilege of doing business within the state's borders. In other words, a natural person who is a citizen has freedom of mobility from state to state without special restriction, whereas a corporation does not.

A corporation is a legal entity separate and distinct from those who created it, own it, or are employed by the organization. Hence the corporation can acquire, own, and dispose of property in its own name. It can sue and be sued, and its continued existence is not affected by the death or the disability of an owner. In short, an entity is one with rights and responsibilities of its own.

One of the primary advantages of the corporate form of organization is, accordingly, limited liability. This means that normally the owners of a corporation are not personally liable for the contracts or the torts of the corporation. A shareholder of a profit-making corporation is not personally financially liable, with some few exceptions, for corporate debts beyond the extent of his contractual investment. Moreover, an employee who is an agent of a corporation is not liable for corporate obligations negotiated by him, so long as he acts within the scope of his authority, since the corporate employer is legally capable as an entity of being responsible.

A corporation is formed by the filing of articles of incorporation with the secretary of state or other designated official of the state in which incorporation is sought. When approved by this official, the corporate charter is said to be issued. Although requirements regarding the proper form of the articles may differ somewhat from state to state, the major contents of the articles are these: the name of the corporation, the address of the corporation's office, and the name of the registered agent who is authorized to receive service of process, the names and addresses of the incorporators, the duration of corporate existence (on which there is usually no limit), the purposes of the corporation, the names of the initial members of the board of directors, and the number of shares as well as the classification of shares of stock of a profit-making corporation. The "incorporators" are those who prepare, sign, and file the articles of incorporation. Some states require a minimum number of incorporators, but many others permit a single individual to act as the incorporator.

POWERS OF A CORPORATION

A corporation must act only within its corporate authority, which means that it possesses only those powers which the state has expressly or impliedly granted to the organization through issuance of the charter and by virtue of the statute under which the corporation is formed.

A power is the legal capacity to execute contracts or enter transactions to carry out corporate purposes. Hence the wording and language of the purpose clause in the articles of incorporation are of utmost significance in determining the extent of corporate power.

Powers are of two kinds: express and implied. Express powers are those specifically designated by charter or by statute. The relevant statute under which the corporation is formed will enumerate various express powers as, for example, the power to buy, lease, or otherwise acquire and hold property and the power to make contracts to effectuate corporate purposes. Implied power flows directly from express powers, and is defined, simply, as the power to enter those transactions which are reasonably necessary or convenient to carry out the express powers. The extent of implied power is generally determined by whether or not the transaction tends directly to further or accomplish the corporation's purposes and objectives.[2]

---

[2] In *Mulvey v. Charlotte Hungerford Hospital*, 26 Conn. Sup. 394, 225 A. 2d 495 (1966), the court held that where the corporate purpose clause provided for "maintaining and supporting a hospital" there was implied power to build, own, and maintain a medical office building for staff physicians, since such a facility would materially aid the hospital in carrying out its purposes.

Similarly, the Missouri State Medical Association, a nonprofit corporation, had the implied power to join with the Missouri Association of Osteopathic Physicians and Surgeons to form an independent corporation, Health Care Foundation of Missouri, for the purpose of conducting reviews of quality and costs of services rendered

Any departure from express or implied corporate power is said to be ultra vires, or beyond corporate authority. Therefore in planning for the future and in making commitments, the governing body of the corporation must keep a close eye on the corporate power to act, and legal advice regarding this issue is of utmost importance. For example, if a nonprofit corporation makes a donation or gift to another institution for a purpose not included in its own charter, the gift would be ultra vires.

An ultra vires transaction should be distinguished from an illegal act. The latter is an absolutely void transaction, such as the employment by the hospital of an unlicensed professional person.[3] In contrast, an ultra vires contract is in general voidable and can be challenged by the state through a suit for an injunction. The corporation itself can issue such a challenge as an entity in a suit against a member or members of the governing body or a corporate officer. A stockholder or member in a membership nonprofit corporation can also file suit for an injunction. In an extreme situation the state could, of course, revoke the corporate charter.

Whether or not the issue of ultra vires can be raised by the parties to the transaction—that is, the corporation and the party with whom it dealt or contracted—as a defense for failure to perform is a matter of individual state law. Aside from statute, the usual common law rule, if an ultra vires contract has not been performed by either party, is that the contract cannot be enforced and there can be no recovery of damages for failure to perform. On the other hand, if such a contract has been performed by one party, the other must also perform. If performed by both parties, the contract will be allowed to stand and cannot be rescinded. Many states, however, have enacted statutes which now provide that the parties to an allegedly

---

by physicians. *Komanetsky, M.D., et al. v. Missouri State Medical Association, et al. and Health Care Foundation of Missouri,* 516 S.W. 2d 545 (Mo. Ct. App. 1975). Compare: *Queen of Angels Hospital, et al. v. Younger,* 136 Cal. Rptr. 36 (Ct. App. 1977). (A charitable corporation formed to maintain and operate a hospital could not lease its premises, abandon hospital operations, and devote proceeds of the lease in order to operate medical clinics in low-income areas, regardless of the worthy purpose of the clinics, since this would constitute a violation of the hospital's articles of incorporation.) See also: *Holt v. College of Osteopathic Physicians and Surgeons,* 40 Cal. Rptr. 244, 394 P. 2d 932 (1964). (Where a corporate purpose clause provided for the establishment and conduct of an osteopathic medical and surgical college, the trustees could not make a decision to delete the word "Osteopathic" and convert the college to an allopathic medical school.)
[3] *Manuel Tovar v. Paxton Community Memorial Hospital,* 29 Ill. App. 3d 218, 330 N.E. 2d 247 (1975). (A physician licensed in Kansas but not licensed in Illinois could not maintain an action for an alleged breach of an employment contract with an Illinois hospital.)

ultra vires contract cannot avoid the accompanying obligations by claiming absence of corporate power as a defense.

One should especially note, however, that members of the governing body of the corporation as well as corporate officers could be held personally liable for losses caused the corporation as a result of an ultra vires transaction, if they acted knowingly or without good faith. There would be no personal liability, however, as long as they acted honestly and the ultra vires transaction was simply due to a mistake of judgment.

Typical transactions which directly raise the issue of corporate power, or ultra vires, can be readily identified. A hospital corporation cannot ordinarily lend its credit or guarantee the debts of another corporation, because such a transaction would be outside the scope of a hospital's purpose. Similarly, it may not in general make loans to corporate trustees, officers, or members. Depending upon local or state law, it may be prohibited from forming a partnership with another corporation or an individual, since such a partnership would remove control from the governing bodies of the participating institutions, or at least require the sharing of control with another entity. Likewise a corporation may lack the power to consolidate with another corporation, although two corporations could always dissolve and transfer their assets to a properly formed new corporate entity, as long as the transfer was consistent with the original purposes for which the property was held.

A few states place express statutory restrictions on the amount or type of property owned and held by a charitable corporation. These restrictions may be expressed in general terms. For example, a statutory statement may provide that a charitable corporation may hold only the amount of real estate or personal property that is "necessary" to accomplish its purposes. Other statutes may be more restrictive, stating a specific monetary limitation on the amount of property held. However defined and interpreted, the holding of property in excess of the limitation may carry as severe a penalty as escheat to the state, although the donor or seller of property to the charitable corporation whose action resulted in exceeding the limit might have a legal right to rescind the transaction and recover the subject matter of the gift or sale.

NONPROFIT CORPORATIONS

Of particular interest here is the concept of a nonprofit corporation as distinguished from a profit corporation. As previously noted, many states do not have general incorporation laws pertaining to nonprofit corporations, and in these jurisdictions such corporations are frequently incorporated under the general business corporation act. This situation is unfortunate, since the general business act will inevitably contain provisions that are inapplicable to nonprofit enterprise; further, these statutes may be silent on many matters that should be in the statute controlling the formation and operation of such nonprofit organizations as hospitals.

To remedy this situation about one-third of the states have enacted the Model Non-Profit Corporation Act or a variation of it, thus codifying in a separate statute the corporate law of nonprofit organization. Before some of the major provisions of the model act are discussed, some general observations about a nonprofit corporation will be useful.

The usual definition of a nonprofit body is that no part of the income or profit of the organization can be distributed for private gain to the members, the directors or trustees, or the officers of the corporation. A profit-making corporation, as is well known, is owned by shareholders who are entitled to receive dividends from the earnings of the corporation and to share in assets should the corporation be dissolved. A nonprofit corporation is often prohibited by local statute from issuing shares of stock, although the corporation may have voting members who are required to contribute capital and may then be given a "stock" certificate evidencing their membership. They may not be paid dividends. A nonprofit corporation can, of course, earn income and actually make a profit without sacrificing its nonprofit status, when it uses that profit or reinvests it for institutional purposes. Moreover it can, without question, pay a salary or wage to corporate members or trustees who are actually employees, or who are professional persons rendering actual service. As long as the compensation paid is reasonable, it is not "private gain" that would jeopardize the corporation's nonprofit status.

In sum, motive is important in determining nonprofit status. In a nonprofit institution, motives of ethical, moral, or social purposes are predominant, and profit is not fundamental to the purpose of the endeavor. Hence a mere declaration of nonprofit purpose in a corporate charter is never conclusive, if in fact the entity is being used as an alter ego for private gain.

Nonprofit status is a necessary first requirement for tax exemption, not only under the federal income tax statutes and regulations but also under the various state taxation statutes providing for taxes on income, real or personal property, and sales. (Much more will be said elsewhere in this book with respect to taxation.) Aside from taxes, many state regulatory laws may make significant distinctions between nonprofit and business organizations.

A nonprofit corporation must be distinguished from a charitable corporation. Although nonprofit organization and operation is a necessary prerequisite to charitable status, a charitable purpose is not necessarily a characteristic of a nonprofit corporation. To put the matter another way, all nonprofit corporations are not charitable. Many social clubs and similar organizations which exist to provide private service as distinguished from public service may well be organized and operated as legitimate nonprofit corporations, yet not be charitable or benevolent or eleemosynary.[4]

In addition to the fact that a private business corporation has shareholders and a nonprofit corporation does not, there are other significant differences. A nonprofit corporation may or may not have "members," depending upon the provisions of the law under which it is incorporated. In a corporation having members, they would normally be entitled to vote, as are shareholders, in an election of persons to serve on the governing body. Shareholders of a business corporation, however, should be permitted to vote by proxy. In contrast, public policy at common law has been opposed to proxy voting in a nonprofit corporation, although some statutes now provide that the corporate bylaws or charter may permit such voting. Furthermore, the directors of a business corporation are always to be elected by the shareholder owners (although voting rights may be denied particular classes), whereas in a nonprofit organization, even one privately owned, there may be good reason in particular situations to have some board members appointed by a public official or perhaps by the donor of a large gift. For these and other reasons a general nonprofit corporation act is needed, although many jurisdictions still lack one.

The directors or trustees of a nonprofit corporation should not be permitted to vote by proxy because such a vote would constitute an unjustified delegation of their duty to exercise individual discretion. Again, however, many statutes do not clarify this point.

At the dissolution of a nonprofit corporation the distribution of assets is frequently a difficult question. Local law must be consulted, and even then the statutes or cases may lack clarity. There are some cases to the effect that assets acquired by gift are to be returned to the donor; others hold that all assets escheat to the state; and still others rule that in a corporation with membership the members

---

[4]Charitable status is reviewed and explained in Chapter III.

are entitled to the assets. Such confusion and uncertainty about
distribution of assets upon the dissolution of a nonprofit corporation
is still another reason why a comprehensive statute pertaining to
nonprofit corporations should be enacted.

INTERNAL MANAGEMENT OF A CORPORATION

Corporate bylaws constitute the rules for the internal management
and government of the corporation. Unless specifically provided
otherwise by statute or by a provision of the articles of incorporation,
the power to adopt and amend bylaws of the corporation lies with
the membership or shareholders. In short, the board of directors
or governing body cannot adopt or amend corporate bylaws unless
it has been granted the power by specific provision in the statute
or charter. The board, of course, can adopt its own bylaws relative
to the conduct of its own meetings and committee structure. The
corporate bylaws define the rights and duties of the corporate
members or shareholders among themselves and their relationship
to the corporation, the powers and responsibilities of the governing
body, and the rights and duties of the major corporate officers.
Corporate bylaws are an internal document, and hence they need
not be filed in any public office or otherwise made available for
public inspection.

In a membership type of nonprofit corporation, the bylaws will
contain provisions for holding meetings of the members. Some of
the statutes specifically require the members to conduct at least an
annual meeting; and even if the relevant statute is silent on mandatory
meetings, the assumption is that meetings will be held. Typically,
a designated corporate officer will be responsible for giving proper
notice of the meeting to the membership. If he should fail to schedule
and give notice of the required meetings, the statutes will empower
a member to do so. Notice of the meeting must also call attention
to any extraordinary matter scheduled for vote. Failure to give proper
notice will invalidate the meeting unless the members of the corporation have waived their right to notice.

Extraordinary matters normally requiring the vote of members
would include decisions on accepting the charter as issued by the
state, adopting corporate bylaws, amending bylaws, electing board
members, and amending the corporate charter. Members would
generally also vote on major transactions such as the sale or lease
of real estate, significant grants to or contracts with other organizations
(assuming that these would be embraced within corporate authority),
voluntary bankruptcy or corporate dissolution, and any other transac-

tions specifically mentioned in the bylaws as requiring the member-ship's decision. In other words, some major decisions are beyond the power of the governing body and must be dealt with by the membership. As noted previously, proxy voting may or may not be permitted, depending upon local law and provisions in the bylaws.

The Governing Board of a Hospital

The governing body of the hospital has three major functions. The first is to develop policy and articulate plans for both short- and long-range institutional goals. Second, the board is directly responsible for the appointment of staff, including the appointment of senior administrative officers and the delineation of individual medical staff members and clinical privileges. Third, the board ultimately controls and evaluates the performance of both lay admin-istration and the professional staff.

COMMITTEE STRUCTURE AND EXECUTION OF POLICY

To fulfill these three major functions properly, the board must ensure the proper organization of its own committee structure, the administrative committee structure, and the medical staff. For ex-ample, the board must be sure that its own executive committee is functioning and operating as it should in its role, which is to execute board policy between board meetings. This committee should not assume the power to make those extraordinary decisions that are legally reserved to the board as a whole or to the membership of a corporation. Moreover the executive committee should not be permitted to delegate its responsibilities to any individual member of the committee.

Other major standing committees of the board are typically the finance committee, building and grounds committee, personnel committee, public relations committee, education committee, and medical advisory committee. As its name implies, the finance commit-tee is delegated authority for the management and investment of hospital funds and the overall supervision of fiscal policies. Similarly, the buildings and grounds committee oversees generally the physical plant; the personnel committee develops policies regarding salaries, wages, and fringe benefits for employees; the education committee recommends programs for the training of personnel; and the medical advisory committee promotes mutual understanding between the lay board and the professional staff. Each committee's role is to offer recommendations and advice to the governing body, since the ultimate responsibility for all decisions must usually remain with the board.

There may be some exceptions to this general rule. For example, regarding the actual investment of financial resources, some states' incorporation statutes may authorize the corporate charter or bylaws to provide that investment of funds may be delegated by the board exclusively to the finance committee, thereby removing possible liability from other board members for improper investment. Investment of funds, however, must be distinguished from application of funds for hospital purposes. The board must always carry the responsibility for the latter on its own shoulders.

Having determined policy for the institution, the board must make certain that the policy is effectively executed by its committees and the staff. As a board and as individual members the trustees should not, of course, become involved in details of day-to-day management. Fundamentally the board delegates authority for formulating recommendations and executing policy to hospital administration and to the medical staff by way of the chief executive officer, the administrator. The board then periodically reviews performance and holds its agents accountable. It is elemental in law that once a delegation of authority is made for implementing policy it can be and should be revoked if performance is unsatisfactory. The board must not delegate and then surrender or abdicate its responsibilities. For example, any agreement by the board to place managerial authority in one person or in a particular group of persons is illegal. Any agreement expressed or implied for an individual trustee to be nominal is illegal. Accordingly, all corporate officers and the medical staff are in fact subordinate to the board.

As previously noted, the corporate bylaws (sometimes called regulations) govern the board structure and the administrative structure of the hospital, control internal operations, and provide for management of corporate property. The bylaws define the powers, duties, and limitations of the board's responsibilities, in accord, of course, with state incorporation statutes. In addition to corporate bylaws, the board is empowered to adopt bylaws for its own government. Medical staff bylaws and rules and regulations govern and control the organization of the hospital's professional staff, its officers and committee structure, and its functions. These medical staff bylaws and subsequent amendments to them must be approved by the board of trustees and incorporated by reference as a part of corporate bylaws.

The corporate law of each state thus vests the governing body with the right and the duty to delegate, coordinate, and control all corporate affairs. A hospital is not two organizations—administrative and medical—but rather a single organization which exists for the purpose of arranging and providing the community with high standards of medical care and service.

In fulfilling the three major functions, the board has the following specific duties. It handles the major financial matters for the hospital, making certain that assets and funds are properly used. It acquires hospital property, preserves it from destruction and loss, and provides for adequate insurance, both casualty and malpractice. It arranges for the repair of plant and equipment and for the payment of debts and taxes, as well as enforcing and collecting payments due the hospital. It selects and appoints the major administrative officers, and it also selects the medical staff and defines each individual's clinical privileges, upon the receipt of appropriate professional advice. The board establishes and regularly reviews the hospital's relations with other hospitals in the community, as well as its relations with other institutions and with governmental agencies. Finally, and above all, it regularly reviews and appraises the hospital's overall accomplishment, including the quality of professional care rendered by the hospital's medical staff.

COMPOSITION AND MEETINGS OF THE BOARD

The size of the board is determined by the articles of incorporation. The corporate statutes will typically provide for a minimum number of board members, usually three or five. In a membership type of nonprofit corporation the members of the corporation ordinarily elect the members of the governing body. Many statutes will permit a nonmember of the corporation to be elected to the board. In a nonprofit corporation without members the board itself may select new members and hence be "self-perpetuating." In some situations a designated number of trustees may be appointed by a public official. Terms of office and qualifications of the members of the board will be determined by charter or bylaw provisions drafted in accord with any statutory requirements. For example, local statutes may require that trustees be of majority age; they may also require that a designated number of trustees be residents of the state of incorporation.

Vacancies on the governing board caused by the death or disability of a member or by a resignation are filled by the members of a membership corporation in a special election, unless the statutes, the corporate charter, or corporate bylaws provide otherwise. Trustees can always be removed from their posts for legal cause or with justification; but generally this must be done by those possessing the power of election. To put the matter another way, the governing board of a membership, nonprofit corporation may not usually vote to remove a fellow member of the board unless the statutes, charter, or bylaws provide for such action. For example, the Ohio law permits a trustee of a nonprofit corporation to be removed from office pursuant to any procedure provided for in the articles of incorporation or the bylaws. The remaining trustees may then fill any vacancy on the board by majority vote for the unexpired term, unless the articles or bylaws provide otherwise.[5] Sometimes, depending on the circumstances and local statute, removal of a board member must be accomplished by court action or action of the state attorney general. Regardless of who has the power of removal, the individual subject to the proceeding has the fundamental rights of due process of law. As a minimum, he is entitled to a statement of the reasons for removal, an opportunity to be heard, and a right to challenge evidence or cross-examine witnesses against him. One who has been the subject of an improper removal may bring an action in court to attain reinstatement.[6]

Commonly members of the governing board cannot be paid or compensated for their ordinary services on the board unless local statutory law permits the corporate charter or bylaws to provide for compensation. This is the general rule with respect to both profit and nonprofit corporations. The rule is particularly relevant to the nonprofit corporation, however, because of the fundamental doctrine that members and trustees of such an institution must not derive any personal monetary gain from the corporation. Hence salaries to board members or special financial benefits, such as a discount for hospital services rendered to board members and their families, are quite improper in the usual situation, even if local corporate law authorizes such payments.

This general prohibition regarding payments to members of the governing board for their services on the board of course excludes salary paid to a corporate officer who is also a voting member of the board. For example, it may be wise practice to place the chief executive officer of the hospital on the board. In most states such an individual could be paid a reasonable salary for his services as the hospital administrator, although (as will be pointed out later) he should not participate in board action which establishes his annual salary. Similarly the hospital attorney, who sits on the board, may

---

[5] Ohio Revised Code 1702.29 (B) (C) (1955).
[6] *Welch v. Passaic Hospital*, 59 N.J. L.142, 36 A. 702 (N.J. 1897).

be paid a retainer fee. In a very few states, however, the nonprofit corporation statutes are so worded that they seemingly prohibit members of the governing body from receiving any compensation, making no distinction between ordinary and extraordinary services. In such a jurisdiction, salaried officers may not be able to sit as voting members of the governing board.

In managing the affairs of the corporation the board must act as a board in a properly constituted formal meeting. Hence independent action by one or even a majority of board members is not effective to bind the corporation. Except for regular stated meetings provided for in the articles of incorporation or corporate bylaws, proper notice of a meeting must be given to each board member, usually in writing. Unless such notice is given, the meeting is invalid, except that if all members have actually attended the meeting it can be said that they have waived the notice requirement. Even so, decisions made at a casual, unannounced gathering of the board may be ineffective. Moreover, unless the statutes provide to the contrary, members must attend in person, and meetings conducted by telephone are not normally permissible.

Needless to say, a formal written record should be made of the action taken at each meeting of the board. Members who object to any proposed action should make certain that their dissents are noted in the written record. The frequency of meetings is a matter of charter or bylaw provision and of particular circumstances. Unless the local statutes, charter, or bylaws provide otherwise, the place of the board meeting may be at the discretion of the board. Meetings may even occur outside the state of incorporation, as long as the place selected is reasonably convenient.

The charter or bylaws will fix the number of board members necessary for a quorum. In the absence of a provision, the rule is that a quorum is a simple majority of the board and that a majority vote of those voting on an issue is sufficient to bind the corporation. Members of the board may not vote by proxy, since each has a fiduciary duty to attend meetings personally and to exercise independent judgment.

ACCREDITATION STANDARDS FOR GOVERNING HOSPITALS

The foregoing general principles of corporate law are reflected in the standards for hospital accreditation issued by the Joint Commission on Accreditation of Hospitals in the following principle and eleven standards relative to the governing body and management:

Principle: **There shall be an organized governing body, or designated persons(s) so functioning, that has overall responsibility for the conduct of the hospital in a manner consonant with the hospital's objective of making available high quality patient care.**

Standard I

The governing body shall adopt bylaws in accordance with legal requirements and with its community responsibility, identifying the purposes of the hospital and the means of fulfilling them.

Standard II

There shall be full disclosure of hospital ownership and control.

Standard III

The governing body shall provide for the election of its officers and for the appointment of committees as necessary to effect the discharge of its responsibilities. In addition, it shall adopt a schedule of meetings, attendance requirements, and methods of recording minutes of governing body proceedings.

Standard IV

The governing body shall appoint a chief executive officer whose qualifications, authority, and duties shall be defined in a written statement adopted by the governing body.

Standard V

The governing body, through the chief executive officer, shall provide for institutional planning to meet the health needs of the community.

Standard VI

The governing body, through its chief executive officer, shall provide appropriate physical resources and personnel required to meet the needs of the patients as well as the health needs of the community.

Standard VII

The governing body, through its chief executive officer, shall take all reasonable steps to conform to all applicable laws and regulations.

Standard VIII

The governing body, through its chief executive officer, shall provide for the control and use of the physical and financial resources of the hospital.

Standard IX

The governing body shall delegate to the medical staff the authority to evaluate the professional competence of staff members and applicants for staff privileges; it shall hold the medical staff responsible for making recommendations to the governing body concerning initial staff appointments, reappointments, and the assignment or curtailment of privileges.

Standard X
The medical staff bylaws, rules, and regulations shall be
subject to governing body approval, which shall not be
unreasonably withheld. These shall include an effective formal means for the medical staff to participate in the development of hospital policy relative to both hospital management
and patient care.
Standard XI
The governing body shall require that the medical staff
establish controls that are designed to ensure the achievement
and maintenance of high standards of professional ethical
practices.[7]

Compliance with all of the requirements of the Joint Commission
enables a hospital to qualify automatically for participation in the
Medicare program of the federal government, as long as it engages
in utilization review and meets health and safety standards of the
state. For nonaccredited hospitals the conditions of participation
promulgated by the Department of Health, Education, and Welfare
contain requirements about hospital governance that are similar to
the standards of accreditation. Even if a hospital participating in
Medicare does not have an organized governing board, the persons
legally responsible for the institution must carry out the functions
of adopting bylaws, meeting regularly, appointing committees where
necessary, appointing a qualified administrator and members of the
medical staff, and providing a suitable physical plant.

FIDUCIARY DUTIES OF A GOVERNING BOARD

The members of the governing board of any profit or nonprofit
corporation are fiduciaries, and breach of a fiduciary duty can lead
to personal liability. As previously pointed out, directors or trustees
of a corporate entity are not agents of the corporation in their capacity
as members of the board; nor are they principals of corporate
employees. Hence the directors or trustees are not personally and
individually liable on corporate debts and contracts. Moreover they
are not personally liable for the negligence or torts of corporate
employees under the doctrine of respondeat superior. When the
corporation enters into a contract within its corporate authority,
negotiated by its duly appointed agent acting within his authority,
the corporation is the solely responsible party. If a corporate employee

---

[7] *Supplement to Accreditation Manual for Hospitals,* Joint Commission on Accreditation
of Hospitals, Chicago, 1977, 75–83, effective September 1, 1977. See also: *Second
Supplement to the Accreditation Manual for Hospitals,* 81–82, published Aug. 1, 1977,
modifying some of the interpretations of the standards.

commits a tort within the scope of his employment, the corporation as the employer and the person who committed the tort are liable to the injured third party.

Nevertheless the members of the governing board can be personally liable for their own breach of duty or failure to carry out properly their fiduciary role. The term fiduciary means simply, in its broadest sense, one in a position of great trust and confidence, and it is historically derived from the Roman law of Europe. Such a person is invested with rights and powers to be exercised solely for the benefit of others. The members of the governing board of a profit-making enterprise owe their fiduciary duties to the corporation and the stockholders. In a nonprofit corporation the duties are owed to the corporation and members. Hence members of the governing board and corporate officers are personally liable for their own torts, or wrongs in which they take part or participate, even if these are carried out in the name of the corporation.

Members of the governing board of a hospital or other charitable corporation are frequently called trustees. Strictly speaking, they are not trustees, however, because a trustee is vested with the title to property which he holds and manages for the benefit of others. In a corporation the title to corporate property is vested, of course, in the corporation. Under trust law the duty of a trustee on particular facts or circumstances may be greater than the duty of a member of the governing body of a corporation. For most purposes the courts will apply the standards of corporate management when determining the duties of hospital trustees and will not apply the more stringent standards of trust laws. Nevertheless both the trustees and the directors of a corporation have custody and control of property which they must manage for the benefit of others, and accordingly they occupy a position of great trust and confidence.

Duty of Loyalty

As fiduciaries the members of a corporate governing body have two paramount duties—loyalty and responsibility. Loyalty means that the individuals must put the interest of the corporation above all self-interest, a principle based on the biblical doctrine that no man can serve two masters. Specifically no trustee is permitted to gain any secret profits for himself, to accept bribes, or to compete with the corporation.

For example, in *United States v. Thompson* the board members were liable both criminally and civilly for breach of fiduciary duty when they accepted "kickbacks" from architects employed by the hospital for a construction project utilizing government funds through the Hill-Burton program.[8] The case actually involved a county hospital but would be equally applicable to a private nonprofit institution.

The duty of loyalty also raises the question of whether or not a trustee can personally contract with the corporation. Can he, for instance, sell his personal property or services to the hospital? In general, the answer to this question for a private nonprofit hospital is that a trustee may contract with the corporation, provided that certain high standards are met. A trustee of a private hospital may usually contract with the corporation he serves if the contract is fair, if full disclosure of all interest is made, and if utmost good faith is exercised.[9] To establish the fairness of the contract, competitive bidding should be used and the interested trustee should not be counted in the quorum of the governing body which decides the issue. Naturally he should neither vote nor participate in the discussion, either directly or through an agent. The burden of proving fairness of a contract and disclosure of interest is always on the individual trustee, and the court will closely scrutinize the transaction. It is therefore more risky for a trustee to buy from a hospital and then resell at a personal profit than it is for him to sell his personal property or services to the institution.

A contract with a trustee which does not meet the above standards is not void but is voidable at the option of the corporation. In *Gilbert v. McLeod Infirmary* the sale of hospital property to a corporation controlled by Aiken, a hospital trustee, was voided, even though there was no actual fraud and in spite of the fact that Aiken had refrained from discussing the matter and had not voted on the transaction. However, the attorney for Mr. Aiken, who was also a member of the board, had favorably discussed the sale and voted in favor of the proposal. Moreover Trustee Aiken had failed to carry his burden of proof to show fair and adequate consideration for the sale of the property.[10]

In some states and in some cases, however, especially if the hospital

---

[8] 366 F. 2d 167 (6th Cir. 1966). With respect to the duty of loyalty, see also *Patient Care Services, S.C. and Martinez, M.D. v. Segal, M.D., and Medical Services, S.C.*, 337 N.E. 2d 471 (Ill. App. 1975). (A corporate officer and director who actively engaged in a rival and competing business to the detriment of a corporation must answer to the corporation for injury sustained. The defendant physician was an officer and director of the professional service corporation bringing the charge. He had established another professional service corporation to perform identical medical planning services for a hospital client, thereby attempting to seize an opportunity due the plaintiff corporation.)

[9] 19 Am. Jur. *Corporations* sec. 1291 (2d ed. 1965).

[10] 219 S.C. 174, 64 S.E. 2d 524 (1951); Accord: *Fowle Memorial Hospital v. Nicholson*, 189 N.C. 44, 126 S.E. 94 (1925).

was at one time legally an actual charitable trust and was later incorporated as a private corporation, trust law may be applied to the issue of contracting with the corporation in order to carry out the original intent of the donor of the property. Trust law will dictate that a member of the governing board is absolutely prohibited from contracting with the corporation, regardless of the fairness of the contract and the adequacy of consideration. In trust law a trustee in his individual capacity cannot buy from or sell to the trust. It is also possible that a corporate hospital, even though it was never a charitable trust, may hold particular funds or property classified as trust funds. Thus, with respect to the management of these funds, the law of trusts will apply.

In a few jurisdictions there are specific state statutes pertaining to the matter of a board member's entering into a contract with the corporation he serves. Wyoming's statute, for example, applicable to private hospital corporations, prohibits all officers and directors of nonprofit corporations from receiving any direct or indirect pecuniary advantage.[11] Pennsylvania forbids the sale or furnishing by an officer or board member of supplies, materials, or services to any institution receiving state moneys, unless full disclosure of interest is made in writing.[12] Maryland's statute requires an officer or trustee of any nonprofit institution to file an annual financial report if he is also an employee, partner, or owner of any firm doing business amounting to more than $10,000 with the nonprofit corporation.[13] Both the Maryland and Pennsylvania statutes provide criminal penalties for violation.

With respect to governmental hospitals and contracts with officers and board members a strict rule is normally applied either as a result of statutes controlling the operation of governmental institutions or simply on the basis of judicially declared public policy. The rule is that the officer or board member may not contract with the hospital in the sale or purchase of property, services, or supplies. Even if full disclosure is made and the contract is fair, the court will set it aside. Hence, in *Warren v. Reed,* a board member who agreed to furnish laundry services to the hospital and was in fact the lowest bidder could not enforce the contract, although the hospital did have to pay for the reasonable value of the services furnished prior to cancellation of the contract.[14]

---

[11] Wyoming Comp. Stat. Ann., sec. 17–122.4(1965). A similar statute exists in the District of Columbia, D.C. Code sec. 32–1007(1969).
[12] Pennsylvania Stat. Ann., Title 18, sec. 4684 (Supp. 1972).
[13] Maryland Ann. Code, Article 43, sec. 568Y (Supp. 1973).
[14] 231 Ark. 714, 331 S.W. 2d 847 (1960).

Whenever a member of a governing board wishes to contract with the corporation he serves, he must therefore seek careful legal advice based upon local law applicable to the particular transaction. Of utmost importance also is current public opinion on these matters of conflict of interest. Currently the trend is to challenge real or imagined conflicts of interest at every opportunity. In addition to making certain that the precise letter of the law is observed, every hospital should carefully draft the appropriate policy declarations pertaining to both direct and indirect conflicts of interest and should closely follow these declarations. Of special concern are such indirect conflicts as that involving a board member who is a major executive of a company from whom the hospital obtains goods or services. Although arm's-length contracts bargained in good faith with such an independent firm (or bank) may be perfectly legal, they invite public charges of self-benefit to the hospital board member. Also of current concern is acceptance by hospital officials of gifts, gratuities, and excessively lavish entertainment offered by companies or organizations doing business with the hospital, and this matter should be the subject of carefully drafted policy statements.

Duty of Responsibility

The fiduciary duty of responsibility means that members of the governing board must exercise reasonable care, skill, and diligence proportionate to the circumstances in every activity of the board. In other words, the trustees can be held personally liable for negligence, which can be an affirmative act of commission or omission. The exercise of reasonable care can be defined as the care that an ordinary, prudent trustee would exercise under similar facts and circumstances. Good faith and honesty are the major tests in determining whether reasonable care has been exercised. A few court cases and a specific statute in Georgia make members of the board personally liable only for gross negligence or willful misconduct, but the usual standard of expected conduct is that a trustee of a nonprofit corporation can be liable for ordinary negligence.[15] This is the same standard of care imposed upon the director of a business corporation.

Embraced within this standard of responsibility is the notion that the trustees or directors of a corporation must actually direct. It is not enough merely to preserve corporate property as caretakers. They

---

[15] *Stern, et al. v. Lucy Webb Hayes National Training School for Deaconesses and Missionaries, et al.,* 381 F. Supp. 1003 (D.C., D.C. 1974). Contrast: *Beard v. Achenbach Memorial Hospital Association,* 170 F. 2d 859 (10th Cir. 1948), where the court held that trustees were liable only for "gross or willful negligence."

must employ corporate property to obtain corporate objectives. Any negligent loss or improper investment of assets can lead to liability. Further, trustees must attend meetings of the board. Excessive absences can be treated as a negligent omission or nonfeasance. The law is perfectly clear that it has no place for "dummy directors." Moreover, as noted previously, trustees must personally vote on issues and cannot ordinarily vote by proxy. Examples of activities which could lead trustees to be held personally liable for negligence are: distributing corporate assets to members of the corporation contrary to law or the articles, knowingly approving ultra vires transactions, improperly dissolving the corporation, making improper loans to trustees or officers, and failing to dissent when improper action occurs. As part of the last item, the individual trustees must make certain that other trustees do not breach their trust.[16]

Also within the fiduciary duty of responsibility is the idea that trustees must exercise reasonable care in selecting and appointing such corporate agents as the administrator, or chief executive officer of the hospital.[17] Trustees must also use reasonable care in supervising the agents whom they appoint and in holding them accountable. Hence trustees have an individual duty to remove an incompetent chief executive officer when they know or should have known of the officer's failure to perform properly. Negligence in regard to the appointment or the subsequent supervision of hospital employees can lead to personal liability. This rule applies with equal force to professional and nonprofessional hospital employees whom the board appoints and to whom it delegates authority.

Still perhaps a somewhat open question is whether or not a member of the governing board is personally liable if he knows a member of the medical staff to be professionally incompetent and fails to move the board toward a solution of the matter. As discussed in detail in a later section, there is clearly a corporate duty to exercise reasonable care in selecting and appointing individuals to the medical staff and in delineating their privileges. Moreover the cases are now clear to the effect that a corporate duty exists to restrict clinical privileges or terminate an appointment when the board knows or should have known of incompetence on the part of a medical staff member.[18] That is, there is corporate liability when the board knew

---

[16] *Hill v. Hill,* 79 N.J. Equity 521, 82 A. 338 (1912). (Liability was found when defendant trustee was aware that a co-trustee had acquired an interest adverse to the trust and did nothing about the matter. This case involved an actual trust.)
[17] See: *Reserve Life Insurance Co. v. Salter,* 152 F. Supp. 868 (S.D. Mississippi, 1957).
[18] See text and cases discussed in Chapter XII.

of evidence of professional malpractice, or when it should have known of this through the action or inaction of the relevant medical staff committees or departments charged with the responsibility of medical audit of each staff physician's clinical performance. Whether or not there could be personal liability in a member of the governing body has not yet been squarely presented to a court for decision. To date, however, the cases involving the individual duty of trustees to remove an incompetent hospital administrator, and the doctrine that trustees have a duty to act when they know of a breach of duty by a fellow trustee indicate that a member of the hospital board could conceivably be personally liable if he had knowledge of incompetence in a member of the medical staff and failed to bring it to the attention of the board for deliberation and decision. In effect, this would simply mean a logical extension of the long-recognized legal doctrine that board members can be held personally responsible when they direct, participate, or acquiesce in a negligent act by a hospital employee.

None of the foregoing means that the individual trustees are to interfere in day-to-day management or the clinical practice of professional staff. No individual on the board is expected to visit the hospital administrator's office daily to question his decisions or to exert minute supervision with respect to his work. Neither are lay persons expected, or indeed competent, to question the clinical practices of the medical staff. The duties discussed above mean rather that board members have a duty to hold corporate agents, including duly organized medical staff committees, accountable for their work. Accordingly, regular reviews of performance, supported by written and documented records, are required for both administrative and professional personnel.

Board members may rely on written, documented reports and recommendations from responsible professional sources such as medical staff committees, hospital accountants, and legal counsel. They need not check out or verify all items in such reports if nothing arouses suspicion or question. The risk of personal liability exists in the failure to obtain documented professional advice when such a need is clearly apparent, for example, in a failure to obtain competent legal counsel when the hospital has a recognizable legal problem.

In general, the trustee of a hospital is not liable personally for honest errors in business judgment. This follows the same concept that is applicable to the directors of a profit corporation and means simply that board members must exercise the judgment that ordinary, prudent directors or trustees would be expected to exercise under similar circumstances. As an example of the lack of honest business judgment, a member of a governing board could be liable personally if he permitted institutional funds to remain in a bank which he knew or ought to have known to be in financial difficulty.[19]

NATURE OF LIABILITY FOR BREACH OF DUTIES

If personal liability is successfully asserted against a board member or members, the liability is joint and several. This means that a plaintiff may sue one, several, or all members of the board; and if his suit is successful each of the defendants against whom a court judgment is obtained is fully liable for the amount of the judgment. As previously noted, certain breaches of fiduciary duty may be deemed by statutory law to create criminal liability as well as civil.

Suits asserting breaches of fiduciary duty can be brought by the corporation itself or by a stockholder or member of the corporation against the corporate trustee or director or officers. An official of the state, usually the attorney general, having the power of regulation of the corporation's affairs, can also initiate action. This has been the traditional legal means of enforcing charitable trusts and controlling the affairs of charitable corporations. With respect to governmental hospitals, a taxpayer probably has the requisite standing to bring suit.

In *Stern*, a very recent landmark case, the court held that patients and prospective patients of the hospital have standing to bring a class action suit against hospital trustees.[20] In the class action the plaintiffs sued on behalf of themselves and all others similarly situated. Alleged was breach of fiduciary duty because of fiscal mismanagement which resulted in higher than necessary hospital charges to the patients and the community it served. Specifically, among other charges the plaintiffs alleged that the trustees deposited large sums of hospital moneys in noninterest-bearing bank accounts, while at the same

---

[19] See: *Epworth Orphanage v. Long*, 207 S.C. 384, 36 S.E. 2d 37 (1945). See also: *Queen of Angels Hospital, et al. v. Younger*, 136 Cal. Rptr. 36 (Ct. App. 1977). (There was an improper exercise of sound business judgment or breach of fiduciary duties when the board of a nonprofit charitable corporation compromised a $16-million claim by a religious order for past services rendered the hospital by members of the order. The settlement agreement provided that the hospital would pay the mother house $200.00 per month for each sister in the order over 70 years of age, whether or not the particular sister performed services at the hospital, plus $200.00 per month for each lay employee who had worked for the congregation for over 20 years, not to exceed ten lay employees at any one time. Although the claim was made in good faith and was not dishonest, the agreement was invalid and constituted a diversion of corporate assets, since there was no lawful obligation on the part of the hospital to pay for past services.)

[20] *Stern, et al. v. Lucy Webb Hayes National Training School for Deaconesses and Missionaries, et al.* 367 F. Supp. 536, (D.C., D.C. 1973).

time the hospital was paying interest on loans to it made by the same financial institutions. Further, some of the defendant trustees were directors or officers of the banks and savings and loan associations with whom the hospital conducted business. In addition to ruling that the plaintiffs had standing to sue, the federal district court first ruled that the appropriate legal remedy would be an injunction to prohibit future injuries to the hospital's service population.

Originally named as defendants were nine trustees, six financial institutions with whom the hospital transacted business, and the hospital. Prior to trial the plaintiffs withdrew the names of four of the individual trustees and one of the financial institutions as defendants, and the court dismissed the other financial institutions from the suit. The case proceeded against five trustees individually and the hospital as a nominal defendant.

The first principal allegation was that the defendants conspired to enrich themselves and the financial institutions by depositing large sums of hospital moneys in noninterest-bearing bank accounts at the same time that the hospital was paying interest on loans made to it by the same institutions. The second principal allegation was that the defendants breached their fiduciary obligations with respect to management of the hospital funds. The defendant trustees were variously members of the board's executive committee, finance committee, and investment committee, some serving on more than one of these bodies. They had permitted the fiscal affairs of the hospital to be managed almost exclusively by two trustees and corporate officers, Dr. Orem and Mr. Ernst. The defendants were also directors, officers, and stockholders in the several financial institutions with which the hospital deposited funds or transacted other business.

Since there was no evidence either that the trustees had mutually agreed to direct or encourage Mr. Ernst in his investment decisions or that the defendants had solicited business for any particular financial institution, the complaint of a conspiracy was dismissed. Trustees cannot be charged with a conspiracy when the proof shows simply that the hospital administrators made the decisions about fiscal management without the direction of the trustees or even their advance knowledge.

Nevertheless, the *Stern* case is important not only because the court did find that the trustees had breached their fiduciary obligations of responsibility and loyalty, but especially because it ruled that trustees can be held personally liable for losses caused by negligent non-management or mismanagement of hospital investments. The care required is ordinary and reasonable care, the same standard as that imposed on the directors of a business corporation. Certainly, failure of the finance and investment committee to meet and to supervise adequately the activities of the administrators constitutes a breach of this responsibility. As to loyalty, full disclosure of any conflict of interest must be made, the contract with another institution in which a hospital trustee has an interest must be fair, and interested trustees must refrain from participating in the transaction whenever they or the other institution they serve contracts with the hospital or accepts a deposit of hospital investment funds. In other words, the court did not prohibit hospital trustees from serving as directors or officers of financial institutions with whom the hospital transacts business, but it clearly indicated that such interlocking directorships would be closely scrutinized.

The *Stern* court did not hold the individual trustees liable for damages; nor did it issue an injunction removing them from the board of trustees of Sibley Memorial Hospital.[21] It did, however, issue an order declaring that a trustee violates his fiduciary duty if he fails to use diligence in supervising the actions of corporate officers or of outside experts to whom investment decisions are delegated, if he knowingly permits the hospital to enter a business transaction with himself or with any other organization in which he is interested without full disclosure of his interest, if he actively participates in or votes in favor of a decision by the board to transact business with himself or any organization in which he is interested, or if he fails to perform his duties honestly, in good faith, and with reasonable care and diligence. The order further provided that a written policy statement governing investment of hospital funds be prepared and that all investments conform to the guidelines to be developed in the policy statement.

PROTECTION AGAINST LIABILITY

Despite all that has been said here, the personal liability of hospital trustees is not a serious financial risk so long as they regularly attend meetings of the governing body and vote personally, avoid conflicts of personal interest, and exercise the utmost good faith and honesty. The best means of establishing good faith and honesty is a written record of all the board's deliberations, including the votes of individual trustees on individual transactions. Whenever one dissents from

---

[21] *Stern, et al. v. Lucy Webb Hayes National Training School for Deaconesses and Missionaries, et al.*, 381 F. Supp. 1003 (D.C., D.C. 1974).

majority action of the board, the dissenting trustee should therefore make sure that his dissent is part of the written record.

Individual trustees and corporate officers can protect themselves against liability by purchasing liability insurance or by having appropriate corporate indemnification provisions and procedures. Because insurance may be expensive and not sufficiently comprehensive, many nonprofit corporations favor appropriate indemnification plans. Indemnification merely means that if a trustee is sued in a civil cause of action alleging violation of his fiduciary responsibilities, or if he is prosecuted in a criminal action, he is then entitled to be indemnified by the corporation for his personal expenses, including attorney's fees and perhaps even amounts paid as a result of the action.

At one time the judicial case law regarding the authority of a corporation to indemnify the members of the governing body produced a split of authority from state to state. Some states, by judicial decisions, permitted the corporation to indemnify trustees in certain types of legal action for certain costs, while others did not. Today most of our states have statutes which authorize a corporation to provide for indemnification. Many such statutes apply both to directors or trustees and to officers of the corporation, and frequently they apply to both civil and criminal actions.

The major point here is that, depending upon local state law, the trustees and officers have the right to indemnification under certain circumstances. On this matter, careful legal advice is necessary to explain to the governing body the circumstances under which indemnification can or should be provided. It is also imperative that the corporate charter or bylaw provisions covering this matter be carefully drafted.

Some statutes—those in New York, for example—are exclusive; that is, a corporation can have an indemnification agreement with its governing board members and officers only to the extent precisely authorized by statute.[22] Most states, however, have permissive statutes and a corporation may thus indemnify to a greater extent than the statutes provide. Delaware is a prototype of this model.[23] In general, the statutes authorize indemnification plans for legal actions against trustees and officers by stockholders or by members on behalf of the corporation, that is, derivative actions, as well as for actions by such third parties as creditors or clients of the corporation, as in the *Stern* case discussed above.

---

[22] New York Business Corporation Law, sec. 721–26 (McKinney 1963) and sec. 727 (McKinney 1969).
[23] Delaware Code Ann., Title 8, sec. 145 (1967).

In all actions, derivative or third party, the defendant can be indemnified for his expenses of defense, including attorney's fees, and amounts paid in settlement of the suit. In third party actions, but not in derivative lawsuits, he may be indemnified for payment of actual court judgments or fines levied against him. To be entitled to indemnification for expenses in a derivative action, however, the trustee or officer must generally show that he acted in good faith without negligence or other breach of duty to the corporation. In other words, a successful defense must be the basis for indemnification. In third party actions, also, the defendant must establish his good faith, even if he is ultimately found liable; and if the legal proceeding is criminal in nature he must show that he acted with no reasonable cause for believing that his conduct was unlawful.

III

Taxation of a Charitable Organization

A tax-exempt corporation or organization is one which is both organized and operated exclusively for religious, scientific, educational, or charitable purposes. To determine charitable status one must generally look not only at the declaration of purpose contained in the corporate charter or other organizational document but also at the actual facts of the organization's operation.

The Nature of a Charitable Corporation

In some states a charity must be actually incorporated. In others, however, incorporation is not required, and other forms of business organization may be utilized: an unincorporated association of individuals, a trust, a community chest, or a foundation. Probably few states require incorporation or any particular form of business organization in order to establish charitable status; but as a practical matter, most charitable hospitals will be incorporated.

Some states require that a charitable corporation be incorporated in the state where tax exemption or other preferred status is sought. Hence foreign corporations, that is, those incorporated in states other than the one where charity status is claimed, cannot successfully assert such a claim.

At the outset of this discussion, however, it is important to note that no single all-inclusive definition of a "charity" is applicable to all situations where a definition is necessary. For example, for federal income tax exemption the qualifications a charitable corporation must meet are determined by the wording of the Internal Revenue Code, by regulations promulgated by the Internal Revenue Service, and by court decisions interpreting the statutory law or the validity of

58

the regulations, a matter discussed specifically in later sections of this chapter. Further, the various state constitutions and statutes providing for exemption from local taxes may differ in their precise language, and local courts may differ in their interpretations of constitutional or statutory provisions. Some state laws, for example, will exempt organizations described as "public charities" from local real estate taxation or other local taxes such as income taxes, sales and use taxes, or taxes on personal property. Other states omit the word "public" from tax exemption requirements. Accordingly, the advice of local legal counsel is crucial in a situation involving any specific taxation issue. Since state taxation of real estate owned or occupied by a hospital or other health care institution is also discussed in greater detail below, this section is confined to a general view of the nature of a charity or charitable corporation and to an identification of the major issues that may determine a decision in a particular situation.

Charity in general refers to benevolent or eleemosynary aims and to public service for the benefit of an indefinite number of persons. Hence a charity exists to promote the welfare of mankind more or less at large, or the welfare of a "community." Although benefits may be restricted to a particular class of beneficiaries—the blind, children, the aged—the class must contain an indefinite number of persons to be served by what is probably the majority rule. To put the matter another way, the charity must usually be open to the public and not restricted to a privileged few. Accordingly, public service organizations must often be distinguished from social service and nonprofit organizations. All charitable corporations will be nonprofit corporations, but not all nonprofit organizations will be charitable. Countless nonprofit corporations—for example, social clubs, fraternal organizations, and labor unions—may provide a significant degree of social service, but they do not exist and operate for charitable purposes. It is, of course, clear in every jurisdiction that the very essence of nonprofit status is that no private benefit can accrue to private individuals. This requirement is analyzed and illustrated in the sections below dealing with federal and state taxation.

The general definition or concept of a charity noted in the foregoing paragraph raises the issue of whether benefits may be restricted to certain segments of a community. In all jurisdictions and for both federal and state purposes, hospitals or other health care institutions which serve only children, for example, or women, or mentally ill individuals are clearly considered charitable, as long as they meet the other relevant requirements. In other words, confining the activity to a specialized purpose and accordingly restricting benefits to a particular age or sex group or to the treatment of a particular illness do not jeopardize charitable status, nor would restrictions necessitated by the available staff and facilities. The class of persons to be served is "indefinite."

May the benefits of a charity be restricted to the members of a particular church, lodge, labor union, or fraternal order, or to the employees of a particular company? Here the answer may be more difficult and may depend upon local law and the precise issue at stake in a given situation. Especially if local law requires tax-exempt organizations to be "public charities," it then follows that the beneficiaries may not be restricted to the members of a given church, fraternal order, or similar group. A leading case, mentioned here solely by way of illustration, is *Philadelphia v. Masonic Home* in Pennsylvania, which denied real estate tax exemption to a home for aged Masons.[1] This is probably the majority rule for the purposes of tax exemption from local state real estate taxes, although in a great many jurisdictions there is no precise authority. At least one can say that this rule might well be expected to prevail, according to the trend in social thinking. In contrast, by court interpretation of the law of Kansas, which does not require a "charity" to be "public," organizations serving, for example, only Masons, Methodist clergymen, or Roman Catholic nuns are categorized as charitable and hence tax exempt.[2] The definition of and limitations on the class of persons to be served by a "charity" thus depend upon local law and are still an open question in many jurisdictions. As noted elsewhere, federal income tax law under Section 501(c)(3) of the Internal Revenue Code does not permit tax exemption to organizations catering only to a closed membership group.

Some state court decisions have permitted charitable status to hospitals or homes which followed policies restricting beneficiaries on the basis of race, color, creed, or national origin.[3] Both the Federal Civil Rights Act of 1964, however, and the local state civil rights

[1]160 Pa. 572, 28 A. 954 (1894). Accord: *Missouri Pacific Hospital Assn. v. Pulaski County*, 211 Ark. 9, 199 S.W. 2d 329 (1947). (A hospital owned by a railroad and open only to railroad employees was not exempt.)
[2]See: *Kansas Masonic Home v. Board of Commissioners*, 81 Kan. 859, 106 P. 1082 (1910). *Accord: Fitterer v. Crawford*, 157 Mo. 51, 57 S.W. 532 (1900). (However, in *Crawford* the home was denied tax exemption for other reasons.)
[3]*Maxwell v. Good Samaritan Hospital Assn.*, 195 So. 2d 255, (Fla. App. 4th Dist. 1967), *aff'd*, 204 So. 2d 519 (Florida 1967). (Statute did *not require* the absence of racial discrimination. The local tax assessor attempted to deny tax exemption on the basis of a hospital policy which discriminated. The court held that the assessor had no such power, thus permitting charity status in spite of discriminatory practices.)

acts applying to "public accommodations" or similarly defined institutions are typically applicable to general hospitals and of course must be consulted whenever racial restrictions are attempted. Further, the Fourteenth Amendment to the federal Constitution might well be applicable and might prohibit such restrictions if the institution receives a significant amount of either federal or state financial aid. Finally, even if the only question in a given controversy or case is the narrow one of defining a "charitable purpose" which is expected to serve the "community," any form of restriction of beneficiaries on the basis of race or national origin is likely to result in a denial of charitable status on the basis of judicially declared public policy. This outcome would be especially likely, of course, in those jurisdictions which specifically provide for charities to be "public."

A few states may attempt to require that a charity restrict its benefits to residents of the state where its property is located or its services performed, denying charitable status to organizations that serve nonresidents to any significant degree. Such a restriction is, of course, highly unrealistic and should be considered contrary to public policy in an era of population mobility. No authoritative case support has been found which thoroughly upholds such residential requirements. The Colorado court in construing the statute of that state permitted charitable status and tax exemption for an organization that served nonresidents, so long as the *primary* benefits were extended to Colorado residents.[4] In contrast and perhaps illustrative of the general rule, a charity incorporated in New York does not jeopardize its status by doing most of its work outside the state and with nonresident beneficiaries.[5]

It is frequently said that a charitable corporation or organization may not restrict its services because of a patient's inability to pay. This matter also requires careful analysis and consideration of particular facts in relation to the precise question being decided. For federal income tax exemption and for most state real estate exemptions, as discussed elsewhere, the statement means as a minimum that a general acute care hospital, for example, with an emergency service facility may not summarily reject a patient who seeks emergency care, if the rejection is solely on the basis of inability to pay. Naturally, however, and in accordance with sound economics and the needs of particular communities, it is not required of all hospitals, even general hospitals, that they provide emergency services.

---

[4] *Young Life Campaign v. Board of Commissioners*, 134 Colo. 15, 300 P. 2d 535 (1956).
[5] *People ex rel. Near East Foundation v. Boyland*, 201 Misc. 855, 106 N.Y.S. 2d 736 (1951).

The point is more obvious with respect to highly specialized institutions, such as hospitals which care only for patients with a particular disease or disability. Charitable status is therefore not lost by restricting benefits according to the institution's ability to serve, given its purpose, facilities, and staff.

Even though a charity may not generally restrict its emergency care to those able to pay, the question still remains whether or not the organization must necessarily render some amount of free care to maintain its status. Charges to those able to pay will never jeopardize charitable status. A few state courts, in cases involving hospitals seeking charitable status, have seemingly required the rendering of *some* free care to those unable to pay.[6] This approach appears to follow the early English law that care of the indigent must be a primary concern of a charitable hospital. By this minority view the hospital must not be entirely self-supporting and must rely to some undefined extent upon public philanthropic support.[7] It follows that a charitable corporation cannot operate at a profit.[8] Still, the organization could require that those able to pay do so as long as it earned no profit and affirmatively served the poor through the receipt of public support to cover deficits. Simply charging off uncollectible debts would not meet this requirement.

Most state courts, however, and federal Internal Revenue Ruling 69–545, promulgated in 1969 and governing federal income taxation of hospitals, have not required that a charitable institution must grant a given amount of free care to maintain charitable status. This Internal Revenue ruling has recently been contested in the courts, and the litigation is reviewed later in this chapter. It is of historical interest that prior to 1969 the federal government did require a tax-exempt hospital to furnish an undefined amount of service below costs.[9]

For the purposes of state tax exemptions and whenever it is necessary to determine charitable status as a matter of local law, the majority rule clearly indicates that a health care institution need not prove that it provides a certain amount of free care. This is a broader and more liberal view of the nature of a charity: relief of poverty is not a necessary prerequisite.[10] As long as there is no

[6]*Cleveland Osteopathic Hospital v. Zangerle*, 153 Ohio State 222, 91 N.E. 2d 261 (1950) and *Vicksburg v. Vicksburg Sanitarium*, 117 Miss. 709, 78 So. 702 (1918).
[7]Bromberg, "The Charitable Hospital," *Catholic University Law Review*, vol. 20, no. 2, Winter 1970, 241–44.
[8]*Oregon Methodist Homes, Inc. v. Horn*, 226 Ore. 298, 360 P. 2d 293 (1961).
[9]Revenue Ruling 56–185, 1956–1 Cum. Bull. 202. This ruling was changed by Revenue Ruling 69–545, 1969–2 Cum. Bull. 117.
[10]Bromberg, *supra* n. 7, at 244–48.

private gain or profit, promotion of health is per se a valid charitable purpose. Accordingly, the institution can be self-supporting and earn a profit as long as the profits are utilized for institutional needs and not distributed directly or indirectly to individuals. Profit can be invested in physical facilities or added to endowment. All patients can therefore be required to pay full costs, although a general hospital with emergency care facilities should not refuse emergency service because the patient cannot pay. Many state court decisions follow this approach, and the philosophy was well stated by the New York court in *Doctors Hospital v. Sexton* as follows:

> Hospitals which are devoted to the care of the sick and injured, which aid in maintaining public health and which make valuable contributions to the advancement of medical science are rightly regarded as benevolent and charitable. A hospital association not conducted for profit which devotes all of its funds exclusively to the maintenance of the institution is a public charity and this is so irrespective of whether patients are required to pay for the services rendered.[11]

The view that care of the indigent is not a necessary condition for charitable status is justified on the grounds that both the wealthy and the poor are appropriate beneficiaries of charity whenever they are the victims of illness or injury, that a requirement of free care is difficult to define in terms of amount and extent, and that modern social welfare programs of government are designed to care for those unable to pay for medical and hospital services.

Finally, although promotion of health per se may be a valid charitable purpose for many organizations, such as health research institutions and specialized hospitals, a general community hospital must actually benefit the community if it is to retain charitable status[12]—hence the requirements mentioned earlier that the hospital must admit patients without regard to race or creed and must welcome emergency room patients, assuming available facilities and staff. In short, a community hospital must not turn away emergency patients on the basis of either their wealth or their poverty.[13] Some voluntary community hospitals have been known to instruct police and ambu-

---

[11] 267 App. Div. 736, 741, 48 N.Y.S. 2d 201, 205 (1944), *aff'd*, 295 N.Y. 553, 64 N.E. 2d 273 (1945). Also see: *Bishop & Chapter of the Cathedral of St. John the Evangelist v. Treasurer of the City and County of Denver*, 37 Colo. 378, 86 P. 1021 (1906). (A hospital may charge fees to all patients and amount received may exceed expenses.)
[12] Bromberg, *supra* n. 7, at 248–51.
[13] *Hart v. Taylor*, 301 Ill. 344, 133 N.E. 857 (1921) and *Natchez v. Natchez Sanitorium Benevolent Association*, 191 Miss. 91, 2 So. 2d 798 (1941). (The *Hart* case involved the validity of a charitable testamentary trust.)

lance companies to take indigent emergency patients to public hospital facilities, and such a policy would violate their status as a charity.[14] Some authorities, including Wilbur Cohen, former Secretary of Health, Education, and Welfare, have suggested that all charitable hospitals should be required to accept some patients eligible for Medicaid benefits.[15] Systematic refusal of admission or services to such persons shows an unwillingness to serve the community, although such a requirement has not yet been firmly established as a matter of law. In the final analysis, each case will be decided on the particular facts, and the ultimate inquiry will always be whether the hospital is serving the community, as defined by state law and taking into account the availability and accessibility of other facilities.

Federal Taxation of Income

To be exempt from federal income taxation under Section 501(c)(3) of the Internal Revenue Code, a private "corporation, . . . must be organized and operated exclusively for religious, charitable, scientific, . . . or educational purposes . . . no part of the net earnings of which inures to the benefit of any private shareholder or individual." It is to be especially observed that hospitals, nursing homes, and other health care institutions are not specifically named as exempt from tax. Nevertheless they can qualify for exemption by meeting the two primary requirements of the Internal Revenue Code set forth above and by following the regulations promulgated by the Internal Revenue Service to implement the code.

The first basic requirement of the code is that the tax-exempt organization must be both organized and operated for a purpose recognized as charitable. The second requirement is that there must not be private monetary gain or benefit to private persons. These matters were discussed earlier in the chapter.

However, it bears repeating here that the public service concept of a charity embraces these rules: services may not be restricted on the basis of race or creed; a hospital's emergency room services may not be refused because of inability to pay; and a hospital may not restrict the use of its facilities to a small, particular group of physicians, thereby excluding other qualified professional personnel from membership on the medical staff.[16] It is recognized, of course,

---

[14] Bromberg, *supra* n. 7, at 250.
[15] Bromberg, *supra* n. 7, at 249–50.
[16] Revenue Ruling 56-185, 1956-1 Cum. Bull. 202. The ruling cited here restated the two code requirements and the necessity of an open medical staff. It does not specifically prohibit discrimination based on race or refusal of emergency care because

that a particular hospital may not have the facilities or the need to extend membership to all physicians who apply for admission to the medical staff; accordingly, a private hospital may reject such an application from even a competent and well-qualified physician without losing its tax-exempt status. Under the judicial law of medical staff privileges, however, the hospital may be obligated to review a physician's application fairly and carefully, provide him or her with an opportunity for a hearing if the application is rejected, and state the reasons for rejection.[17] Perhaps the tax exemption requirement with respect to selection and appointment of medical staff can best be summarized by saying that the hospital must be willing to consider qualified applicants to the extent that facilities for their practice are available. For example, the staff must not be arbitrarily limited to the members of a particular medical partnership.

Formerly, an organization exempt from federal income taxation under Section 501(c)(3) was prohibited from devoting a "substantial part" of its "activities" to the influencing of legislation. The concept of "substantial" was never defined precisely, although from time to time the Internal Revenue Service did challenge legislative lobbying activities of tax-exempt charitable organizations. The prohibition has now, however, been removed by Congress in the Tax Reform Act of 1976. The new statute permits legislative lobbying by certain tax-exempt organizations, although it establishes certain limitations expressed in both percentage and absolute monetary amounts based upon the charity's annual budget.

As explained above, the state law in most jurisdictions does not require that a charitable organization offer a given amount of free care to the community or provide services below cost. Prior to 1969 the Internal Revenue Service through the issuance of Revenue Ruling 56–185 (1956) pursuant to the 1954 Internal Revenue Code did, however, require that a tax-exempt hospital operate insofar as it could for the benefit of those unable to pay. Moreover the hospital was prohibited from denying admission to persons on the basis of

---

of inability to pay. Thus the statement in the text is based on general public policy relative to public charities. In 1970 the Internal Revenue Service announced that it would no longer recognize exempt status for a private corporation that engaged in racial discrimination.

Bob Jones University v. Connally, 472 F. 2d 903 (4th Cir. 1973), denied permanent injunction against the Internal Revenue Service, which had removed the university's tax-exempt status on the grounds that it practiced racial discrimination. This case thus held that the Internal Revenue could not be enjoined from withdrawal of tax-exempt status, pending litigation on the merits of that removal.

[17] See Chapter XIII.

inability to pay. The actual monetary amount or extent of the required free care was, however, never specified.

In 1969 a new Revenue Ruling (69–545, 1962–2 Cum. Bull. 117) was promulgated by the Internal Revenue Service. This ruling removed the requirements of service to those unable to pay, thereby making the federal income tax definition of a charitable purpose consistent with the decisions of most state courts in state taxation cases. However, the legal validity of this regulation was challenged in a recent lawsuit, and the federal district court for the District of Columbia held the regulation to be invalid.[18] The district court first held that the plaintiffs in a class action, several indigent persons, and a Welfare Rights Organization, had proper legal standing to sue in that they had suffered injury as a result of the revenue ruling in question, even though precise proof of the unavailability of medical care to them was lacking. Then the court went on to hold the 1969 regulation invalid on the basis that it was beyond the administrative powers of the Internal Revenue Service to issue the ruling, and the court enjoined the Service from following ruling 69–545. Since Congress had remained silent on the issue of free care by failing to insert into the Tax Reform Act of 1969 a specific tax exemption for "hospitals," the district court judge reasoned that it must have been the intent of Congress to retain previous policy as represented by Revenue Ruling 56–185.

The foregoing opinion, however, was reversed by the circuit court of appeals on the merits of the issue. Specifically, the court held that the provisions of Revenue Ruling 69–545 were consistent with the intent of Congress and constituted a permissible definition of "charitable."[19] The basic issue of federal public policy, of course, is whether or not a hospital is to be regarded in part as an almshouse for the poor or as a community service organization for the ill and injured. Realistically the nearly certain advent of a national health service should result in a decision that tax-exempt hospitals need not provide free care.

The United States Supreme Court arrived at the same ultimate result as the court of appeals but on the basis of quite different reasons.[20] The court failed to render an opinion on the merits of the issue of whether the concept of "charitable" as required by Section

[18]*Eastern Kentucky Welfare Rights Organization v. Shultz, Secretary of the Treasury*, 370 F. Supp. 325 (D.D.C. 1973).
[19]*Eastern Kentucky Welfare Rights Organization v. Simon*, 506 F. 2d 1278 (D.C. Cir. 1974).
[20]*Simon, Secretary of the Treasury, et al. v. Eastern Kentucky Welfare Rights Organization, et al.*, 96 S. Ct. 1917 (1976).

501(c)(3) of the Internal Revenue Code requires a tax-exempt
organization to extend services to patients unable to pay. Rather,
the court ruled that the plaintiffs lacked standing to sue and to
challenge the validity of Revenue Ruling 69-545 (1969). The Eastern
Kentucky Welfare Rights Organization could not establish standing
simply on the basis of its goal to promote access of the poor to
health services in the absence of any injury to the organization.
Further, the individual indigent plaintiffs had not established a "case
or controversy," as required by Article III of the Federal Constitution
before a federal court can redress an alleged injury, for the reason
that the suit was brought against the Secretary of the Treasury and
the Commissioner of Internal Revenue rather than against a hospital.
It was speculative whether or not the alleged denial of access to
hospital services was actually the result of the revenue ruling permitting tax-exempt status without requiring the hospital to provide the
community with a component of free care. Speculative claims do
not suffice to invoke federal judicial power.

The second primary Internal Revenue Code requirement for
tax-exempt status is that there must not be private monetary gain
or benefit to private persons. This requirement goes hand-in-hand
with the concept of public service or benefit. Each case must be
decided on its own individual facts and circumstances, since man's
ingenuity with respect to activity through the corporate form of
business is nearly limitless. No one single factor or set of factors
will decide the issue and hence determine the status of a given
institution. Rather, the court will look to the facts of operation,
applying one criterion or more to determine whether or not a
corporation claiming tax-exempt status is a shield for attaining private
gain.

Bromberg identifies factors which the courts will consider, most
of which flow from or relate directly to the major factor of corporate
control.[21] When control of a corporation rests exclusively with a
small group of individuals, especially when, for example, a group
of physicians who once practiced in partnership or who owned a
proprietary hospital have subsequently incorporated as a nonprofit
corporation, the facts raise an issue regarding their motives for
incorporation and invite close scrutiny. The six specific factors
indicating private gain are: (1) Division of profits among trustees,
members, or officers of a corporation. (2) Private use of corporate
funds or facilities. (3) Free office space for physicians in the hospital,

---

[21] Bromberg, *supra* n. 7, at 252-53.

a specific example of the second factor. A moderately large community hospital with an open medical staff can probably justify granting free office space to some private physicians on the basis that patients benefit by having the doctors in or near the hospital, and that physicians require such space to carry out their medical staff responsibilities on behalf of the hospital. But it is a different matter when a half-dozen physicians, for example, control the hospital and decide among themselves to utilize hospital space rent free to further their private gain. (4) Exclusive privileges to admit patients. As noted previously, a tax-exempt hospital is expected to have an open medical staff to the extent of considering fairly all qualified applicants as far as available facilities allow. (5) Exclusive right to treat patients. Factor four cannot be circumvented by admitting patients of non-members of the medical staff and then placing the right of treatment exclusively in the hands of a small, closed staff. (6) Low charity record. Even if tax-exempt status is granted without requiring free care, the charity record of a hospital is evidence of a willingness to serve the public. To put the matter another way, the absence or near absence of charity work is evidence, depending on all the other factors noted above, of private gain.

The use of the corporate form to gain private benefit is well illustrated in the leading case of *Sonora Community Hospital v. Commissioner,* and later affirmed by the United States Court of Appeals.[22] In *Sonora* two physicians formed a nonprofit corporation to own and operate a 42-bed general hospital. A contract between the hospital and two private medical technologists provided that the latter were to operate the laboratory and x-ray departments and remit one-third of their gross receipts to the physicians personally. In return, the founding doctors provided no supervision of the laboratory or x-ray department and no services of consequence. Moreover the hospital controlled by the doctors provided only a minimal amount of charitable care, ordinarily referring all charity patients to a governmental institution. A large percentage of the hospital patients were those of a four-person "medical group" controlled by the two founding physicians; in other words, the patients of other physicians in the community were in large part denied access to the hospital. In such circumstances, the court had no difficulty in determining that the hospital was in actuality being operated for the private gain of the two founding physicians.

---

[22] 46 T.C. 519 (1966), *aff'd,* 397 F. 2d 814 (9th Cir. 1968). See also: *Harding Hospital v. U.S.,* 505 F. 2d 1068 (6th Cir. 1974).

Since state tax exemptions also frequently depend as a minimum upon the same two primary requirements for federal income tax exemption, the state courts also issue opinions on the question of private gain or benefit. One such case was *City of Corpus Christi v. Roberts Hospital.*[23] Although the hospital was organized as a charity, it contracted with an individual to manage the hospital, the terms being that the corporation would receive $300 net, and all other earnings would inure to the administrator. Clearly, under this arrangement, the institution was being operated for the benefit of the administrator. In *Malone-Hogan Hospital Clinic Foundation v. Big Spring*, a nonprofit hospital corporation which employed doctors on salary adjusted the salaries every three months in accordance with the earnings of the hospital.[24] In addition, the physicians were given free office space, meals, telephone service, and subscriptions to professional journals. State tax exemption was denied. In a third Texas case, which illustrates general principles, the facts showed that five physicians owned a proprietary hospital. They transferred these assets to a new nonprofit, charitable hospital, but excluded four other physicians in the community from membership on the medical staff and also denied admission to the patients of physicians not on the staff. The hospital accepted no charity patients. These facts were sufficient to show that the hospital was being operated for private gain, although in this instance the physicians were not receiving direct monetary gain in the form of salary or other benefits from the hospital.[25] Resolution of the issue of private gain thus involves a consideration of all factors relevant to the balancing of private interests against service to the community.

Contracts between a hospital and a medical specialist under which, for example, a pathologist or radiologist receives a defined percentage of departmental revenue, gross or net, have raised the issue of private benefit. As long as the contract is negotiated at "arm's length," as long as the specialist's income is "reasonable" compared to that of other similar specialists in similar or typical circumstances, and as long as the physician has no significant ownership or control over the hospital, the arrangement does not constitute private gain to jeopardize the hospital's tax status.[26] The hospital may legitimately furnish space, supplies, equipment, and personnel, and it may fix the charges for service jointly with the doctor and then bill the patients. These conditions may be contrasted with the *Sonora Commu-*

---

[23] 195 S.W. 2d 429 (Texas Civ. App. 1946).
[24] 288 S.W. 2d 550 (Texas Civ. App. 1956).
[25] *Raymondville Memorial Hospital v. State*, 253 S.W. 2d 1012 (Texas Civ. App. 1952).
[26] Revenue Ruling 69–383, 1969–2 Cum. Bull. 113.

nity Hospital case and with *Lorain Avenue Clinic v. Commissioner,* in which tax exemption was denied. In *Lorain* a family group controlled the clinic, and the members fixed their compensation under a system which effectively divided the clinic's profits among them.[27]

A recent Internal Revenue ruling dealt with the issue of whether a nonprofit hospital was permitted to pay pensions to retired employees although it had no formally approved retirement plan. The question was whether or not such payments amounted to the disbursement of gifts or gratuities, thus constituting distribution of corporate earnings to private individuals. As has been pointed out earlier, a nonprofit organization may pay reasonable compensation, including fringe benefits of employment, for services rendered. The opinion in this ruling was that the payments were entirely proper, even without a formal plan or contract with all retired employees, since the accepted practice is to view such disbursements as a part of compensation.[28]

A significant advantage of tax-exempt status under Section 501(c)(3) of the Internal Revenue Code is that donors of gifts to the organization may deduct the, value of their gifts from their income tax liability. This is not the case for organizations exempt from income tax liability under Section 501(c)(4) of the code, which grants preferred tax status to certain groups or corporations whose purpose is to promote social welfare in contrast to dispensing charity. Some prepaid group medical practice plans or health maintenance organizations may therefore not qualify for exemption under 501(c)(3), since they may be in essence a closed group of persons who have agreed to associate for their own self-interest rather than for the public or community interest.[29] Thus, if a health maintenance organization, even one organized as a nonprofit corporation, has a closely controlled governing body, if participation is limited, for example, to members of a particular labor union or the employees of a particular employer, or if all members prepay the full costs of services rendered and patients do not represent an economic cross section of the community, the organization may be denied exemption from taxation under Section 501(c)(3). Because it is a 501(c)(4) organization, the donors of grants or gifts to such a prepaid group practice or health maintenance organization could not deduct the value of the grants

---

[27] 31 T.C. 141 (1958).
[28] Revenue Ruling 73-126, 1973-1 Cum. Bull. 220.
[29] Revenue Ruling 56-185, 1956-1 Cum. Bull. 202.

from their own taxes. This fact understandably inhibits the financing of newly created group plans for prepaid medical care.

Most hospitals which are exempt from taxation under Section 501(c)(3) of the Internal Revenue Code must file an annual information return with the Internal Revenue Service. This return will indicate the annual gross income, expenses, and disbursements, the total contributions received, and the compensation paid to "highly compensated" employees.[30] Exempt from this annual filing requirement are hospitals which have annual gross receipts of less than $5,000 and are operated by a religious organization, fraternal benefit society, or an instrumentality of the United States. Hospitals with gross receipts of less than $5,000 that are supported by state or federal governmental funds other than amounts paid by the government for the care of indigents, and institutions primarily supported by public contributions are likewise exempt.

The Tax Reform Act of 1969 distinguishes between public charities and private nonprofit foundations, and public charities are granted preferred status with respect to donations, since these are fully deductible by the donor. To establish status as a public charity the organization must file notice of claim to status with the Internal Revenue Service, in addition to obtaining the original exemption letter from Internal Revenue certifying exemption under Section 501(c)(3). Failure to file the notice of claim as a public charity results in a presumption of foundation status.[31] The purpose of this provision was to encourage donations to public charities and to discourage in a state the accumulation of excessive funds in the hands of private, family-controlled foundations. Accordingly, foundations are made subject to controls and to Internal Revenue scrutiny that are not applicable to public charities: for example, less favorable treatment for donors of funds, additional disclosure of financial condition and operation, and a specially assessed governmental audit fee.

Prior to the passage of Medicare-Medicaid legislation, physicians engaged in private practice and members of a hospital medical staff frequently rendered medical services without charge to hospital patients who might not have a private physician. Enactment of governmental programs for the care of the aged and indigent made these doctors eligible to receive payment for such services. Since historically and traditionally it has commonly been considered an obligation of hospital staff doctors to care for patients who are without

---

[30] Internal Revenue Code of 1954, sec. 6033 (a) and (b).
[31] Internal Revenue Code, sec. 508 (b).

a private physician, the medical staff at many hospitals have organized separate nonprofit organizations or groups whose purpose is to collect and disburse funds derived from Medicare and Medicaid patients, the physicians simply assigning these fees to the organization.

The establishment of such organizations has raised questions under the federal tax law. First of all, is the organization or corporation that collects and disburses the fees exempt from income tax under Section 501(c)(3) of the Internal Revenue Code? The answer is affirmative as long as the organization's purpose is to conduct a charitable program for the benefit of the hospital. For example, the organization might provide financial assistance to interns and residents for their education if the hospital is a teaching institution, purchase new equipment for the hospital, or create medical research grants. If all funds of the organization are utilized in the ways described, then the organization is both organized and operated exclusively for charitable purposes and is serving a public purpose without private gain or benefit.[32] If, on the other hand, most of the funds collected by the organization are returned to the participating physicians, then the organization would not be tax exempt. It would then be operating simply as a collection agency for private purposes, even if some of the funds were used for the hospital. Whether or not the organization can return a relatively small portion of the funds to the physicians and still maintain tax-exempt status appears at the time of writing to be an open question.

A second major issue with respect to the organizations described above is whether or not the fees collected for services rendered to indigent patients are taxable to the individual physicians. Such fees are *not* taxed to the individual and may be excluded from the report of gross income if the participating doctors are engaged in full-time salaried employment by the hospital, or are full-time members of a medical school faculty, and hence earned the fees in the course of that employment. In essence, by virtue of the employment arrangement, the fees are not controlled by the doctor and hence not taxable to him.[33] Such a factual situation is not as frequent or as typical, however, as that described at the outset of this discussion, namely, a situation where hospital staff physicians with a private practice assign their Medicare-Medicaid or insurance fees to the collecting and disbursement organization, which in turn disburses the funds to the hospital for charitable purposes as has

---

[32] Revenue Ruling 69–631, 1969–2 Cum. Bull. 119.
[33] Revenue Ruling 58–220, 1958–1 Cum. Bull. 26 and Revenue Ruling 69–274, 1969–1 Cum. Bull. 36.

been explained. In this factual situation, the arrangement is in essence voluntary on the part of the doctors, who in fact have control over the fees that they have earned. Hence they must report the income on their individual tax returns. In turn, however, the physicians may deduct the amount assigned to the collection organization (which was itself tax exempt), as a charitable contribution subject to any limitations specified in the Internal Revenue Code relative to donations to a charity.[34] Similarly, any fees collected directly by the physician and individually, voluntarily donated to the hospital are included in taxable income but deductible as charitable contributions.[35] Finally, if salaried faculty members of a medical school are permitted to carry on a private practice but required by the university to remit the fees so earned to the school by the terms of their employment contract, the income is includable in the faculty members' gross taxable income; but it is deductible as an ordinary and necessary business expense because of the contractual requirement with the university.[36] Depending upon all the facts and circumstances of the individual taxpayer, deductions as business expenses may produce a more favorable tax situation than deductions as contributions to a charity.

In conclusion, it should be noted that compensation paid to medical students, interns, and residents is considered to be compensation or wages and not educational scholarships or fellowships excludable from taxable income. Accordingly, such payments are taxable income to the recipient.[37] This position of the Internal Revenue Service is based simply on the notion that the primary purpose of a hospital is to care for patients and not to educate students. Students and house staff, when performing patient care responsibilities, are in actual fact performing an employment function. Therefore hospitals making such payments to house staff are obligated to comply with provisions of the Internal Revenue Code with respect to withholding of federal income tax. Only if a "fellow" is a physician studying for an advanced degree at a hospital, who performs no patient care responsibilities in place of other employees or for the benefit of the training institution, are payments made to him considered to

[34] Internal Revenue Code, sec. 170 and Revenue Ruling 70–161, 1970–1 Cum. Bull. 15.
[35] Revenue Ruling 69–275, 1969–1 Cum. Bull. 36.
[36] Internal Revenue Code, sec. 162 (a) and Revenue Ruling 66–377, 1966–2 Cum. Bull. 21.
[37] Revenue Rulings 68–520, 1968–2 Cum. Bull. 58, 65–117, 1965–1 Cum. Bull. 67, 57–386, 1957–2 Cum. Bull. 107. *Anderson v. Commissioner of Internal Revenue*, 54 T.C. No. 148 (1970). (A stipend paid an intern and resident was taxable.)

be in the nature of a nontaxable grant of fellowship.[38] By definition in the Internal Revenue Regulations a "fellowship grant" is "an amount paid or allowed to, or for the benefit of an individual to aid him in the pursuit of study or research."[39] In sum, a nontaxable educational scholarship, grant, or fellowship has no substantial quid pro quo of service to the grantor on the part of the recipient. As said in *Aloysius J. Proskey*, which held that a stipend paid to a resident physician at University Hospital, Ann Arbor, was fully taxable as compensation for services:

> There can be no serious doubt that work as a resident physician provides highly valuable training, particularly in preparing for specialties in the various fields of medicine.
> Yet virtually all work as an apprentice, whether in medicine or law, carpentry or masonry, provides valuable training. Nothing in section 117 requires that an amount paid as compensation for services rendered be treated as a nontaxable fellowship grant, merely because the recipient is learning a trade, business, or profession. Whatever training petitioner received during the years of his residency—and we do not deny that it was substantial—was merely "incidental to and for the purpose of facilitating the raison d'être of the Hospital, namely the care of its patients."[40]

TAXABILITY OF UNRELATED BUSINESS INCOME

A public charity exempt from income tax under Section 501(c)(3) of the Internal Revenue Code which derives income from various sources or activities must face the issue of whether or not the activity is an unrelated trade or business. Income generated by an activity unrelated to charitable status is taxed, just as income is taxed for any individual or corporation engaged in a profit-making endeavor, although the tax-exempt status of the charity itself is not lost. The taxability of income from an unrelated trade or business is provided for by Sections 511–14 of the Revenue Code of 1954.

At the outset it must be noted that a hospital's investment income consisting of dividends, interest, and annuities, as well as income from research, is not taxable as unrelated to charitable purpose.[41] However, income derived from the operation of regularly conducted gift shops, restaurants, parking lots, hospital pharmacies, physicians'

[38]Revenue Ruling 57–560, 1957–2 Cum. Bull. 108.
[39]Regulations, sec. 1.117–3. See: *Bingler v. Johnson*, 394 U.S. 741, 22 L. Ed. 2d 695, 89 S.C. 1439 (1969).
[40]51 T.C. 918, at 925 (1969).
[41]Internal Revenue Code of 1954, sec. 512(b).

offices, residences for interns, nurses, or other staff, and other facilities owned and operated by a hospital presents the question of an unrelated trade or business. The mere fact that all income from such activities is devoted to hospital or charitable purposes does *not* make the income tax exempt. The reason for this general rule is this: a hospital enterprise such as a pharmacy or a parking lot for which charges are made and which is open to the general public should not be permitted an unfair competitive advantage in relation to private business.

Accordingly, the general rule or test of a particular income-producing activity is whether or not it is "substantially related" to the charitable purpose of the tax-exempt institution.[42] Is the pharmacy, restaurant, or parking lot furthering the purpose of the charity? To help answer these questions of substantial relationship and the furthering of charitable purpose the Internal Revenue Code provides for the "convenience rule," which states that the income is not taxable if the hospital can demonstrate that the activity is conducted primarily for the convenience of the hospital's staff, patients, and visitors, in contrast to an enterprise selling goods and services to the general public. Even if a given activity is not "substantially related" to the hospital's purpose, the income from the activity is free from tax if most of the work which generated the income is accomplished by volunteers or if merchandise being sold was donated to the hospital.[43] This rule permits the hospital to engage in fund-raising efforts, even if regularly done, that are supported by volunteer workers and donations.

To illustrate the concept of unrelated business income, one Internal Revenue ruling dealt with the operation of a hospital pharmacy.[44] The pharmacy, located on the ground floor of the building, sold nonprescription and personal items as well as prescription drugs and was open to the general public. Although the primary source of income was derived from hospital patients, the income was deemed to be taxable, because sales to nonpatients on a regular and continuous basis did not meet the test of the convenience rule. A liberal definition of "hospital patients" is recognized, however, and would include outpatients, persons seen in the emergency room and referred to an outpatient clinic, discharged bed patients returning for refills of prescription drug items, patients in a hospital's extended care

---

[42]Internal Revenue Code, sec. 513 and Treasury Regulations, sec. 1.513-1(a).
[43]Internal Revenue Code, sec. 513(a).
[44]Revenue Ruling 68-374, 1968-2 Cum Bull. 242.

facility, and persons enrolled in a home care program.[45] Moreover, "casual pharmaceutical sales" to private patients of physicians on the hospital's medical staff, permitted as a courtesy for the mutual convenience of the physician and patient, would be allowable as long as such sales were not promoted, were relatively infrequent, and constituted an insignificant proportion of total gross receipts.[46] However, if the hospital should own a medical office building leased to private physicians and should maintain a pharmacy there which regularly sold both prescription and nonprescription items to the private patients of the doctors, then the convenience rule again fails of application, and the income from the pharmacy would be taxable.[47] Similar principles of convenience to hospital staff and patients, in contrast to encouragement of the general public to patronize the facility, govern the taxability of income derived from hospital-owned gift shops, restaurants, and parking lots.[48]

Note, however, that if these activities are separately incorporated rather than owned and operated by the hospital, the income might be taxable, since separate incorporation suggests a motive for operation beyond mere convenience for hospital patients and staff. The reason is that such a separate entity might be deemed a "feeder organization" under Sections 501 and 502 of the Internal Revenue Code. By definition a "feeder organization" is a separate business conducted for profit; it is not an integral part of the hospital, which pays its earnings to the hospital or other tax-exempt organization.

To protect the legitimate interests of commercial business, the income of a feeder organization may be taxable if the primary purpose is to earn profit, and if the organization is in competition with private commercial enterprise and has no substantial relation to the conduct of the hospital. As previously indicated, the mere use of profits or earnings for hospital purposes is not in itself enough to establish the activity as a related trade or business. Thus, according to an Internal Revenue ruling, the income of a thrift shop, separately incorporated, would be taxable, even though substantially all labor was by volunteers and the merchandise was donated.[49] In contrast,

---

[45]Revenue Ruling 68–376, 1968–2 Cum. Bull. 246.
[46]Revenue Ruling 68–374, 1968–2 Cum. Bull. 242.
[47]Revenue Ruling 68–375, 1968–2 Cum. Bull. 245.
[48]Revenue Ruling 69–269, 1969–1 Cum. Bull. 160. (An income-producing parking lot used only by patients and their visitors was not an unrelated trade or business.) Revenue Ruling 69–267, 1969–1 Cum. Bull. 160 (gift shop) and Revenue Ruling 69–268, 1969–1 Cum. Bull. 160 (cafeteria and coffee shop primarily for employees and medical staff, even when this service is contracted with a vending company).
[49]Revenue Ruling 68–439, 1968–2 Cum. Bull 239.

a corporation organized to provide specialized purchasing and consulting services to several hospitals was free from tax as a related business, since the facts established that it was not effectively in competition with private interests.[50]

In 1968 Congress affirmatively recognized the merit and value of hospitals' joining together to share various kinds of goods or services through the mechanism of a separate corporation organized to supply goods or services to the participating hospitals. Under Section 501(e) of the 1954 Internal Revenue Code such a corporation can itself be tax exempt under 501(c)(3) of the code if four requirements are met: First, the service corporation must be organized and operated on a cooperative basis evidenced by appropriate bylaws or agreement. Second, if it is a stock corporation, all the stock must be owned by participating hospitals, and all earnings must be paid to the member hospitals. Third, all participating hospitals must themselves be tax exempt or governmental hospitals. Finally, the services or goods supplied must be one or more of those specifically named in the code. Eleven services are enumerated: data processing, purchasing, warehousing, billing and collection, food, industrial engineering, laboratory, printing, communication, record center, and the selection, training, and education of personnel. Such service organizations are thus recognized as organized and operated exclusively for charitable purposes. If these tests are met, the service corporation will not be considered a "feeder organization."

Notably absent from this enumerated list are laundry services, a deliberate omission. The income of a separately incorporated centralized laundry or cooperative would theoretically be taxable, since it cannot qualify under Section 501(e). As a practical matter, however, the enterprise could be organized as a cooperative, paying all of its net income to its patrons on the basis of services performed and thus avoiding taxable income. This procedure is certainly legitimate as long as all the patrons are themselves tax-exempt organizations, either private charitable hospitals or governmental; and contributions to the service corporation by the patrons will not jeopardize the tax-exempt status of the latter. But if a proprietary hospital is included among the members of a central service laundry organization, then any contribution to the laundry by an exempt hospital over and above its proportionate share of benefits received might well jeopardize the tax-exempt status of the contributor, the reason

---

[50]*Hospital Bureau of Standard Supplies v. United States*, 158 F. Supp. 560 (Court of Claims, 1958).

being that it could be benefiting a proprietary institution, representing a noncharitable purpose.[51]

Another method of sharing services is for a particular hospital directly to own and operate a particular service—for example, a laundry or computer service—and then sell the service to other institutions in the community. This does not affect the hospital's tax-exempt status as long as the service is sold only to other tax-exempt hospitals, or to a proprietary hospital above cost, and as long as the service sold to others does not become a substantial part of the hospital's activity. If, however, the hospital sells services to a proprietary institution at less than cost, the provider hospital's tax-exempt status may well be placed in jeopardy, since the institution is not then being operated exclusively for charitable purposes. In any event, the profit earned by the provider institution through the sale of services to others above cost would be taxable as income from an unrelated business.[52]

A third method of sharing services is for a tax-exempt hospital to enter a partnership or joint venture with another hospital or medical care organization to conduct a particular activity such as running a laundry. The first legal issue here is to determine whether local corporate law empowers the hospital to enter into such a partnership or joint venture. As pointed out elsewhere, the provisions of the corporate statutes and the hospital's charter must be consulted. So far as federal income tax status is concerned, the hospital will not be adversely affected, even if its partner is a profit-making proprietary organization, so long as profits shared by the partners are equivalent to assets contributed to the partnership and services received. Of course, income received by the proprietary partner will be taxable to it. Income received by the tax-exempt hospital may or may not be taxable to it as unrelated business income. If such income can be related only to services rendered for the hospital's own patients, the income from the partnership or joint venture will not be taxed.

Income derived from property owned by a tax-exempt hospital and rented to others is specifically excluded in the Internal Revenue Code's definition of unrelated business income, unless the property

[51]Revenue Ruling 69-633, 1969-2 Cum. Bull. 121.
[52]Revenue Rulings 69-160, 1969-1 Cum. Bull. 147 and 69-633, 1969-2 Cum. Bull. 121, Internal Revenue Code, sec. 511 and 513. See also: sec. 513(e) of Tax Reform Act of 1976, which attempts to clarify the circumstances under which a hospital may provide services to other institutions without having income taxed as unrelated business income. The section establishes several severe limitations on the sale of services to other hospitals and health care institutions.

is "debt financed."[53] Generally, therefore, rent received from all real estate that is not debt financed is exempt from taxation. On the other hand, rental income from debt-financed property is generally taxable in proportion to the amount of the debt. A mortgage loan, of course, is the most common example of a debt to finance the acquisition or the improvement of property. Rental income from a "business lease" of more than five years is generally taxable if an indebtedness on the property exists at the close of the taxable year.[54]

There are very significant exceptions to the general rule taxing income from debt-financed property or from business leases of more than five years. If the rental income is derived from using the property in a way that is substantially related to charitable purposes, then it is free from federal tax. Hence the rent from a medical office building built by a hospital on adjacent land and leased only to medical staff physicians for terms longer than five years was considered nontaxable in a recent Internal Revenue ruling.[55] The ruling properly recognizes that the proximity of the physicians' offices to the hospital increases efficiency, encourages fuller utilization of hospital facilities, and improves the overall quality of patient care.

State Taxation of Real Estate

Real estate owned by governmental hospitals, federal or local, is exempt from real estate taxation by the state; the exemption is created by specific provision of the relevant state constitution or by statute. In general, ownership of the property standing alone is sufficient to establish exemption. Some states add the requirement that the property be in use by the "public," but hospitals have little difficulty in establishing that they meet this requirement.

With respect to privately owned hospitals, the real estate that they occupy or own may or may not be tax exempt, depending upon a number of factors. The first requirement of note is that the hospital must qualify as a charity, a matter defined by local state law and discussed previously. Accordingly, real estate owned by a proprietary hospital, or one operated for profit, is fully taxable, just as the property of any other business is taxable.

---

[53]Internal Revenue Code, sec. 512(b)(3)(4).
[54]Internal Revenue Code, sec. 514(f).
[55]Internal Revenue ruling 69-464, 1969-2 Cum. Bull. 132. Internal Revenue Code, sec. 514(b)(3). Similarly, income from the leasing of an adjacent office building to a medical group by a tax-exempt hospital is related income and not taxable. Revenue Ruling 69-463, 1969-2 Cum. Bull. 131.

In some states the source of exemption for real estate owned or occupied by a voluntary hospital that qualifies as a charity is a state constitutional provision which is mandatory. That is, the legislature of the state could not terminate the exemption granted, and neither could the courts, although the judicial branch of government would have the power to interpret the meaning of the constitutional language. Other state constitutions contain permissive tax exemption provisions for charitable organizations; a few states are entirely silent on the matter. In either situation, tax-exempt status will depend upon legislative enactment. The permissive type of constitutional provision thus has the effect of granting sole ultimate power of exemption to the legislature, which may determine the requirements of attaining tax-exempt status—again subject to court interpretation, especially with respect to legislative intent. The distinction between a mandatory constitutional provision and a permissive provision—or no provision at all—becomes increasingly significant in an era when local governments constantly need and are searching for additional revenue and when there is consequently unremitting political pressure to restrict or reduce the tax exemptions for real estate.

In general, every parcel of land owned or occupied by a charitable hospital must be separately qualified for tax-exempt status. Further, each parcel must normally meet two tests: "ownership" by the hospital and "use" for a charitable purpose. The test of ownership is not as simple as it might first appear. Real estate law recognizes various types of estates in land, as well as leasehold interests in land owned by another. All states, so far as the ownership test is concerned, grant exemption to land owned by a charity when the organization holds a fee simple legal title. Nearly all likewise grant exemption to ownership in the form of equitable title, an example of an equitable title being the purchase of land on an installment land contract under which the seller retains legal title until the purchase price is paid in full, or until the buyer has reached a certain equity in property and refinances the balance by mortgage. A very few states will deny exemption to a charity holding an equitable title.

A larger number of states will deny real estate tax exemption to the owner of land who leases it to a charitable corporation. Here, clearly, the land is not owned by the charity which has by virtue of the lease the right of possession and use but has neither legal nor equitable title. On the other hand, some states will exempt such property from taxation, probably on the basis that it is sound public policy to reduce the operating costs of charitable organizations. This matter, of course, is resolved by individual states according to the provisions of their constitutions and statutes.

A typical provision in most states requires that tax-exempt property of a charity be held for the "exclusive use . . . for charitable purposes." Note carefully that this contemplates actual use or occupancy of the property itself, and property owned for investment income would therefore not qualify for exemption. In other words, the use of the property determines the tax-exempt status and not the use of income derived from the property. Moreover, the word "exclusive" in these provisions raises issues with respect to the status of property rented to or occupied by such others as medical staff members who practice as private physicians, hospital interns, residents, and nurses. The usual approach to these situations, which are decided case-by-case and state-by-state, is to examine how closely the use of the property relates to the primary purpose of the hospital, and to analyze the relative benefits to the respective parties.

In general, property rented to private physicians or others at a rental based on its commercial market value, which allows the hospital to earn a profit in excess of overhead, will be subject to real estate taxation. This follows either from an express statutory provision forbidding rental of property held by a charity, or from judicial interpretation of the "exclusive use" provision. Some states, however, would probably allow exemption for property rented to medical staff physicians for their private offices, or to hospital personnel for their residences, if rental covered only the overhead cost. The rationale would be that the hospital and its patients benefit by having the staff close at hand at all times, and public policy should hence serve the interests of the charity unless there is an express provision forbidding any rental. On the other hand, some courts will deny exemption to facilities such as physicians' offices or residences for staff, even if rental does not exceed the costs of maintenance and amortization of investment. They do so either on the grounds that the primary benefit is a private, not charitable, benefit, and therefore the "exclusive use" test is not met, or on the grounds that local statutes require *hospital occupancy* for all tax-exempt land.[56]

Although it has been held, by way of further example, that a residence building for student nurses who paid no rental at all was

---

[56]For example: *Milton Hospital v. Board of Tax Assessors*, 271 N.E. 2d 745 (Massachusetts 1971), and *Medical Center of Vermont, Inc. v. City of Burlington*, 131 Vt. 196, 303 A. 2d 468 (1973): (Case remanded to determine facts of whether the physician's offices represented private or public use). *White Cross Hospital v. Warren*, 6 Ohio St. 2d 29, 215 N.E. 2d 374 (1966): (Offices leased to physicians are not exempt).

tax exempt, the same state denied exemption for rent-free housing furnished to married residents and interns. The residence for nurses was exempt on the grounds that such a facility enabled the hospital to attract these persons for professional training and they paid for their nursing education.[57] On the other hand, because married house staff were paid a stipend, housing for them was primarily a private and not a charitable use, even though they paid no rent.[58] These two cases are mentioned here to illustrate how one jurisdiction has applied the statute requiring "exclusive use for charitable purposes" to qualify for tax exemption, and also to illustrate the distinctions that courts draw in particular cases between a private and charitable benefit.

It is believed, however, that most states would allow tax exemption for facilities rented to nurses and house staff, especially if rent is not in excess of overhead, on the theory that the primary purpose is public or charitable. The hospital should be able to document, if challenged by local tax authority, that patients benefit when personnel are housed close to the institution.[59]

Recent litigation in New York illustrates the issues of public policy which come into play with respect to hospital-owned real estate. Genesee Hospital constructed an office building adjacent to the hospital for lease to private physicians. Rental paid by the doctors was established at currently competitive prices but, initially at least, did not cover operating costs. The hospital is a teaching institution with a full-time staff of salaried physicians, together with resident physicians and interns. The private attending staff participate actively with the house staff in patient care and medical education. As in many other states, the New York statute requires that real property "owned by a corporation or association organized or conducted exclusively for . . . hospital . . . purposes . . . and used exclusively for carrying out . . . such purposes . . . shall be exempt from taxation. . . ." Further, however, the statute provided that "if any portion of such real property is not so used exclusively to carry out . . . such purposes but is leased or otherwise used for other purposes, such portion shall be subject to taxation and the remaining portion only shall be exempt." At issue, then, was whether the office building was "used exclusively" for hospital purposes.

The trial court rendered an opinion favorable to the hospital and

---

[57] *Aultman Hospital Association v. Evatt,* 140 Ohio St. 114, 42 N.E. 2d 646 (1942).
[58] *Doctors Hospital v. Board of Tax Appeals,* 173 Ohio St. 283, 181 N.E. 2d 702 (1962).
[59] For example, a leading case: *Oakwood Hospital Corporation v. Michigan State Tax Commission,* 374 Mich. 524, 132 N.W. 2d 634 (1965).

held that the building was exempt from taxation.[60] Rather than applying a literal interpretation of the word "exclusively," the court, citing precedent, applied the standard of whether the office building was "reasonably incident to the major purpose" of the hospital. Since the evidence clearly established that the hospital's concern was to maintain a "first-rate" medical center for both patient care and medical education rather than to benefit the private physicians personally, the trial court judge, in essence, concluded that the hospital, its house staff, and patients benefited relatively more from the use of the building than the private physicians did. The public policy involved was made evident when the trial court concluded that the community views a modern hospital working together with a highly trained staff of attending physicians as an important investment.

On appeal, however, the decision was reversed, and the space leased to the private practicing physicians was held to be subject to taxation. The appellate division recognized that the concept and development of a professional building is an admirable addition to the community and doubtless enhanced the patient care and teaching functions of the hospital. Nevertheless, the facility was in direct competition with privately developed professional office buildings serving an identical function of providing space for the private practice of medicine. Accordingly the leased space did not qualify for exemption under the language of the New York statute.[61]

Issues similar to those relating to physicians' offices and nurses' residences are sometimes raised regarding hospital-owned and -operated cafeterias, gift shops, pharmacies, parking lots, and the like. Again, the legal issue is whether or not these activities are consistent with the requirement of "exclusive use for charitable purposes." If such an activity is not conducted for commercial profit, and if it takes place in a part of the hospital building or the immediate premises not open to the general public, the granting of tax-exempt status is likely.

The hospital must be able to document that the activity is carried on primarily for the good of the hospital. Hence a parking lot limited to hospital staff and visitors, where the fees charged were all devoted to maintenance and improvement of the lot, was held to be exempt.[62]

---

[60]*Genesee Hospital v. Wagner*, 76 Misc. 2d 281, 350 N.Y.S. 2d 582 (Sup. Ct. 1973).
[61]*Genesee Hospital v. Wagner*, 364 N.Y.S. 2d 934, 47 App. Div. 2d 37 (1975), *aff'd mem.*, 39 N.Y. 2d 863, 386 N.Y.S. 2d 216, 352 N.E. 2d 133 (1976). Accord: *Greater Anchorage Area Borough v. Sisters of Charity of the House of Providence*, 553 P. 2d 467 (Alaska 1976).
[62]*Bowers v. Akron City Hospital*, 16 Ohio St. 2d 94, 243 N.E. 2d 95 (1968) and *Maine Medical Center v. Lucci*, 317 A. 2d 1 (Maine 1974).

On the other hand, if any of the criteria noted above are violated, or if the facility is operated by an organization independent of the hospital through a lease arrangement whereby the hospital earns a profit, then tax-exempt status may well be jeopardized.

If tax-exempt status for a cafeteria, gift shop, parking lot, or similar facility cannot be maintained, it then becomes crucial to determine whether or not the local state statute permits split-listing of property for purposes of real estate taxation, since the activity under discussion most frequently takes place in part of the hospital building itself. Split-listing means, essentially, that the local tax authorities will list as taxable the actual space used for the activity that is not exempt, while listing the remainder of the hospital building as exempt. In most jurisdictions split-listing is permitted, and a hospital's loss of real estate tax exemption for a minor portion of the total building is not too serious. Some states do not allow it, however, and in these jurisdictions it is especially important to seek competent legal advice regarding the activities named above, or similar ones.

Many hospitals own vacant land or recreational land for employees, which is often geographically separated from the institutions. With respect to vacant or unoccupied land there is a diversity of judicial opinion, depending upon the exact language of local state statute and judicial interpretation of that language. For tax exemption some states may provide that the land be "occupied" as well as "used for charitable purposes." Even if being "occupied" is not a statutory requirement, one must determine the meaning of "used." Vacant land which is held simply for possible use in the indefinite future and for which no plans for development exist would normally be taxable.[63] On the other hand, if plans for construction and development are well along, fund raising is under way, and actual bids have been received for construction, then the land, although not yet in actual use, is exempt in some jurisdictions.[64] Some states, however, may require actual use and occupancy before granting exempt status.

Land owned for employees' recreation is, of course, being used in the literal meaning of that term, and thus the legal issue is whether or not such a facility relates primarily to the hospital's purposes. The leading case on the question held that tennis courts and other

---

[63]For example: *Oak Ridge Hospital v. City of Oak Ridge*, 57 Tenn. App. 487, 420 S.W. 2d 583. (1967) and *Cleveland Memorial Medical Foundation v. Perk*, 10 Ohio St. 2d 72, 225 N.E. 2d 233 (1967).
[64]For example: *Good Samaritan Hospital Association v. Glander*, 155 Ohio St. 507, 99 N.E. 2d 473 (1951) and *Cleveland Memorial Medical Foundation v. Perk, supra* n. 63.

recreational areas for employees, as well as housing for interns, residents, nurses, and other personnel, and land used for a nurses' training school were exempt.[65] On the other hand, a building under construction for housing student nurses, and a thrift shop where donated merchandise was sold for the benefit of a free children's clinic maintained jointly by the hospital and a Community Chest agency, were held to be taxable in the *Cedars of Lebanon Hospital* case.

As mentioned earlier, most state courts do not require that an institution render a certain amount of free care, or care below cost, and be partly subsidized by public contributions before it can be exempt from real estate taxation. This rule and the accompanying discussion of the nature of a charitable corporation are now to be applied specifically to nursing homes and homes for the elderly, since issues of real estate taxation are frequently raised with respect to such institutions.

Illustrating the general rule that an undefined amount of free care is not necessary to qualify for state real estate tax exemption is the Nebraska case of *Evangelical Lutheran Good Samaritan Society v. County of Gage.*[66] A home for the aged was organized as a nonprofit corporation. It required all residents to pay if they were able. The rates were nearly the same as those charged by proprietary homes, and the home operated at a profit in some years and at a deficit in others. The court held the real estate to be exempt, ruling in effect that "charity" should be defined in broader terms than almsgiving and the relief of poverty.

In *Central Board on Care of Jewish Aged, Inc. v. Henson,* the Court of Appeals of Georgia ruled that a home for the elderly was exempt, and said:

> For the appellant to be tax exempt it must be purely charitable and public. . . . A familiar meaning of the word "charity" is alms-giving, but as used in the law it may include substantially any scheme or effort to better the condition of society, or any considerable part thereof . . . "charity," as used in tax exemption statutes, is not restricted to the relief of the sick or indigent, but extends to other forms of philanthropy or public beneficence, such as practical enterprises for the good of humanity, operated at moderate

---

[65] *Cedars of Lebanon Hospital v. Los Angeles County,* 35 Cal. 2d 729, 221 P. 2d 31, (1950).
[66] 181 Neb. 831, 151 N.W. 2d 446 (1967).

cost to the beneficiaries, or enterprises operated for the general improvement and happiness of mankind.

Neither would the fact that the residents paid rent according to their ability destroy the charitable nature of the institution. . . . The purpose of the home is to care for the aged and provide for their physical and mental welfare. As is stated in *Bozeman Deaconess Foundation v. Ford,* 439 P 2d 915, 917: "The concept of charity is not confined to the relief of the needy and destitute, for aged people require care and attention apart from financial assistance, and the supply of this care and attention is as much a charitable and benevolent purpose as the relief of their financial wants."[67]

In the *Henson* case the home was maintained for elderly persons of the Jewish faith, with an average age of nearly 83. Each resident paid a monthly charge based upon his financial ability, the maximum being $450. No applicant was ever refused admission because of inability to pay, and at all times a few residents were permitted to remain without payment. Deficits in annual operating expenses were covered by contributions from time to time by the Jewish Welfare Fund or by individuals. The home provided medical and nursing services.

In similar fashion the Iowa Supreme Court exempted a church-supported retirement home which charged those able to pay but did not reject anyone unable to pay. In essence, tax-exempt status is not lost by relying primarily for financial support on those residents who pay a monthly charge or are otherwise able to make gifts or contributions.[68] Adequate housing, care of the aged, and general promotion of a pleasing environment are valid charitable purposes, without its being necessary to establish relief of poverty per se as the primary goal of the institution.

On the other hand, some retirement communities are categorized as "luxurious" and serve only those able to pay a substantial nonreturnable entrance fee as well as monthly charges for housing and perhaps board. These will not, as a rule, qualify for exemption from state real estate taxation. Thus, in *Presbyterian Homes v. Division of*

[67]120 Ga. App. 627, 629, 171 S.E. 2d 747, 479 (1969). Compare reinterpretation of Georgia Constitution and Code requiring that a tax-exempt organization be "purely charitable and public": *St. Joseph Hospital of Augusta v. Bohler,* 229 Ga. 577, 193 S.E. 2d 603 (1972): (when a hospital's costs were borne by patients who were encouraged to pay, and its policies were not directed toward persons destitute and without economic means, it was not exempt from taxation even though its emergency room was open at all times to the general public, its available annual surpluses are utilized to improve facilities, and during some years the hospital operates at a deficit. The court made no reference to the *Henson* decision).
[68]*South Iowa Methodist Homes, Inc. v. Board of Review,* 173 N.W. 2d 526 (Iowa 1970).

Tax Appeals, the New Jersey court rejected exemption for a home for the elderly, where the corporation specifically reserved the right to terminate the residence of a person who could not continue to pay the monthly charge, or who became ill and unable to care for himself.[69] As previously stressed, mere organization as a nonprofit corporation under local state law is not sufficient to justify tax exemption.

---

[69] 55 N.J. 275, 261 A. 2d 143 (1970).

PART THREE

The Physician–Patient Relationship–Professional Liability

George J. Siedel III

IV

Breach of Contract and Intentional Tort

An understanding of the physician-patient relationship is essential to sound hospital management, since hospital liability is often based on a breach of duty arising from the relationship. More specifically, as it becomes harder to initiate a malpractice action against physicians, claimants increasingly think of the hospital as a possible defendant. One bar association has even suggested that only hospitals, excluding physicians, be liable for malpractice committed on the hospital premises.[1] If adopted, this proposal would cover most malpractice claims, because 74 percent of all alleged malpractice occurs in hospitals, according to a 1973 HEW report on malpractice.

Three theories are commonly used in an action brought by a patient against the physician: breach of contract, liability based upon intentional tort, and negligence. In this chapter, after an introductory overview of the creation and termination of the physician-patient relationship, the first two theories will be examined. Actions based upon these theories are few; but they may have disastrous consequences for the physician and hospital, especially if the defendants are not covered by a malpractice policy, as is often the case with intentional tort. The negligence theory, treated in the following chapter, is by far the most common theory for recovery used by plaintiffs. Most commentators use malpractice only in reference to negligence, although a few experts feel that the term also covers breach of contract and intentional torts.[2] One unfortunate conse-

---

[1]"Urge Malpractice Liability Shift," 54 *Mich. St.B.J.* 184 (1975).
[2]See, e.g., J. Waltz and F. Inbau, *Medical Jurisprudence* 41 (1971).

91

quence of these conflicting definitions has been that many physicians
and hospitals believe they have complete professional liability coverage
under their malpractice insurance policies, when in fact they are
covered only for negligent acts.[3] To obviate such confusion, the
discussions here will avoid using malpractice as a synonym for
negligence.

The Physician-Patient Relationship

Professional liability of the physician is in most cases founded
upon a breach of duty. The duty, in turn, arises from the contractual
relation between physician and patient. In the absence of a contract,
the law imposes no duty on the physician to treat a patient.

Assume, for example, that a physician driving down a country
lane sees a child beside the road who has fallen off a bicycle and
sustained a compound fracture as well as serious abrasions. The
physician, like most passersby, has an ethical duty to help the child.
The physician's ethical duty is even codified in Section 5 of the
"Code of Ethics of the American Medical Association," which states
that in an emergency the physician should do his best to render
service. But, also like any other passerby, the physician has no legal
duty to help the child or call for help. The law will not require
him to be a Samaritan.

This principle is illustrated by *Childs v. Weis*.[4] A Dallas woman
seven months pregnant was visiting another town when she began
to suffer labor pains and bleeding. At a local hospital emergency
room she was examined by a nurse who called the defendant physician
and then advised the woman to go to her doctor in Dallas. About
an hour after the mother left the hospital, the baby was born in
a car. Twelve hours later the infant died. The court held that the
physician had no duty to the woman because no physician-patient
relationship had been established by contract.

Establishing the Relationship

Although a contract is necessary before the physician-patient
relationship can exist, there is no requirement that the physician
and patient expressly agree on its terms. In the purchase of an
automobile one of the parties makes an offer, which is accepted

---

[3]In *Security Insurance Group v. Wilkinson*, 297 So. 2d 113 (Fla. App. 1974), for example,
the court held that a hospital's professional liability policy did not include coverage
for breach of contract to treat the plaintiff's wife.
[4]440 S.W. 2d 104 (Tex. Ct. Civ. App. 1969). This case is discussed in greater detail
later in conjunction with hospital emergency care.

by the other party. Such details as price, terms of payment, date of delivery, and identity of the car are expressly agreed upon by the parties, thus creating an *express* contract. On the other hand, a person may enter a bookstore, pick up the latest bestseller, pay a clerk, and leave the store without saying a word. This would be an *implied* contract because the terms of the contract were not expressly manifested by the parties.

The physician-patient relationship may be established by an express or implied contract. A typical situation would be one in which a patient goes to a doctor's office after stepping on a rusty nail. By going to the office the patient is making an offer to enter into a contract. A physician who sends the patient away, as in *Weis,* has rejected the offer and owes no duty to the patient. But if the physician begins to examine the injured foot, he has accepted the offer, and an implied contract is created. An express contract could be created just as easily in this situation if the physician and patient manifestly agreed on the terms of the contract before the examination, including what the patient was to pay and what the physician was to do for the payment.

In most cases the physician-patient relationship will be established by an express or implied manifestation of mutual assent. There are, however, exceptional cases in which informed consent is often the issue. These arise when the patient is unconscious and unable to give even an implied assent to treatment. Despite the lack of mutuality of assent, there are at least two possible bases for finding a duty on the part of the physician to the unconscious patient. First, a court might find that the contract was actually made with another party, usually a close relative of the unconscious person acting for his benefit. Under such an arrangement the unconscious party, as the beneficiary of the contract between the physician and the relative, acquires the same rights as if he had been a primary party to the contract. Secondly, even when not contracted with another person, the law will treat the rendering of services to an unconscious person as a contract implied in law. Such a contract, in addition to preventing "unjust enrichment" by requiring the patient to pay for the services, also imposes the same duties on the physician that would arise under an express or implied-in-fact contract.[5]

The basic principles of contract law discussed above are difficult to apply in the widely varying circumstances which arise in medical practice. Illustrating a few of the more troublesome situations are

---

[5] Waltz, *supra* n. 2, at 170.

the following variations on a theme in *Childs v. Weis*. While in that
case the court decided that no contract was formed when the physician
talked to the nurse on the telephone and advised the patient to
call her own doctor, it does not follow that a contract cannot be
formed over the telephone. In *O'Neill v. Montefiore Hospital*, for
example, a man who had symptoms of a heart attack went to a
hospital emergency room where he advised a nurse on duty that
he was a member of a prepaid medical group.[6] The nurse told
him that the hospital did not treat members of the group, but she
called one of the group's physicians so that the patient could describe
his symptoms over the telephone. There was a conflict in testimony
regarding what the physician told the patient. The physician testified
that he offered to come to the emergency room to examine the
man but that the patient declined, saying that he would prefer to
wait and see another doctor. The patient's wife testified that the
physician told her husband to go home and return to the hospital
when another physician in the group would be available. The man
died of a heart attack shortly after going home. In the suit brought
by the wife, the complaint was dismissed at the close of the evidence.
According to the appellate court, however, a jury might have
concluded, from the evidence in the record, that the physician
undertook to diagnose the ailment of the deceased, and therefore
the case should have gone to the jury.

The *Weis* decision also raises the question of whether an emergency
room physician has a duty to treat all patients who enter the emergency
room. The majority rule is that if a doctor is employed as an emergency
room physician, or is a staff member serving in the emergency room
as required by hospital regulations, he does not have the right
to refuse emergency patients. This issue was not discussed by the
court in *Weis*, although the opinion indicates that the court would
not follow the majority rule. At one point, for instance, the court
hints that Dr. Weis was serving on the emergency service but that
this service did not create a physician-patient relationship because
the hospital did not require physicians to see all patients who came
to the emergency room for treatment.[7]

Another variation of *Weis* involves the contractual duty of a
physician to an outsider rather than to the other party to the contract.
The *Weis* decision was based in part upon *Lotspeich v. Chance Vought*

---

[6] 11 App. Div. 132, 202 N.Y.S. 2d 436 (Sup. Ct. 1960). This case is discussed later
in greater detail in connection with hospital emergency care.
[7] *Childs v. Weis*, 440 S.W. 2d 104, 106 (Tex. Ct. Civ. App. 1969). See, generally,
A. Holder, *Medical Malpractice Law* 7–8 (1975).

Aircraft, which considered this issue. Before being employed by the
company, the plaintiff in *Lotspeich* underwent a physical examination,
which included an x-ray examination. Three years later she was
found to be seriously ill with tuberculosis and was hospitalized for
a lengthy period. Plaintiff's suit was based upon alternative theories:
(1) the physician had discovered her tubercular condition and was
negligent in his failure to disclose it to her; or (2) the physician
was negligent in failing to discover the condition. The appellate
court decided that the condition had not been discovered but that
the doctor owed the patient no duty to discover the disease. In
the words of the court: "This [examination] was wholly for the
benefit of the company, and the doctor owed to it alone the duty
to perform [the examination] efficiently. . . . She [the plaintiff]
had no legal right to demand that he exercise any care whatever
in conducting the examination, except to avoid injuring her."[8]

Similar third party situations arise when a life insurance company
employs a physician to examine an applicant for life insurance, and
when a physician is asked by a court to examine a plaintiff in an
action for personal injuries. As in *Lotspeich*, the rule in these situations
is that a physician-patient relationship is not established between
the physician and the applicant or the plaintiff in the action.

In a number of states, however, there is a trend toward imposing
liability when the physician has not used due care in treating a third
party, at least in giving physical examinations prior to employment.[9]
The right of action in such cases might be limited to recovery allowed
by workmen's compensation statutes, the result ultimately reached
by the *Lotspeich* court.

Another situation where a physician might be liable to the third
party would be created by a contract between a pregnant mother
and her physician. In *Sylvia v. Gobeille*, for example, a baby was
born with serious defects because the physician failed to prescribe
gamma globulin for the mother, even though he knew that she
had been exposed to german measles.[10] The court held that these
facts stated a cause of action for recovery of damages by the third
party—the baby.

As discussed later in connection with defamation, the contractual
relation between the patient and the physician in some states not
only allows the physician but gives him the duty to warn certain

[8]369 S.W. 2d 705, 710 (Tex. Ct. Civ. App. 1963).
[9]Holder, "Creation of the Physician-Patient Relationship," 230 *J.A.M.A.* 278 (1974).
[10]101 R.I. 76, 220 A. 2d 222 (1966).

persons when a patient has an infectious disease. A physician might
also be subject to liability when his patient injures a third party.
In *Freese v. Lemmon* a pedestrian was injured by an automobile driver
who lost consciousness during a seizure.[11] Both the driver and the
driver's physician were sued by the injured person. The physician
was sued on the theory that he was negligent in diagnosing an earlier
seizure and in advising the driver that he could operate an automobile.
The trial court dismissed the complaint against the physician on
the grounds, among others, that the pedestrian did not rely on the
diagnosis and was not known to the physician. The Supreme Court
of Iowa reversed and remanded the case for trial, however, on the
theory that the physician is subject to liability to third persons when
he negligently treats or gives false information to a patient.

In another case, the well-publicized *Tarasoff v. Regents of the
University of California,* the California Supreme Court ruled that
despite his confidential relation to his patients a doctor has a duty
to use reasonable care to warn persons threatened by a patient's
condition.[12] The patient in *Tarasoff* had indicated to his psychotherapist that he intended to kill a certain person and later carried
out his threat. On these facts the court determined that the victim's
parents had a cause of action against the psychotherapist.

One case, not discussed in *Weis* but bearing on the nature of
the doctor's relation to his patients, involved a professor of medicine
at the University of California at Los Angeles who had spoken to
a group of physicians at a medical meeting.[13] One of the physicians
in the audience described a patient's medical history to the professor,
who advised surgery. Later the patient sued the professor, claiming
that the surgery had not been necessary. The court concluded that
the professor had no duty to the plaintiff because there was no
physician-patient relationship.

This decision should be compared with another case in which
a physician, examining patients before selecting them to participate
in clinics at a city hospital, advised a resident that one patient's
leg should be amputated. In the suit against the party alleged to
have caused the original injury, the physician was not allowed to
testify because Missouri statutes prohibited physicians from testifying

[11] 210 N.W. 2d 576 (Iowa 1973). See: *Kaiser v. Suburban Transportation Systems,* 65
Wash. 2d 461, 398 P. 2d 14 (1965) where passengers in the patient's bus were allowed
to recover damages from the defendant physician.
[12] 118 Cal. Rptr. 129, 529 P. 2d 553 (1974), *aff'd,* 131 Cal. Rptr. 14, 551 P.2d 334
(1976).
[13] *Ranier v. Grossman,* 31 Cal. App. 3d 539, 107 Cal. Rptr. 469 (1973).

about information acquired in treating a patient, and the court held that a physician-patient relationship had been established.[14]

The final example of the physician-patient relationship is the situation where a patient receives the services of a physician, typically a radiologist or pathologist, who never comes into contact with him. Like physicians who give advice over the telephone, these have a contractual relationship with the patient, and it poses similar questions of liability.[15]

SCOPE AND TERMINATION OF THE RELATIONSHIP

Once the physician-patient relationship has been established by express or implied contract, the scope of the duty which the physician has assumed is frequently in question. Must the physician who has agreed to treat a patient cater to all his whims at the risk of being held liable if he refuses?

The general rule is that a physician may limit the scope of the contract to a designated geographical area or medical specialty.[16] In *McNamara v. Emmons* a woman sustained a bad cut, which was treated by an associate of the defendant physician.[17] The next morning she left for a vacation in a town twenty miles away. While there, believing she needed further treatment, she called the physician and asked him to come to the vacation town. The physician refused but gave her instructions, including the name of a local physician whom she might call. The court held that in these circumstances the physician was justified in limiting his practice to his own town. In other cases the courts have decided that, at least when no emergency exists, the physician has no obligation to make house calls, but instead may require the patient to come to his office for treatment.

In addition to these contractual limitations, as a general rule the primary physician is relieved of his duty when he calls in a consultant to take over treatment of the patient. The consultant normally does not undertake continuing treatment of the patient after the consultation but has only the duty to treat the patient for the specific purposes relating to the referral. The primary physician would be liable, however, if he was negligent in his selection of a consultant or if he worked with the specialist in treating the patient.[18]

As with any other contract, the contract between the physician and patient must sometimes be terminated. Termination may occur

---

[14] *Smart v. Kansas City,* 208 Mo. 162, 105 S.W. 709 (1907).
[15] Holder, *supra* n. 7, at 6.
[16] *Id.* at 31–32, Waltz, *supra* n. 2, at 149.
[17] 36 Cal. App. 2d 199, 97 P. 2d 503 (1939).
[18] Holder, *supra* n. 7, at 33.

when the patient is cured (or dies), when the physician and patient mutually consent to termination, when the patient dismisses the physician, or when the physician withdraws from the contract. The first three methods of termination are usually legally uneventful; the fourth has been the subject of frequent litigation.

Withdrawal by the physician before the patient is cured often results in a claim of abandonment by the patient. There has been a good deal of confusion about whether abandonment is properly classified as a breach of contract, an intentional tort, or negligence. In many cases, grounds for all three causes of action might exist, especially when the physician thought the patient had been cured and prematurely discharged him from the hospital.[19]

The confusion has been compounded by failure to draw the line between abandonment and lack of diligence in treating a patient— which, as will be seen later, is negligence. The distinction between a claim of abandonment based upon negligence and one based upon breach of contract or intentional tort is especially critical in regard to burden of proof, since plaintiffs relying on the latter two theories often do not have to present expert testimony.[20]

Abandonment may be either express or implied. Express abandonment includes those cases where a physician expressly tells a patient he is withdrawing from the case, without giving the patient enough time to locate another physician. As an example of express withdrawal, the plaintiff in *Norton v. Hamilton* went into labor several weeks before her baby was due.[21] According to her allegations, the physician examined her and concluded that she was not in labor. Later, after the patient's husband had called twice to say that his wife was still in pain, the physician said he was withdrawing from the case. While the husband was looking for a substitute physician, the patient delivered her child alone. The court held that the patient's allegations, if proven, constituted abandonment.

Implied abandonment occurs when the physician's conduct makes it obvious that he has abandoned the patient. In *Johnson v. Vaughn,* Dr. Vaughn initially admitted the patient to the hospital, treated him, and then went home, leaving word that he was to be called if the patient's condition grew worse.[22] Since the patient seemed dangerously ill when Dr. Vaughn left, the patient's son called a

---

[19] D. Louisell and H. Williams, *Medical Malpractice* Section 8.08, at 219 (1973); Holder, *supra* n. 7, at 376.
[20] Holder, "Abandonment: Part I," 225 *J.A.M.A.* 1157 (1973).
[21] 92 Ga. App. 727, 89 S.E. 2d 809 (1955).
[22] 370 S.W. 2d 591 (Ky. 1963).

Dr. Kissinger who "gave such attention as appeared to be most urgent," but felt that he could not proceed further without a release from Dr. Vaughn. On being told on the telephone by Dr. Kissinger that the patient was dying and needed immediate attention, Vaughn became irate and vulgar, called Dr. Kissinger a "louse" for trying to steal his patient, and hung up. A call from the patient's son produced more abuse. Finally Dr. Vaughn said he would release the patient if he was paid $50 by nine o'clock the next morning. Thirty or forty minutes had passed before Dr. Kissinger operated, and the patient later died. The court held that these facts were sufficient to show negligence on the part of Dr. Vaughn.

Most physicians can raise a number of defenses to claims of abandonment. If the physician gives sufficient notice of withdrawal so that the patient may obtain the service of another physician of equal ability, the claim will fail. As previously noted, he may also assert his right to limit his practice to a certain specialty or geographical area. A physician who is too ill to treat a patient or to find a substitute also has a valid defense to an abandonment claim. If a physician obtains a substitute physician who is not his agent or employed by him, he has a valid defense so long as the substitute is qualified or the patient has been given enough time to find another physician if the substitute is unacceptable.[23]

Limitations to the last defense were noted in *Stohlman v. Davis.* In that case a child with osteomyelitis was being treated by a physician who was an expert on the subject. The physician went to Arizona to recuperate from an illness and in his place substituted his son, who had practiced medicine for four years. The illness did not constitute an emergency. Since the patient and his father did not learn of the physician's absence until two weeks later, the court held the primary physician liable for abandonment because he had not given notice of the substitution in time for the plaintiff to locate another physician. In the words of the court: "The clear duty, under the circumstances, was imposed upon him either to secure the patient's acceptance of the substitution of his son, Doctor Herbert Davis, or to give him notice so as to secure another physician or surgeon of his own choice."[24]

Other defenses to abandonment claims might also fail. A physician cannot rely on a claim that he stopped treating the patient because the patient was remiss in paying bills.[25] Nor was a physician successful

[23]Wasmuth, *Law for the Physician* 26–29 (1966); Siegal, *Forensic Medicine* 5 (1963).
[24]117 Neb. 178, 220 N.W. 247, 250 (1928).
[25]Holder, "Abandonment: Part I," 225 *J.A.M.A.* 1157, 1158 (1973).

in claiming as a defense that he was attending another patient, when it was shown that he had already given the plaintiff medicine to induce labor.[26]

Furthermore, a physician may not in every instance abandon a patient simply because he is told that another physician is handling the case. *Maltempo v. Cuthbert* is an example.[27] The plaintiff's diabetic son was in a county jail awaiting transportation to a state prison to serve a sentence for a drug violation. In jail the son's health deteriorated, and his mother called her family physician for assistance, but could only reach the defendant physician who was taking his calls. This man told the mother that he would investigate the matter and call back if there were any problems. He then called the jail, learned that the son was being treated by the jail physician, and did nothing further. The boy died while being transported to the state prison. The appellate court affirmed an award of $45,000 for the plaintiff, holding that the fact that it was not ethical for the physician to interfere with the jail physician's treatment of the patient did not excuse the defendant's failure to keep his promise to the mother.

Liability for Breach of Contract

In the typical physician-patient contract, as has been pointed out, the physician expressly or impliedly agrees to perform a service. His failure to perform the service with reasonable skill and care will give the patient a cause of action not only for negligence, the usual allegation, but also for breach of contract. Several cases in which the patient's breach of contract action was based upon abandonment have already been discussed in connection with the scope and termination of the physician's contractual duty. *Alexandridis v. Jewett* offers one more example.[28] Two obstetricians impliedly promised to be available when the plaintiff went into labor. When the woman did go into labor one of the obstetricians notified his partner, who was on call. When the partner did not arrive on time, an episiotomy was performed by a first-year resident in obstetrics. The operation resulted in injury to the patient. In the suit which followed, the appellate court found that there was enough evidence to go to a jury on the issue of negligence; furthermore the court held that the partners would be liable for breach of contract if their

---

[26] *Young v. Jordan*, 106 W. Va. 139, 145 S.E. 41 (1928).
[27] 504 F. 2d 325 (5th Cir. 1974).
[28] 388 F. 2d 829 (1st Cir. 1968).

superior skill would have protected the patient from injury.

A physician who promises to use a certain procedure in performing the contract and uses a different procedure instead will also be liable for breach of contract. In *Stewart v. Rudner and Bunyan*, the physician promised to arrange for an obstetrician to deliver a child by Caesarean section.[29] The patient was a 37-year-old woman who had had two previous stillbirths and was extremely anxious to have a "sound, healthy baby." When the patient was in labor, the physician told an obstetrician to "take care of this case" but did not tell him about the promise to perform a Caesarean section. After a lengthy labor, the baby was stillborn. The appellate court upheld a jury verdict for the patient on the grounds that the physician breached his promise that a Caesarean operation would be used to deliver that baby.

The physician is especially susceptible to liability when he not only promises to perform a service, or to perform it in a certain manner as in *Stewart*, but also guarantees a specified result. Such a warranty does not exist unless expressly stated by the physician; consequently the physician who guarantees a result gives the patient a separate cause of action if the treatment is not successful. In *Sullivan v. O'Conner* a professional entertainer entered into a contract with a physician to have cosmetic surgery on her nose, which she felt was too long.[30] The physician promised that the surgery would "enhance her beauty and improve her appearance." In fact, the surgery was unsuccessful and after two additional operations the nose looked worse than in its original form. The appellate court, although recognizing that physicians do not guarantee results simply by agreeing to perform an operation, and that it is often difficult to draw the line between opinion and warranty, upheld a jury verdict for the plaintiff.

Another much publicized case is *Guilmet v. Campbell*. The plaintiff in that case had a bleeding ulcer. He talked with one of the defendant surgeons regarding a possible operation and alleged that he was told (as summarized by the court):

> Once you have an operation it takes care of all your troubles. You can eat as you want to, you can drink as you want to, you can go as you please. Dr. Arena and I are specialists, there is nothing to it at all—it's a very simple operation. You'll be out of work three to four weeks at the most. There is no danger at all in this operation. After the operation you can throw away your pill box. In twenty years if you

---

[29] 349 Mich. 459, 84 N.W. 2d 816 (1957).
[30] 296 N.E. 2d 183 (Mass. 1973).

figure out what you spent for Maalox pills and doctor calls, you could buy an awful lot. Weigh it against an operation.[31]

With this alleged assurance, the plaintiff underwent the operation. Diagnosis after the surgery showed that the patient had suffered a ruptured esophagus, his weight dropped from 170 pounds to 88 pounds, and he developed hepatitis. He then sued the physician on both a negligence theory and a warranty theory. The jury decided that the physicians were not negligent but had breached their promise to cure. This was affirmed by the state supreme court, which decided that the question was properly one for the jury. In an emotional dissent one justice observed:

> In these early weeks of 1971 an exuberant new majority of a once great appellate Court prepared to launch an unwarned, unprecedented, wholly gratuitous and destructively witless war of "contract liability" upon a brother profession which, by the multifold harassment of malpractice actions, has been forced already to undertake what is professionally known as "defensive medicine."[32]

Apparently the Michigan legislature agreed with the dissenting opinion. In an action which underscores the fact that hospital and professional liability law is derived from statutes as well as common law, the legislature in effect overruled *Guilmet* by passing the following statute in 1974:

> In the following cases an agreement, contract, or promise shall be void, unless that agreement, contract, or promise, or a note or memorandum thereof is in writing and signed by the party to be charged therewith, or by a person authorized by him:
> (g) An agreement, promise, contract, or warranty of cure relating to medical care or treatment. Nothing in this paragraph shall affect the right to sue for malpractice or negligence.[33]

The *Guilmet* decision touched on another issue which is especially relevant in breach of contract cases: the necessity for consideration. If a person is to be held to a contractual promise, that person must receive something in exchange, something in consideration for the

[31] 385 Mich. 57, 68, 188 N.W. 2d 601, 606 (1971).
[32] *Id.* at 76, 188 N.W. 2d at 610.
[33] Mich. Comp. Laws Ann., sec. 566.132 (Supp. 1975), *amending*, Mich. Comp. Laws Ann., sec. 566.132 (1967).

promise. In the physician-patient contract, the physician will not
be held to his promise to perform a medical or surgical procedure
unless the patient gives something in return, usually a promise to
pay the physician. In *Guilmet* the court decided that there was
sufficient consideration because the physician promised to perform
the surgery and to cure the patient in return for payment from
the patient. If, however, the physician first promises to perform
surgery, for which the patient promises to pay, and later adds an
additional promise to cure or a guarantee of a particular result,
the courts will not allow the patient recovery for failure to perform
the additional promise or warranty unless there is additional consideration to support the promise.[34]

If there is no express warranty, as in *Guilmet,* does a physician
nevertheless give an implied warranty that products he prescribes
for a patient are reasonably fit for their intended use? This was
the issue faced by the court in *Texas State Optical, Inc. v. Barbel,*
when a patient who had suffered eye damage after being fitted
for contact lenses brought suit against his optometrist. The court
held that the optometrist gave no implied warranty of fitness because
"only a strained view of the professional relationship between an
optometrist and his patient could class the optometrist as a salesman
of lenses."[35]

Liability for Intentional Tort

A second basis for professional liability of physicians is intentional
tort. A tort is a wrongful act which results in injury to another
person, or to another person's property or reputation. Traditionally,
torts have been divided into three categories, each of which involves
a different standard of proof for the plaintiff. An intentional tort,
as the name implies, results when a person intends to do the wrongful
act. Negligence occurs when a person commits a wrongful act because
he fails to do what a reasonably prudent person would do in the
same circumstances. Strict liability results when an act is wrongful,
not because the agent intended the wrong or was negligent, but
because the act involved a high risk of harm to others. As noted
earlier, most malpractice actions are based on negligence, which will
be examined in the next chapter.

Actions based upon intentional tort, while rare, are important

[34]61 *Am. Jur.* "Physicians, Surgeons," sec. 110 (1972).
[35]417 S.W. 2d 750, 751–52 (Tex. Ct. Civ. App. 1967). For a similar holding, see
Magrine v. Spector, 100 N.J. Super. 223, 241 A. 2d 637 (1968).

because they allow a plaintiff procedural flexibility not otherwise available. Perhaps more important, however, are the multiple consequences for the physician who commits an intentional tort. Because intent is usually an essential element in proving both the intentional tort and a crime, many intentional torts such as assault and battery entail criminal as well as civil liability. The commission of a criminal act could lead to a third consequence for a physician: revocation of the license to practice medicine. The following classes of intentional torts committed by physicians while rendering health care are considered alphabetically, not in order of frequency.

ASSAULT AND BATTERY

An assault and battery is a combination of two intentional torts. An assault is conduct which places a person in reasonable apprehension of being touched in a manner that is insulting, provoking, or physically injurious. A battery is the actual touching. Both assault and battery denote acts done without lawful authority or permission. A threat to kiss someone without implied or express consent is an assault, and the act of kissing in such circumstances is an assault and battery. If the person were asleep when kissed there would be a battery without the assault. But kissing someone with express or implied permission is not an assault or a battery.

In regard to medical or surgical treatment the question of permission or consent is complex and is treated more completely in a later chapter. For present purposes, assault and battery cases involving physicians may be grouped into three categories. First are the intentional acts committed by the physician with no consent whatever. In *Burton v. Leftwich*, for example, a physician who was removing sutures from the toe of a 4-year-old child and having trouble controlling his patient hit the child's thigh several times with his open hand, leaving bruises that were visible for three weeks.[36] An appellate court upheld a jury verdict that the physician had committed an assault and battery, although it reduced the jury's damage award. This case should be compared with *Mattocks v. Bell*, where a 23-month-old girl, whom a medical student was treating for a lacerated tongue, clamped her teeth on the student's finger.[37] After trying unsuccessfully to free his finger by forcing a tongue depressor into the child's mouth, the student slapped her on the cheek. A suit by the parents for assault and battery failed, the court holding that the force used was proper under the circumstances.

---

[36] 123 So. 2d 766 (La. Ct. App. 1960).
[37] 194 A. 2d 307 (D. C. Ct. App. 1963).

In these situations a physician's liability for striking a person is similar to the liability of a layman. The case is no different when a physician performs an operation without consent. In the oft-cited *Schloendorff v. Society of New York Hospital,* a doctor was held liable for intentional tort after he had operated on a patient who, according to the jury's finding, had consented only to an examination under ether and had given no consent for an operation.[38]

In the second category of assault and battery the duty to obtain permission has been met, but the physician goes beyond the scope of the permission. In the third category the physician acts within the scope of the consent; but because he does not exercise ordinary care in advising the patient of the risks of the treatment, the patient's consent is not an informed one and the permission is invalid. As will be seen in a later chapter, suit can be brought in both these situations on either a negligence or an assault and battery theory. In recent years negligence has been used in most cases, but there are decisions where liability is based upon assault and battery.[39] *Mohr v. Williams,* although not recent, illustrates these latter cases.[40] In *Mohr* the plaintiff consented to an operation to remove a polyp from her right ear. After she was anesthetized, the defendant surgeon discovered that her left ear needed surgery more than the right ear and operated on the left ear instead. On the grounds, among others, that his conduct amounted to a technical assault and battery, the appellate court upheld a trial court decision to deny the surgeon's motion for judgment.

Although the surgeon in *Mohr* should have consulted with the patient before operating on the other ear, a surgeon will sometimes be justified in operating beyond the scope of the consent, for instance when an emergency prevents him from obtaining the patient's consent. In *Barnett v. Bachrach,* a surgeon who was operating on a patient diagnosed as having an ectopic pregnancy discovered that the pregnancy was normal but that the woman had acute appendicitis.[41] He removed the appendix and later sued the patient for his fee. The patient defended the suit by alleging that the appendix was removed without her consent. In holding for the surgeon, the court noted that if he had not taken out the appendix the patient and child might have been endangered.

---

[38] 211 N.Y. 125, 105 N.E. 92 (1914).
[39] W. Prosser, *Law of Torts* 165 (1971).
[40] 95 Minn. 261, 104 N.W. 12 (1905).
[41] 34 A. 2d 626 (D. C. Mun. Ct. App. 1943).

DEFAMATION

Defamation is the wrongful injury of another person's reputation. Written defamation is libel and oral defamation is slander. One element of proof that is unique to defamation is publication, which requires that the defamatory statement be made to a third party and not to the defendant alone. This point was made in *Shoemaker v. Friedberg,* in which a physician wrote the patient, telling her that she had venereal disease, and the woman showed the letter to two or three other women.[42] Later, in the presence of a friend, she discussed the diagnosis with the physician but brought suit against him, alleging a breach of confidentiality. The court held that no recovery should be allowed, the patient having "published" the diagnosis herself.

A number of defenses to defamation are particularly relevant to an action against a physician. The demonstrated truth of a defamatory statement is an absolute defense, although the defendant has the burden of proving that the statement was true. Certain statements, such as those made during the course of a judicial proceeding, or those by one physician to another in discussing a patient's treatment, are said to be absolutely privileged, thereby providing the physician with an absolute defense. In *Thornburg v. Long,* for example, a specialist incorrectly reported to a family physician that a patient had syphilis.[43] When the patient sued the specialist for libel, the court held that the statement was privileged because the specialist had a duty to communicate the information to the family physician.

Certain statements, while not absolutely privileged, are at least entitled to a qualified privilege if they were made to protect a private interest of the physician, the patient, or a third party. In *Simonsen v. Swenson* a physician believed that a patient had syphilis.[44] While he was awaiting additional tests, he advised the patient's hotel proprietor that the patient might have a contagious disease, and the proprietor forced the patient to move. It was later discovered that the patient did not have syphilis, but the court held that the physician was not liable for defamation because he had a duty to disclose the information.

FALSE IMPRISONMENT

The intentional tort of false imprisonment involves the unlawful restriction of a person's freedom. The physician who forces a patient

---

[42] 80 Cal. App. 2d 911, 183 P. 2d 318 (1947).
[43] 178 N.C. 589, 101 S.E. 99 (1919). See: Waltz, *supra* n. 2, at 263–67.
[44] 104 Neb. 224, 177 N.W. 831 (1920).

to remain in the office until he pays a bill, for example, or signs certain forms, faces possible liability for false imprisonment.

Many false imprisonment actions involve patients who have been involuntarily committed to a mental hospital. In *Stowers v. Wolodzko*, a psychiatrist was held liable for damages of $40,000 for his treatment of a woman who had been involuntarily committed to a mental institution.[45] Although her commitment was allowed by a state statute, the court held that because the psychiatrist kept the woman incommunicado by preventing her from calling an attorney or a relative his actions constituted false imprisonment arising from the unlawful restraint on her freedom. The court also held the psychiatrist liable for assault and battery for giving the patient involuntary medication beyond what was permitted by statute.

Closely related to false imprisonment is an action for abuse of process brought against a physician who wrongfully uses a commitment statute to commit a patient without justification. In *Maniaci v. Marquette University* a 16-year-old college freshman obtained her parent's permission to leave school.[46] College officials learned that she was leaving and, without asking whether she had parental permission, had her committed to a hospital in order to stop her. In the hospital, attendants removed the girl's clothes, bathed her, and gave her a housecoat to wear. Later she was locked in a room with several other female patients who engaged in sexual activities which shocked the girl. Eventually she established contact with her family through a social worker and was released. On these facts the trial court awarded plaintiffs $20,001 on a false imprisonment theory. The Wisconsin Supreme Court reversed the decision on the ground that there was no "unlawful" restraint of freedom, the statutory procedures having been complied with. The court also determined, however, that the evidence showed a cause of action for abuse of process and remanded the case for trial on that theory.

INVASION OF PRIVACY

In discussing defamation it was noted that truth is an absolute defense in a defamation action based upon a physician's statement to third parties. There are, however, two additional bases for possible liability even when the statement is true: invasion of privacy and wrongful disclosure of confidential information. In actions for malpractice invasion of privacy occurs when a patient is subjected to unwanted publicity. A Michigan physician was held liable for invasion

[45] 386 Mich. 119, 191 N.W. 2d 355 (1971).
[46] 50 Wis. 2d 287, 184 N.W. 2d 168 (1971).

of privacy when he allowed a lay friend to observe the delivery of a baby in the patient's home.[47]

Wrongful disclosure of confidential information is especially important to physicians, because the tort could result in the triple consequences noted earlier: civil damages, loss of license, and criminal penalties.[48] Some disclosures, however, are not subject to an action involving privacy or a wrongful disclosure because they are privileged. Physicians have a duty to disclose child abuse, for example. But they must be cautious in exercising supposed privileges, as illustrated by *Griffin v. Medical Society of New York.*[49] In *Griffin* a plastic surgeon photographed a patient's nose before and after surgery, and published the pictures in a medical journal, under the title "The Saddle Nose." The patient sued the surgeon and the journal. The surgeon defended this publication on the grounds that under the New York privacy statutes the disclosure was privileged because it was not "for advertising purposes." The judge refused to dismiss the action before trial, however, noting that even an article published for scientific purposes could be an advertisement in disguise.

MISREPRESENTATION

Misrepresentation is another tort for which physicians have been held liable. Misrepresentation is properly classified as either intentional—that is, fraudulent or deceitful—or negligent. In both cases it must be shown that a false representation of a present or past fact was made and that it was relied on by the person claiming injury.

Whether intentional or negligent, misrepresentation cases involving physicians fall into two other distinct categories: representations to induce a patient to undergo treatment, and later representations concerning the results of the treatment. Preoperative misrepresentation is discussed in a later chapter in connection with consent. Here it is enough to note that the misrepresentation theory in preoperative cases may be used more often in the future, since injured patients are now more likely to have heard recent charges by the doctors and laymen that a great deal of unnecessary surgery is being performed.

A physician who misrepresents the nature or results of treatment he has rendered would be liable for fraud, even though he was not negligent in rendering the treatment, and the presence of fraud

---

[47]*DeMay v. Roberts,* 46 Mich. 160, 9 N.W. 146 (1881).
[48]Holder, *supra* n. 7, at 268.
[49]7 Misc. 2d 549, 11 N.Y.S. 2d 109 (1939).

sometimes enables a patient to bring suit after the statutory time limit. In *Hundley v. Martinez* a physician repeatedly assured his patient, an attorney, that his eye would be all right after a cataract operation.[50] In fact, the attorney became virtually blind in one eye. Although suit was brought after the statute of limitations had run, the court held that the limitation was suspended if the jury found that the physician had obstructed the plaintiff's right of action by fraud or other indirect ways.

OTHER THEORIES

Finally, two intentional torts recognized in recent years should be mentioned. One of these was explained by the Supreme Court of Washington in *Grimsby v. Samson.*[51] A husband sued a physician and a hospital for abandoning his wife, claiming that as a result of abandonment he was forced to witness the pain and agony of his dying wife. The court allowed the claim on the theory that the tort of "outrage" had been committed by the defendant, whose reckless and wanton conduct had resulted in the husband's having to watch his wife die. The court listed four requirements for recovery on an outrage theory: (1) The act must be intentional or reckless; (2) the conduct must be outrageous and extreme; (3) the conduct must result in "severe emotional distress"; and (4) the plaintiff must be an immediate member of the family and present at the time of such conduct.

The other relatively recent intentional tort is illustrated by a California case, where a physician was held liable for failing to fulfill his agreement to treat a patient.[52] Since the refusal was said to be on racial grounds, liability was based upon the state civil rights statute, the court holding that medical practice is a business under the statute.

Distinctions Between Grounds for Action

The third basis for professional liability, negligence, is treated in the next chapter, but the chief distinctions between actions based upon a breach of contract, intentional tort, and negligence may be indicated at this point by a hypothetical example. A patient, operated on for appendicitis, experiences intense pain and consults the surgeon. The doctor tells him nothing is wrong and withdraws from the case. The patient then goes to another surgeon and learns that complica-

[50] 151 W. Va. 877, 158 S.E. 2d 159 (1967).
[51] 85 Wash. 2d 52, 530 P. 2d 291 (1975).
[52] *Washington v. Blampin*, 226 Cal. App. 2d 604, 38 Cal. Rptr. 235 (1964).

tions have developed from the surgery and that these should have
been treated earlier. The patient then visits an attorney to discuss
a possible malpractice action.

As is often true in such circumstances, the action can be based
upon abandonment as a breach of contract or as negligence; in
either case the patient would probably allege that the surgeon failed
to exercise reasonable skill and care. The action on these particular
facts could also be based upon abandonment as an intentional tort.
While many attorneys would plead all three theories as alternative
claims for relief, the choice will often be limited because of four
possible distinctions between these actions.[53]

First, statutes of limitations vary depending on the type of action.
Statutes of limitations set forth the period within which actions must
be brought. The times vary from state to state; even within a state
they vary according to the type of action. If the action is not
commenced within the specified time, a plaintiff is normally precluded
from recovering damages. To illustrate, if the patient in our example
visited the attorney one year and one week after he learned of the
complications, and if the incident took place in Ohio, it would be
too late for him to sue for malpractice, since Ohio statutes provide
that an action claiming malpractice, defamation, assault and battery,
or false imprisonment must be brought within one year. However,
a personal injury action in Ohio must be brought within two years;
an action based upon an oral contract within six years; one based
upon a written contract within fifteen years; and one for wrongful
death within two years of the date of death. Unless a court determined
that malpractice includes all theories which could be used against
a physician, it would theoretically be possible to bring the contract
action any time before the end of the six- or fifteen-year period,
and some intentional tort actions could be brought before the end
of the two-year period.[54]

A second major distinction between the three possible grounds
for relief relates to the availability of damages. Damages are often
classified as actual, nominal, or punitive. Actual damages are the

[53]For example, Dr. Thomas Harris, the author of *I'm OK—You're OK*, paid $50,000
in settlement of a $1.2 million damage suit brought by a woman who charged Dr.
Harris with malpractice, breach of contract, and intentional tort. The woman claimed
that Dr. Harris kept her as a mistress, under the influence of liquor and drugs.
New York Times, Oct. 24, 1974, at 50.
[54]Apparently the Ohio statute is intended to cover all malpractice actions except
those based upon written consent. 42 O. Jur. 2d Section 132 (1960). A similar decision
was reached under a Maine statute in *Merchants National Bank v. Morriss*, 269 F.
2d 363 (1st Cir. 1959). Statutes of limitations are subject to a variety of interpretations
which will be discussed in the following chapter.

damages awarded to a plaintiff in compensation for past and future medical costs, past and future loss of income, physical pain, and mental anguish. Nominal damages are those awarded when a plaintiff has proved the elements of his case but cannot prove actual damages. Punitive damages are awarded to punish a defendant for conduct that the court considers willful or malicious. Punitive damages are analagous to the fine levied against a person convicted of a crime, except that the money goes to the plaintiff, not the state.

A plaintiff's right to recover any of the three types of damages will depend upon the nature of the action. If the action is for intentional tort, all three classes of damages will be available to a plaintiff. In an assault and battery case where a physician has struck a patient, the patient may recover both nominal and punitive damages even though there are no actual damages.[55] In an action for breach of contract, nominal damages are allowed but punitive damages are rare. Actual damages are, of course, allowed in contract actions, but they are often inadequate because pain and suffering is not considered compensable. In a negligence action, nominal damages are not allowed, punitive damages are rarely allowed, but actual damages may include compensation for pain and suffering.[56] These generalizations will ordinarily be true, but the rules vary. In *Sullivan v. O'Conner*, discussed above, the court allowed damages for pain and suffering in the breach of contract action.

The third distinction between grounds for action rests on the need for expert testimony. In most negligence cases and in many contract cases, expert testimony is necessary to prove that the defendant did not exercise the requisite care and skill. Expert testimony is not necessary, however, in proving an intentional tort or in some contract actions, like the hypothetical case where the patient claimed to have been abandoned by the physician.[57]

One other consideration in the choice of grounds for action is that medical malpractice insurance does not cover all conduct commonly referred to as malpractice. A malpractice policy, for example, might not provide coverage for many of the intentional torts discussed above. For this reason, a plaintiff's attorney might choose to use a negligence or breach of contract theory so that whatever damages were awarded would be collectible from the malpractice carrier.

---

[55]Waltz, *supra* n. 2, at 154.
[56]Louisell and Williams, *supra* n. 19, sec. 8.03, at 198.
[57]Holder, "Abandonment: Part I," 225 *J.A.M.A.* 1157 (1973).

V

Negligence

In recent years the word "crisis," already overworked in other contexts, has become extremely popular in commentaries on medical malpractice. Tangible evidence that a crisis exists can be found across the country. For example, on the East Coast a 12-year-old boy who broke his arm in gym class recently had to wait six hours in an emergency room because New York physicians were seeking to dramatize their malpractice problems by refusing to perform ordinary services, while on the West Coast a 13-year-old boy was awarded over $4 million in damages because a doctor did not detect a brain injury resulting from a fight at school.

The problem of malpractice is not new. A section of the "Code of Hammurabi," promulgated around 2250 B.C., was directed toward malpractice: "If a physician operates on a man for a severe wound with a bronze lancet and causes a man's death, or open an abscess [in the eye] of a man with a bronze lancet and destroy the man's eye, they shall cut off his fingers."[1] In medieval England, the existence of malpractice problems is illustrated by the following writ of trespass.

> The King to the sheriff greeting etc. as in Trespass to shew:—wherefore whereas he the said X undertook well and competently to cure the right eye of the said A, which was accidentally injured, for a certain sum of money beforehand received, he the same X so negligently and carelessly applied his cure to the said eye, that the said A by the fault of him the said X totally lost the sight of the said eye, to the damage of him the said A of twenty pounds, as he saith, and have there etc.[2]

[1] Harper, *The Code of Hammurabi* 79 (1904).
[2] Maitland, *Equity and the Forms of Action* 385 (1909).

112

And in the early years of American history Dr. Benjamin Rush, who signed the Declaration of Independence, was involved in a malpractice controversy when he brought a libel suit against an Englishman who had charged him with malpractice in treating yellow fever victims.

Despite this long history, only recently has malpractice been thought to represent a crisis, marked by battle between practitioners of two venerable and learned professions, medicine and the law. The physicians blame the malpractice crisis largely on the legal system and such legal practices as the use of a contingency fee, by which a lawyer retains a percentage of his client's judgment as his fee. Attorneys, on the other hand, claim that the crisis has been caused by inept medical treatment and by the failure of the medical profession to police itself. A popular saying, especially among leaders of the bar, has been, "The cause of the medical malpractice crisis is medical malpractice." Attorneys and physicians alike are critical of the insurance industry, because the crisis was precipitated when insurance companies raised their premiums or even completely withdrew medical malpractice coverage.

Somewhat overlooked amidst the recriminations by physicians, attorneys, and insurance companies has been the consumer of medical services, the patient, although he has the most at stake in the crisis, since he faces the risk of injury at the hands of physicians. He also pays for the malpractice insurance at a rate estimated to be as high as $1.60 for every $10 received in fees by physicians, not to mention the additional charges incurred when physicians are forced to practice defensive medicine.

The focus of this chapter will be on the patient and the way the law decides which of the many patients who are not cured are entitled to compensation from a physician or insurance carrier. Specifically, this chapter will examine the negligence theory of liability, a theory that deserves special attention because its frequent use has made it synonymous with malpractice. Negligence is also important because the standard of care used in a negligence action will often be applied in breach of contract actions, especially those which are not based upon an express promise to perform a particular procedure or to effect a specific result.[3]

It might be well first to take a different view of the malpractice crisis from that usually offered by news sources, attorneys, physicians, and insurers. A 1973 report of an HEW Commission on Medical

---

[3]D. Louisell and H. Williams, *Medical Malpractice*, sec. 8.03, at 196 (1973).

Malpractice, based on a study of claim files closed in 1970, offers a more objective summary of the magnitude of the so-called crisis to date:

> Despite the publicity resulting from a few large malpractice cases, a medical malpractice incident is a relatively rare event: claims are even rarer and jury trials are rarer still.
>
> In 1970, a malpractice incident was alleged or reported for one out of every 158,000 patient visits to doctors.
>
> In 1970 a claim was asserted for one out of every 226,000 patient visits to doctors.
>
> Fewer than one court trial was held for every 10 claims closed in 1970.
>
> Most doctors have never had a medical malpractice suit filed against them and those who have, have rarely been sued more than once.
>
> In 1970, 6.5 medical malpractice claims files were opened for every 100 active practitioners.
>
> A 10-year survey, from 1960 to 1970, of the claims experience of 2,045 physicians in Maryland indicated that 84 percent had not been sued, 14 percent were sued once, and 2 percent were sued more than once.
>
> Most hospitals, no matter how large, go through an entire year without having a single claim filed against them.
>
> Sixty-nine percent of 4,113 hospitals surveyed from June 1971 to June 1972 had not had a malpractice claim, 10 percent had one, and 21 percent had two or more.
>
> Most patients never suffered a medical injury due to malpractice and fewer still have made a claim alleging malpractice.
>
> If the average person lives 70 years, he will have, based on 1970 data, approximately 400 contacts as a patient with doctors and dentists. The chances that he will assert a medical malpractice claim are one in 39,500.[4]

The Standard of Care

A common basis for tort liability is negligence, where the wrongful act resulting in injury is the failure of the wrongdoer, the tort-feasor, to exercise due care. Normally four elements are essential to the proof of a negligence case: a duty of due care, the breach of the duty, causation, and damages. In the following sections, each of these elements will be defined generally and discussed specifically with regard to the professional liability lawsuit.

---

[4]HEW, *Report of the Secretary's Commission on Medical Malpractice* at 12 (1973).

The duty of care requires that each person conduct himself as an average, reasonable person would do in similar circumstances. A person who fails to meet this standard has breached his duty, and if the breach causes injury to another person or property he will be liable for resulting damages. The most common negligent tort is that committed when the operator of a motor vehicle becomes liable for damages because he fails to do what the average, reasonable automobile driver would do and thus causes an accident.

The "average, reasonable person" standard, while adequate in tort cases involving an average tort-feasor, is unsuitable for cases where the defendant is a physician. In cases of negligence involving automobiles, most members of the jury have driven cars themselves and can rely on their own experience, training, and common sense to determine whether the defendant was acting like an average reasonable person. In regard to medical malpractice, however, members of the jury do not have the requisite knowledge, skill, or experience to judge whether a physician has acted reasonably. As a result, courts have adopted a special standard by which physicians are to be judged. Depending on one's viewpoint, this standard favors the plaintiff patient because it makes higher demands on the physician than the usual defendant must meet; or it shields the defendant physician because the standard is established by and defined by physicians themselves.

The standard of what a reasonable person would do, as used in malpractice cases, has been succinctly stated: "A physician is bound to bestow such reasonable and ordinary care, skill, and diligence as physicians and surgeons in good standing in the same neighborhood, in the same general line of practice, ordinarily have and exercise in like cases."[5] This standard is a combination of three tests.

First, the standard requires such "reasonable and ordinary care, skill, and diligence as physicians and surgeons in good standing . . . ordinarily . . . exercise in like cases." This means that physicians are not held to the same standards as the most knowledgeable, highly skilled physicians. Rather the test is whether the physician has exercised the skill and care of other physicians in the same line of practice. In determining the requisite standard, the skill and care of unlicensed physicians is not taken into account, for the test is limited to the skills of physicians "in good standing." In the words of one court:

---

[5] 61 *Am. Jur.* 2d, "Physicians and Surgeons," sec. 110 (1972). See also: T. Roady and W. Andersen, *Professional Negligence* 71 (1960).

While this rule, on the one hand, does not exact the highest
degree of skill and proficiency attainable in the profession,
it does not, on the other hand, contemplate merely average
merit. In other words, in order to determine who will come
up to the the legal standard indicated, we are not permitted
to aggregate into a common class the quacks, the young
men who have had no practice, the old ones who have dropped
out of practice, the good, and the very best, and then strike
an average between them.[6]

Whether reasonable and ordinary care was used is the question
in many cases where a physician has been forced to choose between
two methods of treatment, or where a physician has used experimental
techniques. When the physician must choose between two or more
alternatives adopted by competent physicians, he will not be guilty
of malpractice if he chooses one which he feels best meets the patient's
needs. It is sometimes stated that if the course of treatment is followed
by a "respectable minority," there will be no liability.[7] In one case
the physician, in using one of two methods for performing a
thyroidectomy, severed the patient's laryngeal nerves.[8] The patient
did not claim that the physician was not careful in applying the
procedure, but that he should have chosen another method. The
court rejected this argument because both methods were acceptable.
A more difficult problem arises when the physician chooses a
method of treatment beyond what even a respectable minority would
deem acceptable, that is, treatment that verges on experimentation.
In some situations a physician is clearly justified in using innovative
techniques. An experimental procedure should not result in liability
when standard methods have failed and the condition is serious.
In one case a surgeon performed an unorthodox operation on an
ankle after standard techniques had failed and other physicians had
advised amputation.[9] The court held that the operation was justified
as a last resort. But if the doctor follows an experimental procedure
before attempting standard methods of treatment, he is likely to
be considered negligent. In one instance a physician treated an infant
for a curvature of the spine by using a surgical procedure which

[6]*Holtzman v. Hoy*, 118 Ill. 534, 536, 8 N.E. 832, 832 (1886). It is indeed misleading
to speak in terms of average at all, for "only those in good professional standing
are to be considered; and of these it is not the middle but the minimum common
skill which is to be looked to." W. Prosser, *Law of Torts* 163 (4th ed. 1971). See
also: Roady, *supra* n. 5, at 23.
[7]*Baldor v. Rogers*, 81 So. 2d 658 (Fla. 1955), *rehearing* 81 So. 2d 661 (Fla. 1955);
A. Holder, *Medical Malpractice Law* 44 (1975).
[8]*DiFillipo v. Preston*, 53 Del. 539, 173 A. 2d 333 (1961).
[9]*Miller v. Toles*, 150 N.W. 118 (Mich. 1914).

he had developed but which no one else used. This procedure resulted in a severe hemorrhage which caused the child's death. The intermediate appellate court found both the doctor and the hospital liable for not disclosing to the child's parents that the procedure was novel and unorthodox. The decision against the hospital was reversed, however, the court of appeals deciding that the hospital had no obligation to disclose or to make certain that disclosures were made unless it knew or should have known that informed consent was lacking and that the operation was not permissible under existing standards.[10]

The second test of the physician's standard of care compares the treatment he uses to that exercised by physicians and surgeons "in the same neighborhood." Commonly referred to as the locality rule, this test traditionally has measured the standard of care in a given instance solely by the practices of other physicians in the same locality. In one early action, resulting from the negligent extraction of a tooth, a Kentucky court held that the locality rule was to be used, even though the community (Louisville) was much larger than the villages where the rule was normally applied.[11]

The traditional locality rule, still adhered to by some nineteen states, has been broadened in a number of jurisdictions.[12] One variation, adopted in approximately fourteen states, has been not only to consider practices in the same locality but to include practices in similar geographic areas.[13] Such an expansion of the rule is especially appropriate where there are few, if any, physicians in the same locality whose practices would offer a basis for comparison. This variation, however, does not require an examination of practices in larger towns. In the 1880 Massachusetts case of *Small v. Howard*, the defendant, a physician in a town of 2,500, undertook treatment of a serious wound in the plaintiff's wrist.[14] The trial court's decision that the defendant need only possess the skill of physicians in similar localities was upheld by the supreme judicial court for the reason, among others, that a small-town physician would "have fewer chances to observe others in practice."

Another variation adopted by a few courts is to expand the definition of locality to include the standard of care in medical centers which are readily accessible for treatment of the patient. In Massachusetts

[10]*Fiorentino v. Wenger*, 272 N.Y.S. 2d 557 (1966), *rev'd on other grounds*, 19 N.Y. 2d 403, 227 N.E. 2d 296 (N.Y. 1967).
[11]*Tanner v. Sanders*, 247 Ky. 90, 56 S.W. 2d 718 (1933).
[12]P.L.I., *Doctor and Hospital Liability Today* 8 (1972).
[13]*Ibid.*, at 9.
[14]128 Mass. 131, 35 Am. R. 363 (1880).

the supreme judicial court overruled the "similar locality" rule of
the *Small* decision in *Brune v. Belinkoff*, decided in 1968. In *Brune*
an anesthesiologist in New Bedford administered a spinal injection
of eight milligrams of pontocaine in a solution of glucose during
childbirth. The plaintiff's left leg subsequently became numb and
weak. The trial court, on the basis of *Small*, decided that the defendant,
the woman's physician, should be judged on the basis of practices
in New Bedford instead of Boston, where good medical practice
restricted the dosage in such cases to four milligrams or less. The
supreme judicial court, in reversing the trial court, decided that
the *Small* rule was no longer suitable:

> We are of the opinion that the "locality" rule of *Small v.
> Howard* which measures a physician's conduct by the standards
> of other doctors in similar communities is unsuited to present
> day conditions. The time has come when the medical profes-
> sion should no longer be balkanized by the application of
> varying geographic standards in malpractice cases. Accord-
> ingly, *Small v. Howard* is hereby overruled. The present case
> affords a good illustration of the inappropriateness of the
> "locality" rule to existing conditions. The defendant was a
> specialist practicing in New Bedford, a city of 100,000 which
> is slightly more than 50 miles from Boston, one of the medical
> centers of the nation, if not the world. . . .
> One holding himself out as a specialist should be held
> to the standard of the profession practicing the specialty,
> taking into account the advances in the profession. And . . .
> it is permissible to consider the medical resources available
> to him.[15]

The change in Massachusetts from the "similar locality" rule of
Small to the rule based on availability of medical resources in *Brune*
illustrates a current trend. It is the logical result of what the *Brune*
court called "present day conditions," under which improved transportation and communications systems enable small-town physicians
to keep abreast of medical advances in urban areas. As a Washington
court asked in a telling analogy, why should a small-town doctor
be treated more favorably than other small-town tort-feasors? The
small-town automobile driver has no right to be more negligent than
one in a big city; nor should a small-town doctor be allowed to
be more negligent than his urban counterpart.[16]

---

[15]354 Mass. 102, 108–9, 235 N.E. 2d 793, 798 (1968).
[16]*Douglass v. Bussabarger*, 73 Wash. 2d 476, 438 P. 2d 829 (1968); Holder, *supra*
n. 7, at 54.

Despite the adoption of the *Brune* test of accessibility of medical centers, practices in the local area may still be a factor, though not the controlling one. In *Pederson v. Dumouchel* a physician who was attending a victim of an automobile accident called in a dentist to treat a fractured jaw, but left before the dentist carried out the work.[17] When the patient suffered a convulsive seizure in the recovery room, no physician could be located for an hour and a half. The patient remained unconscious, and because he was thought to have suffered brain damage he was taken to Seattle, nearly 110 miles away. He did not regain consciousness for a month. In the suit brought by the patient, a trial court decided for the defendants, but the appellate court held that a medical or dental practitioner is liable if he fails to exercise the standard of care established in readily accessible medical centers. According to the court, the locality rule constituted only one of the elements which must be considered to determine the degree of skill and care exercised in a given instance.

A few courts have adopted a third variation of the locality rule, which looks to minimal national standards in determining the standard of care. In a case involving a claim against a Charleston, West Virginia, ophthalmologist for negligently performing a cataract operation, the plaintiff introduced the testimony of a New York City ophthalmologist.[18] The New York physician testified as to the procedure for cataract operations and noted that these were standard throughout the country. The appellate court, in remanding the case for further trial, decided that the testimony was proper, although the witness was not personally familiar with the standards of practice in Charleston, because Charleston practitioners would be held to the standard procedure used elsewhere.

As a final variation from the traditional locality rule, even those courts which follow the rule in its strictest form will not utilize a standard of care established locally, if the standard itself is negligent. In *Favalora v. Aetna Casualty and Surety Company* a 71-year-old patient fell to the floor while being x-rayed and suffered a number of injuries, including a fractured femur.[19] The consequent prolonged hospitalization brought on pulmonary embolism and a kidney infection. In bringing suit, the patient claimed that the fall would not have occurred if her radiologist had examined her medical records, which cited her history of sudden fainting spells. A lower court decision for defendants was reversed on the grounds that the community

---

[17] 72 Wash. 2d 73, 431 P. 2d 973 (1967).
[18] *Hundley v. Martinez*, 151 W. Va. 977, 158 S.E. 2d 159 (1967).
[19] 144 So. 2d 554 (La. App. 1962).

standards, which did not require a radiologist to take into account the patient's history, were negligent. In making this determination the court looked to teaching institutions, which required radiologists to examine the history of their patients.[20]

The third and final test applied to the standard of care is whether the care is comparable to that of physicians and surgeons "in the same general line of practice." This rule, sometimes called the "school rule," is a throwback to the days of different recognized schools of treatment: the allopathic school, which utilized a method of treating diseases by using agents which produced effects different from the agent of the disease treated, for example; and its opposite, the homeopathic school. Many of the schools have now become merged into what is known as the regular practice of medicine. Osteopathy is one of these. The practice of osteopathy still differs substantially from the practice of medicine in some states where osteopaths are not allowed to use drugs or perform surgery. In these states osteopaths would be judged by standards within their own school of medicine. In other states, however, where an osteopath can perform surgery and use drugs, the osteopath has been held to the standards established

---

[20] At times it is difficult to determine which of the four tests a court is applying. Consider the statement of the court in *Faulkner v. Pezeshki*, 44 Ohio App. 2d 186, 189, 190, 192, 337 N.E. 2d 158, 162 (1975):

> There has developed in malpractice actions, generally, what is known as the "locality rule," in considering the qualifications of an expert witness who has offered to testify upon the medical standards that should have been observed in a particular case. Such rule developed in early years upon the theory that doctors in a rural area should not be held to the same standards of medical expertise as doctors in urban areas because of the difficulties of communication and travel, with restricted opportunities to be kept abreast of medical advances, and the necessity of practicing in often inadequate hospital facilities. For a leading case developing the rule, see *Small v. Howard* (1880), 128 Mass. 131. Basically, four standards are involved: (1) the standard used in the community in which the defendant practices, (2) the standard used in a similar community, (3) one followed in the vicinity where the physician works, or (4) one based upon general professional practice, rather than a practice limited to a specific geographic locality, with community practice bearing on the issue of due care. As a consequence, expert witnesses are qualified only if they possess the requisite familiarity with the applicable proper standard, local, similar or vicinity, since the jury will be instructed as to such standard. See annotation, 37 A.L.R. 3d 420, 422.
>
> The locality rule is being increasingly eroded by judicial decisions, as being antiquated in light of present-day means of communication, travel, and the techniques available to the medical profession to keep abreast of modern developments. . . .
>
> Irrespective of the continuing validity of the same or similar locality standard in Ohio, we are of the view that the standard should not exclude testimony of an expert witness where the standards to which he proposes to testify are minimum standards applicable wherever medicine is practiced. The question, to us, is not whether the proffered witness practices in Portsmouth or a similar locality, but if he knows what the applicable standards are. See *Ardoline v. Keegan* (1954), 140 Conn. 552, 102 A. 2d 352. To the extent that minimum standards are involved, the standards of practice in Portsmouth and elsewhere are within his scope of knowledge.

in the regular practice of medicine.[21]

Despite the disappearance of several schools, the school rule is still important today because of the continued existence of a few such branches of medicine, and more importantly because of the trend toward specialization in the medical profession. The standard for judging practitioners in these specialities or schools is established by the practices of others in the same school or specialty. And increasingly, at least for a specialty within the medical profession, the specialist is being judged by standards beyond the confines of a particular geographic locality.[22]

In applying the school rule, courts have faced two major problems: What practices can be considered part of a legitimate school of treatment? And what limitations, if any, should be placed on the use of standards of a recognized school of treatment? *Nelson v. Harrington* answers the first question.[23] In that case a spiritualist, sued by the parent of his patient, wanted to defend the action on the ground that the treatment was in accord with the practices of other spiritualists. The court held that a school requires rules and principles of practice set up to guide the members in treating patients. The spiritualist school did not meet this test because the only principle followed uniformly by the school was to diagnose and treat the disease by means of a trance. Consequently the defendant was held to the standards of medical practice.

Illustrating a possible trend toward rejecting the idea that certain practices, at least those on the outer fringes of medical treatment, may constitute a school are two decisions involving a so-called drugless healer. In the first the drugless healer diagnosed as "inflammation of the spine and congestion of the bowels" what turned out to be appendicitis.[24] The patient, an 8-year-old child, subsequently died of peritonitis. The appellate court, in affirming a judgment for the parent of the child, noted that a drugless healer is entitled to be judged by the standard of care of other drugless healers, although this court also decided that regular medical practitioners could testify regarding the standard of diagnosis of appendicitis. Unfortunately the drugless healer in this case failed to learn his lesson: twenty-seven years later he was sued again for failure to diagnose appendicitis.[25]

---

[21] J. Waltz and F. Inbau, *Medical Jurisprudence* 54 (1971).
[22] Holder, *supra* n. 7, at 56.
[23] 72 Wis. 591, 40 N.W. 228 (1888).
[24] *Wilcox v. Carroll*, 127 Wash. 1, 219 P. 34 (1923).
[25] *Kelley v. Carroll*, 36 Wash. 2d 482, 219 P. 2d 79 (1950). This decision and the *Nelson* and *Wilcox* cases are discussed in Roady, *supra* n. 5, at 24–29, and in Waltz, *supra* n. 21, at 49–54.

In this case the healer deterred the patient from calling in a medical doctor and prescribed a laxative and "sine wave" treatment. The patient died and his widow sued the healer. This time the appellate court went beyond the earlier decision, deciding that the defendant did not belong to a school of medicine and was therefore to be judged by standards applicable to regular medical practice.

The question regarding limitations in the use of standards of recognized schools has been raised in cases involving chiropractors. If a chiropractor is charged with malpractice, he will normally be measured by the rules and practices of his own school and not those of a medical doctor.[26] If he exceeds what he is licensed to do, however, he will be held to the standards of physicians who are entitled to practice medicine. The same principle would of course apply to persons not practicing according to any school who might attempt to practice medicine: nurses, medical students, or the growing number of paramedics. In *Thompson v. Brent* a "medical assistant" working in an orthopedist's office was held to the standard of care required of physicians in using a Stryker saw to remove a cast.[27]

One might wonder whether the same reasoning would apply when a general medical practitioner engages in specialized medical treatment normally practiced by board-certified specialists, in other words, whether the general practitioner who occasionally does surgery would be held to the standards of board-certified surgeons. Although the question rarely arises now that hospitals generally limit their facilities to board-certified specialists, at present most courts do not hold the general practitioner to the standards of the specialists, despite a growing sentiment in favor of a stricter measure.[28] In *Sinz v. Owens* the appellate court held that a physician who did not use skeletal traction in treating a double comminuted fracture of a patient's leg would be held to the skill of a specialist only if he should have known that more than a general practitioner's skill was necessary.[29] If a physician presents himself as a specialist, however, he will be held to a higher standard of care than that of a general practitioner.

To conclude this analysis of the standard of care traditionally used to determine whether a physician was negligent, a recent decision of the Supreme Court of Washington, *Helling v. Carey*, may be noted.[30] The plaintiff had been treated by two ophthalmologists from 1959

---

[26] *Sheppard v. Firth*, 215 Ore. 268, 334 P. 2d 190 (1959).
[27] 245 So. 751 (La. App. 1971).
[28] Waltz, *supra* n. 21, at 52. See also Roady, *supra* n. 5, at 30.
[29] 33 Cal. 2d 749, 705 P. 2d 3 (1949).
[30] 83 Wash. 2d 514, 519 P. 2d 981 (1974).

until 1968. During this time she experienced difficulty with her contact lenses, but not until 1968, at age 32, was she told by one of the ophthalmologists that tests of her eye pressure and field of vision showed she had glaucoma. She then sued the ophthalmologists alleging permanent damage to her eyes as a result of the defendants' negligence in not carrying out these tests nine years earlier. The trial and appellate court decisions were for the ophthalmologists. In reversing these decisions, the Supreme Court of Washington noted that according to medical experts for both plaintiff and defendants professional standards did not require routine testing for glaucoma for patients under age 40, a group in which the disease afflicts only one out of 25,000 persons. The court concluded, however, that because the test was simple, inexpensive, and painless the standard adopted by the profession was itself negligent.

If other courts follow *Helling*, it is conceivable that the special standard of care used to determine a physician's negligence will fall by the wayside, and courts will rely on other methods to decide what is reasonable and prudent. But even more ominous in *Helling* was the concurring opinion of three judges that physicians should be held liable without fault. According to the rationale, physicians should bear the loss because they are in a financial position to shift the burden to society through higher fees.

Proving the Standard of Care and Breach of the Standard

When a special standard of care is used to determine a physician's negligence, a plaintiff patient must first prove the standard and then show that it was breached by the defendant physician. This proof is accomplished by the use of expert testimony, which normally comes from the defendant's fellow practitioners since they alone know the meaning of the standard. Moreover, unlike lay witnesses, physicians and other experts are not limited to testifying to facts they have observed, but may give their opinion on the nature and cause of a patient's illness or injury.

It is often claimed that admitting a physician's opinion as evidence is of little help to a patient needing expert testimony, because a conspiracy of silence is believed to exist among physicians, making them reluctant to testify against fellow members of the profession.[31]

[31] In *Faulkner v. Pezeshki*, 44 Ohio App. 2d 186, 193, 194, 337 N.W. 2d 158, 164 (1975) the court noted: "Locating an expert to testify for the plaintiff in a malpractice action is known to be a very difficult task, mainly because in most cases one doctor is reluctant and unwilling to testify against another doctor. Although doctors may complain privately to each other about the incompetence of other doctors, they are extremely reluctant to air the matter publicly."

One manifest example was a California case where a county medical society threatened to expel members and cancel their insurance if they testified for the plaintiff. This threat, a court held, did not give the plaintiff ground to recover from the medical society in tort.[32] If the conspiracy theory is valid a plaintiff might find it impossible to offer the required expert testimony, for courts have held that a plaintiff may not use a subpoena to force a physician not related to the case to testify.[33]

Although not developed specifically to relieve a plaintiff of the necessity for expert testimony in proving the standard of care or breach of the standard, six possible methods are available to a plaintiff to lessen the difficulty of obtaining expert testimony under present rules.

First, the plaintiff might use the physician's out-of-court statements as admissions of negligence. Statements made out of court are hearsay and traditionally excluded from evidence, but an admission made out of court will be accepted as evidence. Courts face a difficult task in determining whether the statement was really an admission of negligence, or whether it was merely a statement of sympathy for the patient.

In one case, for instance, a physician stated after a patient's death, "I don't know, it never happened to me before, I must have gone too deep or severed a vein." This, the court held, was too vague and indefinite to establish negligence.[34] In another case a physician doing a sigmoidoscopic examination tore the patient's large intestine.[35] While walking out of the operating room he stated to another physician, in the presence of the patient's husband, "Boy, I sure made a mess of things." When questioned by the husband, the physician stated, "In inserting the sigmoidoscope into the rectum, I busted the intestine." The court held that this admission could take the place of expert testimony because a jury could infer that the physician had not exercised the requisite degree of care.

Physicians should be especially careful about their statements when offering to settle claims. The law tries to encourage settlements and will not allow into evidence an offer of settlement if the case goes to court. If the offer of settlement includes an admission of negligence, however, the admission itself can be used as evidence.

---

[32] *Agnew v. Parks,* 172 Cal. App. 2d 756, 343 P. 2d 118 (1959).
[33] *Id.*
[34] *Scacchi v. Montgomery,* 365 Pa. 377, 75 A. 2d 535 (1950).
[35] *Wickoff v. James,* 150 Cal. App. 2d 664, 324 P. 2d 661 (1958). Both of these cases are discussed in Long, *The Physician and the Law* 28–29 (1968).

Second, even when the defendant physician makes no out-of-court admissions, a court will allow the plaintiff to call him as a witness. Unlike a criminal defendant, who can invoke the privilege against self-incrimination, the defendant physician, or any other defendant in a civil case, must testify as to the facts within his knowledge. Most courts feel it is unfair to require that the physician not only testify as to such facts but also provide the expert testimony needed by the plaintiff to establish the standard of care. A growing trend to the contrary, however, is illustrated by the New York decision in *McDermott v. Manhattan Eye, Ear and Throat Hospital.*[36] The defendant physicians, one of whom was one of the world's leading ophthalmologists, advised the plaintiff to undergo a series of operations to correct a corneal condition in her left eye. The operations resulted in blindness, and plaintiff claimed that the surgery was not approved by accepted medical practice, given the original diagnosis. At the trial the plaintiff presented no expert witness of her own, but instead called on the defendant to testify as to the standard of care required and the deviation from the standard in her case. The appellate court stated that plaintiff had the right to require the defendant to testify both as to his actual knowledge of the case and, if he was so qualified, as an expert to establish the generally accepted medical practice.

Third, the expert testimony requirement may be made less onerous by the rule that if the negligence is so obvious that it is within "common knowledge," expert testimony will not be required. One example would be the negligence of a surgeon who amputates the wrong leg. A more subtle example was presented in *Hammer v. Rosen,* where three witnesses, not experts, testified that the defendant had physically beaten an incompetent patient. Although the defendant physician claimed that expert testimony was necessary to show that the beatings deviated from standard psychotherapy treatments, the court held otherwise because "the very nature of the acts complained of bespeaks improper treatment and malpractice."[37]

Fourth, the need for expert testimony and especially the effect of the so-called conspiracy of silence are lessened when a plaintiff is permitted to introduce medical books to prove the standard of care. Medical publications are generally not admissible for this purpose. Publications are hearsay—that is, they are out-of-court statements made by an author who is not present to explain or

---

[36] 15 N.Y. 2d 20, 203 N.E. 2d 469 (1964). See: Waltz, *supra* n. 21, at 82.
[37] 7 N.Y. 2d 376, 165 N.E. 2d 756 (1960). See: Long, *supra* n. 35, at 31.

qualify his statements under direct or cross-examination—and in most states their use is limited to testing the credibility of an expert witness or reinforcing the opinion given in evidence by the expert.[38] In a few states, however, by statute or court decision, the medical books can be used as direct evidence to prove the standard of care. In a Wisconsin case the court took judicial notice of the standard of care set forth in a looseleaf reference service, "Lewis' Practice of Surgery," to determine whether an orthopedic surgeon was negligent in performing a laminectomy and diskectomy.[39] Even in states using the Wisconsin approach, however, the author must be proved to be a recognized expert or the publication to be a reliable authority.

Fifth, perhaps the most complex exception to the expert testimony rule is res ipsa loquitur, which means "the thing speaks for itself." The doctrine goes back to an English case decided in 1863, *Byrne v. Boadle.*[40] The plaintiff, Byrne, was walking down the street and was hit on the head by a barrel of flour which had rolled out of a warehouse owned by Boadle. The court found that Boadle was negligent because barrels of flour do not normally fall out of windows unless someone has been negligent.

Three conditions are essential to the use of res ipsa loquitur: (1) The accident must be of a type which normally would not occur without someone's negligence; (2) the defendant must have control of the apparent cause of the accident; and (3) the plaintiff could not have contributed to the accident. Whether the doctrine should be applied in a particular case is determined by the judge. Once a judge decides that res ipsa loquitur is applicable, most states have ruled that a permissible inference of negligence has been created; this in turn means that the case must go to the jury, which can then decide for plaintiff or defendant. In a few states the doctrine creates a presumption of negligence which requires the judge to enter a verdict for the patient unless the physician rebuts the presumption.[41]

In malpractice cases the first condition makes res ipsa loquitur difficult to apply, because it precludes use of the doctrine unless a layman can tell whether the injury is one that would not normally occur if a physician had not been negligent. In one example, a

[38] Bergen, "Medical Books as Evidence," 217 *J.A.M.A.* 527 (1971).
[39] *Burnside v. Evangelical Deaconess Hospital,* 46 Wis. 2d 519, 175 N.W. 2d 230 (1970).
[40] 2 H. and C. 722, 159 Eng. Rep. 299 (1863).
[41] W. Prosser, *Law of Torts* 214, 229–30 (4th ed. 1971).

patient underwent surgery for resection of the sigmoid colon.[42] The incision was closed with sutures; but it opened eight days later, and a second operation was required to close it once more. The court held that res ipsa loquitur did not apply because a layman would not know whether the separation of the incision was likely to be due to negligence. Thus the doctrine cannot be used simply because the results of the treatment are bad.

Leaving foreign objects in a patient after surgery is negligence within the common knowledge of laymen, however, and in such cases res ipsa loquitur is frequently used. In *Jefferson v. United States* the plaintiff was a soldier who had undergone a gall bladder operation in 1945.[43] Eight months later, after he had been suffering spells of nausea and vomiting, another operation was performed which disclosed a towel which had eroded into the duodenum. The towel, thirty inches long and eighteen inches wide, was marked "Medical Department U.S. Army." These facts, the court held, showed negligence on the part of the defendants.

The task of proving that the apparent cause of the accident was within the control of the defendant, the second of the three essential conditions, can also become complicated in medical malpractice cases where the negligence of any one of a group of persons could have caused the injury. A common rule is that the doctrine cannot be applied in an action against several defendants, any one of whom could have caused plaintiff's injury.[44] A major departure from this rule, however, was the California case of *Ybarra v. Spangard.*[45] After an appendectomy, the plaintiff felt sharp pains in his right shoulder and later suffered paralysis and atrophy of the shoulder muscles. The subsequent suit went to the California appellate court, which allowed the use of res ipsa loquitur against all of the defendants who had had any control of the patient while he was anesthetized. These included the surgeon, the consulting physician, the anesthesiologist, the owner of the hospital, and several hospital employees, even though some of the defendants were probably innocent of negligence.

To illustrate the third condition, that the plaintiff could not have contributed to the accident, a hospital employee in one case went away after leaving a cup, saucer, teabag, and hot water on a table

[42]*Jamison v. Debenham*, 203 Cal. App. 2d 744, 21 Cal. Rptr. 848 (1962).
[43]77 F. Supp. 706 (Md. 1948), *aff'd*, 178 F. 2d 518 (4th Cir. 1949), *aff'd*, 340 U.S. 135 (1950).
[44]Waltz, *supra* n. 21, at 100.
[45]25 Cal. 2d 486, 154 P. 2d 687 (1944).

beside a patient who was recovering from surgery and under the influence of pain-killing drugs.[46] The patient was later found suffering from burns. It was claimed that res ipsa loquitur should be applied because the injury occurred when she was under the influence of the drugs and did not understand what was going on. The court held that the doctrine did not apply in this case because according to witnesses the plaintiff admitted that she had spilled the water on herself and that she was awake and alert at the time.

The sixth exception to the rule requiring expert testimony involves the use of statutes, regulations of governmental agencies, standards of private agencies, and hospital rules to determine the standard of care.[47] In *Landeros v. Flood* a physician was held not liable at common law for failing to diagnose a "battered child syndrome," but a civil damage action was allowed on the theory that the physician breached his statutory duty to report intentional or criminal injuries to a child.[48]

Causation and Damages

To prevail in a negligence action, a plaintiff must prove that a physician has been negligent in exercising the required standard of care and that the patient has been injured. There must also be proof of causation, a vital connecting link between the negligence and the injury. First, plaintiff must prove that the defendant's negligence in fact caused the injury. This means showing that the injury would not have occurred but for the defendant's act. This "but for" test, applied alone, would often produce an unfair result, however, especially when some intervening force increased the injury. As a result, courts also require that the negligence be the cause in law, or the proximate cause, of the injury. In those difficult cases where part or all of the injury has not resulted directly from the defendant's negligence but is rather the indirect consequence of an intervening force, the factor which usually determines proximate cause is the foreseeability of the injury. An injury is considered foreseeable if the average reasonable person in the defendant's place would have foreseen that outside forces would intervene.

In applying these general principles to malpractice cases, a major problem has been the determination of whether the physician's

---

[46] *Rice v. California Lutheran Hospital*, 158 P. 2d 579 (Cal. App. 1945), *rev'd on other grounds*, 27 Cal. 296, 163 P. 2d 860 (1945).
[47] *Darling v. Charleston Community Memorial Hospital*, 33 Ill. 2d 326, 211 N.E. 2d 253 (1965). This topic will be covered in greater detail in later chapters dealing with hospital emergency care and coronary care units.
[48] 50 Cal. App. 3d 115, 123 Cal. Rptr. 713 (1975).

negligence was the cause in fact of the injury. At times the courts have decided that some, but not all, of a patient's injuries resulted from the negligence. In one case a physician-patient relationship had been established between a woman and her obstetrician. Later she suffered a miscarriage alone in her home, which was near that of the obstetrician. In the suit charging him with negligence in failing to treat her the court decided that the obstetrician's negligence did not cause the miscarriage, because his presence in the house would not have prevented it. The physician, however, was held liable for the patient's pain and suffering which resulted from being left alone in the house.[49]

In a number of cases physicians have been completely absolved from liability, despite their negligence, because of inadequate proof of causation. In one such case a 16-year-old boy was treated at an emergency room after being hit by a truck.[50] A physician in the emergency room examined the boy and sent him home, where he died early the next morning. The cause of death was a basal skull fracture. The appellate court found sufficient evidence that the physician was negligent in not taking vital signs himself and not ascertaining whether anyone else had taken them. According to the court, however, there was inadequate proof that the alleged negligence was the cause of death. One expert witness testified, "There is no possible way for a physician or anyone else to ascertain with any degree of certainty whether with medical intervention, the individual would have survived or died." Another expert noted, "There certainly is a chance and I can't say exactly what—maybe someplace around 50 percent—that he would survive the surgery."[51] The court held that these statements did not show the defendant's negligence to have been the probable cause of death. A similar result has been reached when one physician made an improper diagnosis which was later corrected by another physician. For example, in *Henderson v. Mason*, the defendant physician failed to discover a piece of steel imbedded in the patient's eye. The steel was eventually discovered and removed by another physician. Recovery was denied because it was shown that the infection and loss of vision suffered by the patient would have resulted even if the defendant's diagnosis had been correct.[52]

---

[49] *Mehigan v. Sheehan*, 94 N.H. 274, 51 A. 2d 632 (1947).
[50] *Cooper v. Sisters of Charity of Cincinnati, Inc.*, 27 Ohio St. 2d 242, 272 N.E. 2d 97 (1971).
[51] *Id.*, at 247, 272 N.E. 2d at 101.
[52] 386 S.W. 2d 879 (Tex. Civ. App. 1964).

In these decisions, which are representative of cases dealing with the causation issue, the courts have not precisely indicated the defect in the proof of causation. Consequently it is difficult to draw general conclusions regarding the reason for denial of recovery. However, while courts often speak of proving proximate cause, in most cases the real issue is clearly whether the patient's injury would have occurred "but for" the physician's negligence. That is, most often the courts have not even reached the proximate cause problem because of an initial determination that the negligence was not the cause in fact.

In one type of malpractice case, courts deal more explicitly with the proximate cause issue. That is where the negligence of the physician is an intervening force which might relieve the original tort-feasor of responsibility for the resulting injuries. It is generally agreed that the original tort-feasor would be liable because treatment of the injury would be reasonably foreseeable, and negligence by a physician is a normal risk in such treatment. The related question of whether the physician must reimburse the tort-feasor for part of the damage award was answered in a recent Ohio decision.[53] The patient had sustained an injury to his spine from an explosion caused by the tort-feasor. Later, allegedly as the result of the negligence of his physician, he suffered a contusion of the spinal cord, paralysis of his lower extremities, and loss of bowel and bladder control. The patient recovered $290,000 from the original tort-feasor, who then sued the physician for his independent acts of negligence. The court, following a majority rule which it considered to be "just and equitable," held that the tort-feasor would be entitled to recovery if the physician was negligent.

Whenever the necessary causal link between the negligence of the physician and the patient is established the patient is entitled to damages. As noted in the previous chapter, actual damages—and in some cases punitive damages—are allowable in a negligence action. Actual damages include compensation for past and future medical expenses, past and future loss of income, physical pain, and mental anguish.[54] Actual damages are often difficult for a court to estimate in malpractice cases. Consider a case where the defendant physician was held liable on the basis of his guarantee to make "a hundred per cent perfect hand," and imagine the difficulty of a jury trying

---

[53] *Travelers Indemnity Co. v. Trowbridge,* 41 Ohio St. 2d 11, 321 N.E. 2d 787 (1975).
[54] Recovery of future loss of income, however, was denied in a recent case where a patient claimed that his doctor was negligent in wrongly diagnosing his illness as terminal. As a result of the diagnosis, the patient took early retirement from his job. *Greinke v. Keese,* 82 Misc. 2d 996, 371 N.Y.S. 2d 58 (1975).

to apply the rule: "We, therefore, conclude that the true measure of the plaintiff's damage in the present case is the difference between the value to him of a perfect hand or a good hand, such as the jury found the defendant promised him, and the value of the hand in its present condition."[55]

In the same case the court discussed another loss which is difficult to recompense, "pain and suffering." The court concluded that plaintiff's suffering was a necessary part of the treatment, regardless of the success of the operation. If recompense for pain and suffering is allowed, some courts leave the assessment of damages entirely to the jury. Other courts allow the plaintiff to figure a per diem sum for pain and suffering and multiply this by his life expectancy. The trial court in one Florida case allowed an attorney for a 9-year-old amputee to use the following chart in making his argument for damages:[56]

"Mike" Braddock

Age 9	Expectancy 56 years

Pain and Suffering to date	395 days	
Experience of accident		5,000.00
Hospital 3/25-4/5/52		1,200.—
First 30 days at home		300.—
To date 353 days		700.—
Inability to Lead Normal Life		
3/25-5/31/52 crutches		340.—
6/1-10/31/52 pylon		459.—
11/1/52 to date artificial limb		348.—
Humiliation and Embarrassment		1,915.—
		10,262.—

20,440 days		*Future 56 yrs.*
Medical		
Checkup by doctor once a year		440.—
Artificial legs		3,600.—
Repairs and Maintenance		2,640.—
Stump socks		985.—
Extra pants, shoes and socks		4,400.—
Limb adjustment every 2 weeks		2,912.—
		14,977.—

---

[55] *Hawkins v. McGee,* 84 N.H. 114, 118, 146 A. 641, 644 (1929).
[56] *Seaboard Airline R. Co. v. Braddock,* 96 So. 127 (Fla. 1957).

Pain and Suffering 20,440 days		20,440.—
Humiliation and Embarrassment		
20,440 days		40,880.—
Inability to Lead a Normal Life		
20,440 days		40,880.—
Loss of Earning Capacity		121,000.—
5500 × 50% × 56	Total	248,439.—

The jury returned a verdict for $248,439. The verdict was over-ruled, among other reasons, because a number of items on the chart overlapped, especially the damages for "Pain and Suffering," "Humil-iation and Embarrassment," and "Inability to Lead a Normal Life."

Two methods of figuring pain and suffering are not allowed. A court will not allow the plaintiff's attorney to ask the members of the jury how much payment they would demand before they would allow someone to perform the negligent act on themselves. And courts will not allow "Golden Rule" arguments that ask the jurors to award the plaintiff what they would want to receive if they were in the plaintiff's shoes.[57]

In recovering actual damages, a patient might be receiving a windfall if expenses have already been paid by a health insurer. Courts generally frown on the double recovery of damages, but under the "collateral source" rule followed in most states the patient will be allowed to recover, even though he received payments from a collateral source and hence suffered no out-of-pocket losses. The rationale usually given is that the plaintiff should be allowed to benefit from his own foresight in obtaining insurance and that the negligent party should not receive credit for injuring someone who happened to be insured.[58]

Punitive damages are rarely allowed in malpractice actions. In *Ebaugh v. Rabkin* one patient was to undergo a breast biopsy; another was scheduled for a gall bladder operation.[59] The charts of the patients were switched and the patients were taken to the wrong operating rooms. The mistake became apparent when the physician performing the gall bladder operation discovered that the organ was healthy. A jury awarded this patient $7,500 in actual damages and another $75,000 in punitive damages. The appellate court, however, reversed the award of punitive damages, deciding that, even in cases of gross

[57]Waltz, *supra* n. 21, at 289.
[58]Comment, "An Analysis of State Legislative Responses to Malpractice Crisis," 1975 *Duke L. J.* 1417, 1447–48.
[59]22 Cal. App. 3d 891, 99 Cal. Rptr. 706 (1972).

negligence, punitive damages may be awarded only when the defendant has acted intentionally and with malice.

The size of malpractice awards has become a controversial topic in recent years, especially such verdicts as the $4 million awarded to the boy with brain damage. The 1973 HEW report summarizing the distribution of amounts paid on the malpractice claims closed in 1970 helps to put damage awards into perspective.[60]

Total settlement costs of incidents, in dollars	Percent of incidents	Cumulative percent of incidents
1–499	21.1	21.1
500–999	16.0	37.1
1,000–1,999	12.3	49.4
2,000–2,999	10.1	59.5
3,000–3,999	3.0	62.5
4,000–4,999	2.7	65.2
5,000–9,999	13.4	78.6
10,000–19,999	10.0	88.6
20,000–39,999	5.3	93.9
40,000–59,999	1.3	95.2
60,000–79,999	1.0	96.2
80,000–99,999	0.8	97.0
100,000 and up	3.0	100.0
	100.0	

It is worth noting that approximately 55 per cent of all claimants received no payment at all. The largest number of successful claimants received less than $3,000. According to this report, probably not more than seven claimants each year are paid $1 million or over, but the report concluded in what might be considered an understatement: "There is little doubt that the number of large awards or settlements has been increasing dramatically within the recent past."[61]

To limit a damage award when the jury has been too generous with an injured patient, the defendant's attorney can ask the trial judge either to lower damages or to order a new trial to redetermine the amount of damages. Although courts do not like to interfere with a jury's exercise of discretion in determining damages, they will modify a damage award which is so large that it suggests passion,

[60] HEW, *supra* n. 4, at 11.
[61] *Id.*, at 10.

prejudice, or partiality on the jury's part.[62] In *Larson v. Lindahl* a patient was awarded $15,000 for having been hospitalized sixty days beyond her original hospitalization because of a wrong diagnosis.[63] The appellate court decided that this award was excessive and ordered a new trial.

Common Instances of Malpractice Liability

A 1969 study of medical malpractice, prepared for the Senate Committee on Government Operations, included a ranking of the nine major reasons why patients sue physicians.[64] While the ranking may be subject to change, the reasons offer typical situations that have involved physicians in malpractice litigation.

1. *Foreign body left in patient during surgery.* Examples of this type of negligence were given during the discussion of res ipsa loquitur, one typical case being *Jefferson v. United States,* where the physician had left an army towel inside the patient.[65] It should be remembered, however, that physicians are not liable in all cases where foreign objects are left in patients.[66]

2. *Untoward results of tight casts.* In *Vann v. Harden* the patient, a high school football player, had complained to his physician that a cast on his leg was painful.[67] The physician ignored the complaints and went on vacation. Later the patient's leg had to be amputated, and a jury found the physician negligent in failing to investigate the complaints.

3. *Technical surgical errors.* In *Gluckstein v. Lipsett* cosmetic surgery had been performed on the breasts of a 50-year-old woman.[68] After the surgery one breast was larger than the other and the breasts were scarred and disfigured. The patient was allowed to recover $115,000 in damages.[69]

4. *Lack of informed consent.* Examples are given in a later chapter.

5. *Errors of a resident, intern, or nurse.* A surgeon, for example, will be liable if a nurse, following his directions, administers an

---

[62]Holder, "Excessive Damages," 228 *J.A.M.A.* 937 (1974).
[63]167 Colo. 409, 450 P. 2d 77 (1968).
[64]Sen. Subcomm. on Executive Reorganization, "Medical Malpractice: The Patient vs. the Physician," 91st Cong., 1st Sess. 452 (1969).
[65]77 F. Supp. 706 (Md. 1948), *aff'd,* 178 F. 2d 518 (4th Cir. 1949), *aff'd,* 340 U.S. 135 (1950).
[66]*Dietze v. King,* 184 F. Supp. 944 (E.D. Va. 1960).
[67]187 Va. 555, 47 S.E. 2d 314 (1948).
[68]93 Cal. App. 2d 391, 209 P. 2d 98 (1949).
[69]This case was well publicized after the plaintiff was exhibited to the jury by her attorney Melvin M. Belli.

overdose of ether which results in the patient's death.[70]

6. *Adverse reaction to penicillin or tetanus shots.* These cases exemplify a physician's liability for not using due care in administering or prescribing drugs. Due care includes determining whether the patient is allergic to the substance. For example, a physician administered penicillin to a patient who suffered from conjunctivitis and who subsequently went blind in one eye. He was not liable because he had followed the required standard of due care in questioning the patient about possible reactions to the drug.[71]

7. *Abandonment of an obstetrical patient.* Abandonment was discussed in the previous chapter. Claims of abandonment are frequent in actions involving obstetricians. In one such case, *Norton v. Hamilton,* a physician who left his patient shortly after she went into labor was held liable for abandonment.[72]

8. *Burns due to x-ray, diathermy, or chemicals.* For example, an antiseptic solution, applied to a patient before delivery, collected in pools on the rubber sheet where the woman was lying and caused burns. This was determined to be compensable injury.[73] Burn cases, like those involving foreign objects, often entail the use of res ipsa loquitur.

9. *Neglecting to give proper treatment in a surgical cardiac arrest.* A surgeon will not be liable for a cardiac arrest during surgery unless he could predict beforehand that the arrest was likely or unless he did not act instantly to treat the arrest. When a cardiac arrest occurred during the delivery of a baby, an obstetrician who opened the patient's chest and massaged the heart within one minute after the arrest was held to have followed the standards of due care and was not liable.[74]

In addition to these nine most common reasons for bringing a malpractice action, other factual situations recur with some frequency. A physician who fails to make a correct diagnosis will be liable if he does not exercise the proper standard of care. In *Fortner v. Koch* a physician examining a patient with a swollen knee and other symptoms did not follow the standard of care in the locality, which required a blood test, biopsy, and x-rays.[75] The physician was held liable for failing to take these tests.

---

[70] *Jackson v. Joyner,* 72 S.E. 2d (N.C. 1952).
[71] *Johnston v. Brother,* 190 Cal. App. 2d 464, 12 Cal. Rptr. 23 (1961).
[72] 92 Ga. App. 727, 89 S.E. 2d 809 (1955).
[73] *Woronka v. Sewall,* 320 Mass. 362, 69 N.E. 2d 581 (1946).
[74] *Dunlap v. Marine,* 242 Cal. App. 2d 162, 51 Cal. Rptr. 158 (1966).
[75] 272 Mich. 273, 261 N.W. 762 (1935).

Another common basis for liability is a physician's failure to consult a patient's prior doctor or to refer the patient to a specialist. In one case a physician treating a patient for asthma damaged the optic nerve and caused a loss of sight.[76] He had been advised that the patient had undergone nasal surgery but had not consulted the former physician. Had he done so, he would have discovered that the patient's optic nerve was unprotected. The physician's failure to consult with the earlier physician constituted negligence. In another case, as the result of a general surgeon's attempt to do vascular surgery without consulting a specialist, the leg of a teenage boy had to be amputated.[77] A jury verdict for the patient was upheld on appeal.

Finally, liability can arise when the physician fails to give proper instructions to a patient. For example, a physician instructing an immigrant with a serious heart condition was held liable for the patient's death, because the patient was not made to understand that he could not return to work.[78]

Defenses to Malpractice

Given the theoretical bases for a malpractice claim and the factual illustrations discussed above, what defenses, if any, can a physician raise if he is sued on a negligence theory? The following definitions and illustrations of a number of defenses, listed in alphabetical order, are especially relevant in malpractice actions. Other defenses, such as the res judicata theory discussed in Chapter I, are of course available, but have no special significance in malpractice cases.

1. *Assumption of risk.* A defendant in a tort action can occasionally raise assumption of risk as a defense. In many jurisdictions a person who voluntarily exposes himself to a known risk will be precluded from recovering damages caused by incurring the risk. In medical malpractice cases the risk is often in a new method of treatment, and an important issue is whether the possible effects of such treatment were made known to the patient. This issue is closely related to informed consent, for a physician who has informed the patient of the risk will not only be relieved of liability for failure to state that the treatment may be dangerous, but he will also be able to assert in his defense that the patient knowingly assumed the risk. In *Karp v. Cooley,* for example, the surgeon was not held liable

---

[76]*Langford v. Kosterlitz,* 107 Cal. App. 175, 290 P. 80 (1930).
[77]*Wilson v. Gilbert,* 25 Cal. App. 3d 607, 102 Cal. Rptr. 31 (1972).
[78]*Krusilla v. United States,* 287 F. 2d 34 (2d Cir. 1961).

for the death of a patient after a heart transplant because the patient had consented to the operation after being fully informed of the dangers.[79] Normally, however, the risks that the patient has assumed do not include the physician's negligence in treating the patient. In *Karp*, if death had resulted from the surgeon's failure to exercise the standard of care required in heart transplants, the surgeon would probably have been liable.

2. *Contributory negligence.* Even if a physician himself is negligent, contributory negligence is a complete defense in many states. Under this theory if the patient failed to act as a reasonable, prudent person would, and if his negligence contributed to the injury, he cannot recover damages for the physician's negligence. In one case a physician who was grossly intoxicated negligently treated a patient.[80] The court refused to hold the doctor liable on the grounds that the patient was negligent in accepting treatment from a physician who was obviously drunk.

It is important that cases where the patient's negligence contributed to the injury be distinguished from those where the contributory negligence merely aggravated an injury caused by the physician's negligence. If the contributory negligence aggravates an injury that would have occurred despite due care by the patient, he will be allowed at least a partial recovery. In a Wisconsin case, *Schultz v. Tasche*, an 18-year-old girl was negligently treated for a fracture of the right femur.[81] As a result the right leg was one and one-half inches shorter than the left and was deformed and painful. The appellate court decided that the girl could recover for the doctor's negligence despite her own negligence in leaving the hospital early, driving fifteen miles to her home, and failing to return for additional treatment. The girl's negligence, the court decided, merely aggravated the existing injury, and its only relevance was to reduce the damage award.

The *Schultz* case was based upon a contributory negligence theory which has since been replaced, in Wisconsin and most other states, by a "comparative negligence" approach. Although there are different theories of comparative negligence, in all cases the attempt is made

---

[79] 349 F. Supp. 827 (S.D. Tex. 1972). This case is discussed in greater detail in the chapter on consent for treatment. See also: Holder, *supra* n. 7, at 306–9.
[80] *Champs v. Stone*, 74 Ohio App. 344, 58 N.E. 2d 803 (1944).
[81] 166 Wis. 561, 165 N.W. 292 (1918). See also: *Heller v. Medine*, 377 N.Y.S. 2d 100, 102 (1976): "A patient's failure to follow instructions does not defeat an action for malpractice where the alleged improper professional treatment occurred prior to the patient's own negligence. Under such circumstances, damages are reduced to the degree that the plaintiff's negligence increased the extent of the injury."

to compensate the injured party to some extent despite his contributory negligence. In one variation, illustrated by a later Wisconsin case, a hospital patient slipped while taking a shower and was injured.[82] The jury decided that the hospital was 20 per cent negligent, possibly for failing to install safety devices in the shower, but that the patient was 80 per cent negligent. As a result the patient was awarded only $4,500.

   3. *Exculpatory contract.* Occasionally a physician will raise as a defense a contract clause to the effect that the patient agrees to forfeit his right to sue the physician for negligence. The general rule that such exculpatory contracts are invalid has been applied to physician-patient contracts. The same rule applies to hospitals. In *Tunkle v. Regents of The University of California* the court held that a contract between a hospital and a patient which freed the hospital from all liability was against public policy.[83]

   4. *"Good Samaritan" statutes.* "Good Samaritan" statutes, discussed more completely in a later chapter, offer the physician another defense. Although such statutes vary a good deal among the forty-two states which have them, they commonly provide that a physician rendering emergency care at the scene of an accident will not be held liable for his negligence. This defense is of doubtful utility because, as noted in the 1973 HEW report cited earlier, there has never been an officially reported court decision where a physician acting as a Good Samaritan has been sued for negligence.

   5. *Release.* A so-called release may operate as a defense for a physician. If a physician and patient reach a settlement on a malpractice claim, a release given by the patient to the physician will bar a later suit for injuries arising from the same negligent act. A more complicated factual setting results when a tort-feasor injures a patient and the injury is aggravated by the negligence of the physician treating the patient. If the patient settles with the tort-feasor and gives him a release, does the release also cover the physician? Although most states would probably require that the physician must be named specifically in the release before he can assert the release as a defense, some states have decided that even if the release is phrased in general terms it frees the physician. *Whitt v. Hutchison* is an example of the latter approach. In that case the plaintiff, who was injured at a ski resort, claimed that his injuries were aggravated by the negligence

---

[82]*Schuster v. St. Vincent Hospital,* 45 Wis. 2d 135, 172 N.W. 2d 421 (1969).
[83]60 Cal. 2d 92, 32 Cal. Rptr. 33, 383 P. 2d 441 (1963). See: 61 Am. Jur. 2d "Physicians, Surgeons," sec. 107 (1972).

of the physicians treating him. The plaintiff settled with the ski resort for $6,000 and signed a form releasing the resort

> from any and all liability . . . and any and all other loss and damages of every kind and nature sustained by or hereafter resulting to the undersigned . . . from an accident which occurred on or about the first day of March, 1969, at Clear Fork Ski Resort, Butler, Richland County, Ohio, and of and from all liability, claims, demands, controversies, damages, actions, and causes of action whatsoever, either in law or equity, which the undersigned, individually or in any other capacity, their heirs, executors, administrators, successors and assigns, can, shall or may have by reason of or in any wise incident [to] or resulting from the accident hereinbefore mentioned.[84]

The court held that this release was broad enough to include malpractice claims and upheld a dismissal of the suit against the defendant physicians and hospital.

6. *Statute of limitations.* The statute of limitations is a defense commonly raised in malpractice cases. As noted in the previous chapter, statutes of limitations set forth the period within which actions must be brought. The period for malpractice actions is generally shorter than for other actions, although the statutory provisions vary greatly from state to state.[85]

In malpractice cases the major problem is determining the time when the statutory period begins. If the statute of limitations for a particular state provides that the period during which a malpractice suit may be brought is two years, three major points in time might trigger the statute of limitations, depending on the state and the factual circumstances.

First, many states interpret the statute literally and have decided that the two-year period begins when the negligent treatment is performed.[86] Second, a number of other states use the discovery rule and begin counting the time on the day when the patient discovers or should have discovered the alleged malpractice. In a recent Michigan case an appellate court decided that the two-year statute of limitations began when the plaintiff discovered that a surgical needle had been left in her abdomen, even though the needle had

---

[84] 43 Ohio St. 2d 53, 54, 330 N.E. 2d, 678, 679–80 (1975).
[85] A summary of statutes of limitations may be found in A. Moritz and R. Morris, *Handbook of Legal Medicine* 212–14 (1970). See the preceding chapter for examples of the Ohio statutes of limitations.
[86] *Id.* at 211; *Hill v. Hays,* 193 Kan. 443, 395 P. 2d 298 (1964).

been there since 1949, twenty-five years before the court's decision.[87]
Some courts limit such exceptions to cases where a foreign object
is found in the patient. The third possibility is the termination rule,
under which the period begins when the treatment ends, or in a
few states when the physician-patient relationship ends.[88]

Other possibilities would apply in many states in particular factual
settings. For example, if a physician fraudulently conceals the malpractice, the statutory period will be delayed until discovery of the
negligence.[89] The period often begins later when the patient is a
minor. In *Chaffin v. Nicosia* a physician's negligent use of forceps
during a childbirth resulted in almost complete loss of sight in the
child's right eye.[90] Suit was allowed twenty-two years later because
the action was commenced within two years after the injured person
reached the age of majority. Moreover some courts have decided
that, despite the discovery rule, an action for wrongful death accrues
at the date of the death.[91]

Some have cited such variations from the literal interpretation
of the statutes of limitations as a significant cause of the malpractice
crisis. According to malpractice insurers, for instance, it is very difficult
to determine rates because potential losses for a policy year are
made so uncertain by the possibility of malpractice claims twenty
to thirty years after the negligent treatment.

In fairness it should be noted that the statute of limitations defense
can be raised by the patient as well as the physician. In one case
in which a surgeon sued a patient for payment covering services
rendered, the patient's attorney pointed out that the statute of
limitations had run.[92] The surgeon then wrote to the patient's
employer, charging that "having no other defense, [he] cowardly
slinks behind the defense of statutory limitation." As a result the
employee lost his job and sued the physician for libel. The surgeon's
letter, an appellate court decided, gave the patient a sufficient cause
of action, and the surgeon was held liable for damages.

7. *Workmen's compensation.* A final defense is a no-fault statute,
workmen's compensation, adopted in one form or another by all
states. Under state workmen's compensation statutes, employees
injured on the job may be compensated even though their injuries

---

[87] *Cates v. Bald,* 54 Mich. App. 717, 221 N.W. 2d 474 (1974).
[88] 1970 *Wis. L. Rev.* 915, 918; 6 *Akron L. Rev.* 265, 267–68 (1973).
[89] *Barrer v. Bowen,* 63 N.J. Super. 225, 164 A. 2d 357 (1960).
[90] 261 Ind. 698, 310 N.E. 2d 867 (1974).
[91] *Hubbard v. Libi,* 229 N.W. 2d 82 (N.D. 1975).
[92] *Hollenbeck v. Restine,* 114 Iowa 358, 86 N.W. 377 (1901).

were not caused by the negligence of their employer or fellow employees. On the other hand, if the injury resulted from the negligence of the employer or fellow employees, the worker will not be allowed to recover damages in a negligence action because workmen's compensation is normally the exclusive remedy. Thus if the physician and patient have the same employer, the patient in most states could not recover damages caused by the physician's negligence.[93]

Although one or more of the above defenses might be useful to a physician in a particular case, perhaps the best defense for doctors as for others is a good offense. That is, the most obvious way for physicians to avoid liability is to exercise the required standard of care in treating their patients. Physicians need also to be careful in other matters. They should avoid offhand criticism of other physicians; such loose talk is often a major cause of malpractice actions. In the words of the late Dr. Louis J. Regan, an authority on malpractice, "Various authorities have estimated that 50 to 80 per cent of all the suits for malpractice would be eliminated if such destructive criticism [by succeeding physicians of the work of a predecessor] could be stopped."[94] Although careless accusations are dangerous, the physician who justly criticizes a colleague does a great service to his profession in helping to prevent malpractice and in changing the public's belief in a conspiracy of silence.

Physicians should also keep accurate medical records. The importance of accurate records is illustrated by a survey done in conjunction with the 1973 HEW report on medical malpractice. According to this survey, one-fourth of the defense and plaintiff attorneys who were interviewed felt that evidence of falsified records had a significant influence on jurors.[95]

Finally, and perhaps most important, physicians should take a personal interest in each patient. Despite the impersonality prevalent in our society, patients still have high expectations of sympathetic treatment when they visit their physicians, probably bolstered by what has been called the "Dr. Welby syndrome." When the physician fails to meet the high standard of personal concern established by Dr. Welby, symptoms of a revenge syndrome manifest themselves. In the words of Eli P. Bernzweig, the executive director of the HEW Commission on Malpractice:[96]

---

[93]*Proctor v. Ford Motor Co.*, 36 Ohio St. 2d 3, 302 N.E. 2d 580 (1973).
[94]Averbach, "Rx. for Malpractice," 19 *Clev. St. L.R.* 20, 24 (1970).
[95]HEW, *supra* n. 4, App. at 112.
[96]*Medical Malpractice* 4 (D. McDonald, ed. 1971).

In this whole field of malpractice litigation there is a strong
get-even, or revenge factor. I have heard plaintiffs' attorneys
say that their clients did not really want to sue for money.
What they really wanted was a chance to be alone in the
room with the defendant doctor for about fifteen minutes.
When a physician has maltreated you in a psychological sense,
the revenge motive arises. If we ever had a tort in this country
known as psychological malpractice we would not have enough
courthouses to take care of all the cases.

Liability for Acts of Others

In a number of cases physicians who are not personally negligent
have been held liable for the negligence of others. Liability in these
cases is often based on the principle of respondeat superior: that
is, let the superior be responsible for the negligence of his agents
or employees, or "Look to the man higher up."[97] Questions regarding
respondeat superior often arise in hospitals when the issue is whether
the physician or the hospital must answer for the negligence of
hospital employees, an issue thoroughly discussed in a later chapter.
Outside of the hospital, in the physician's office, the physician is
responsible for the negligent acts of nurses, paramedics, x-ray
technicians, and other physicians in his employ. As was mentioned
earlier, in *Thompson v. Brent* a physician was held liable because
a "medical assistant" in his employ was negligent in removing a
cast with a Stryker saw.[98]

There are exceptional cases, however, where a physician would
not be liable. A physician who had ordered an attendant to place
hot irons in a patient's bed to keep her warm was not liable for
burns caused by the attendant's negligence, because the attendant
was the employee of the patient not the physician.[99]

In addition to possible liability for the acts of his employees a
physician might also be held liable when he refers cases to other
physicians not in his employ. In general a physician is not liable
when a substitute physician or a specialist takes over a case; but
if he is careless in selecting the substitute or the specialist he will
be liable for his own negligence. If he continues to participate in
the treatment of the patient, his legal status will be that of a joint

---

[97]W. Prosser, *Law of Torts* 458–59 (4th ed. 1971).
[98]245 So. 2d 751 (La. App. 1971).
[99]*Malkowski v. Graham*, 169 Wis. 398, 172 N.W. 785 (1919).

venturer, and he will be liable for the negligence of the other physician.[100]

Furthermore when a physician is in partnership with other physicians he will be liable for the torts of his partners, as long as the acts were committed within the scope of the partnership business. If partnership assets are insufficient to pay a judgment, the physician's personal assets may be used to satisfy the judgment.

In one extreme case a man sued a medical partnership for alienation of affections, claiming that his wife had an affair with one of the partners.[101] The court decided that the partnership would be liable if it were shown that the partners did not use reasonable means to prevent the errant partner from committing a tortious interference with the plaintiff's family relations. Liability of this type could be limited by incorporating the partnership. The corporation would then have to respond in damages, although the physicians who personally committed the tort would of course still be individually liable for their own wrongful acts.

Up to this point a number of issues frequently raised in malpractice litigation have been discussed. Helping to put these into perspective is a table from the 1973 HEW report, which illustrates how frequently the issues have been significant to the outcome of malpractice cases on appeal.[102]

Reforms of the Tort System

In response to the malpractice crisis, a number of states have taken action in recent years in an attempt to alleviate the problem. Three major approaches have been utilized to date. First, much effort has gone toward treating one of the symptoms as well as a precipitating cause of the crisis: the tremendous increase in insurance rates and the termination of malpractice insurance coverage. Many states have provided for the creation of a joint underwriting association (JUA). This is essentially an insurance mechanism designed to apportion malpractice risks among carriers writing malpractice insurance, although the term has been applied to a wide variety of insurance arrangements. In New York, for example, a JUA of personal injury liability insurers was established in 1975.

---

[100]*Morrill v. Komasinski*, 256 Wis. 417, 41 N.W. 2d 620 (1950). See: Waltz, *supra* n. 21, at 119–21.
[101]*Kelsey-Seybold Clinic v. Maclay*, 456 S.W. 2d 229, 466 S.W. 2d 716 (Tex. 1971).
[102]HEW, *supra* n. 4, App. at 130.

Rank (1961–71)	Issues or Doctrines Most Significant to Case Outcomes	Percentage of Cases		
		1961–71	1950–60	Pre-1950
1.	Burden of Proof	19.0	26.1	31.1
2.	Standard of Care	16.8	13.3	14.8
3.	Expert Testimony—need for, locality rule, adverse witness	13.4	8.5	16.6
4.	Statute of Limitations	11.9	6.9	7.4
5.	Proximate Cause	8.5	5.9	6.4
6.	*Res Ipsa Loquitur*	8.0	8.0	2.1
7.	Procedural Issues	5.1	5.3	3.9
8.	Informed Consent/Consent	4.6	2.7	1.1
9.	*Respondeat Superior*	4.1	6.4	7.1
10.	Instructions to Jury	4.1	4.8	8.8
11.	Charitable Immunity	3.2	3.7	3.9
12.	Warranty/Contract Breach	2.7	1.6	.7
13.	All Other	11.6	19.2	13.2
	Average Number of Doctrines Significant to Outcome of Case	1.13	1.12	1.17

The association operates when the superintendent of insurance determines that no private coverage is available. Although the association terminates automatically after six years, at that time a state insurance fund becomes operative, which all physicians must join. The law also permits participation in a federal reinsurance program and allows the New York State Medical Society to set up its own insurance company.[103] In addition to providing for a JUA and self-insurance plan like the one adopted in New York, other states have established insurance plans which would cover judgments in excess of the primary liability coverage. Such plans are usually financed through added premiums collected from health care providers.[104]

Using a second approach, a number of states attack the longer-range problem of protecting the public from incompetent physicians. In Michigan, for example, more licensing requirements have been adopted, and a doctor who wishes to renew his license must attend continuing education courses totaling at least 50 hours in the year preceding the application for renewal.[105] Recent Michigan statutes also require that state medical societies and hospitals report to the licensing board any disciplinary action taken against physicians. Hospitals, for example, must report the removal, resignation, or suspension of any person from the medical staff.[106] Another Michigan statute provides that malpractice insurance carriers report certain data within thirty days after filing an answer on behalf of an insured party in a malpractice action.[107] Finally, recent Michigan statutes provide immunity from liability for those making the required reports. The immunity applies, for instance, to persons or organizations having knowledge about the quality of health care rendered a person when they report this information to a review body, such as a peer review committee or a professional standards review committee, or if they

---

[103] N.Y. Ins. Law, Sections 681–695 (McKinney Supp. 1975). See: Trout, "New York State Malpractice Legislation," 3 *J. Leg. Med.* 26 (1975) for an outline of New York malpractice legislation.

[104] Miike, "State Legislatures Address the Medical Malpractice Situation," 3 *J. Leg. Med.* 25 (1975). The Supreme Court of North Carolina has determined that the North Carolina statute creating a Health Care Liability Insurance Exchange is unconstitutional because it forces all liability insurers to participate, in violation of the due process clause. "By reason of this constitutional provision, the simple statement, 'I don't want to,' is still a sufficient answer to some governmental demands of this State." *Hartford Accident and Indemnity Co. v. Ingram,* 226 S.E. 2d 498 (1976).

[105] Mich. Stat. Ann., sec. 14.542(10) (Supp. 1976). See: Siedel, "Malpractice Reform in Michigan," 1976 *Det. C.L.R.* 235 for a review of the events leading to malpractice reform in Michigan and a summary of that state's comprehensive malpractice legislation.

[106] Mich. Stat. Ann., sec. 14.542(11a) (Supp. 1976).

[107] Mich. Stat. Ann., sec. 24.12477 (Supp. 1976).

assist the Medical Practices Board in any of its duties.[108] In addition
to adopting statutes similar to the Michigan legislation, other states
have given licensing agencies the power to act against incompetent
physicians and have added new grounds for the exercise of disciplinary
powers.[109]

The third approach, more directly related to this chapter, is to
reform or replace the method of deciding which patients among
those who have not been cured are entitled to compensation. Reforms
which have been adopted or proposed can be grouped into four
categories: (1) Prelitigation reforms, including the use of screening
panels, the requirement of a notice of intent to sue, and the imposition
of penalties for persons who sell medical information; (2) procedural
and substantive changes in the litigation process, including mediation,
giving priority to malpractice cases, limiting the use of ad damnum
clauses, limiting the statute of limitations, and changing the standard
of care; (3) modifying damage awards by limiting the amount of
awards; and (4) changes in the contingency fee system.

PRELITIGATION REFORMS

Among the most important of the reforms modifying prelitigation
procedures is the use of screening panels. Screening panels are
ordinarily composed of members selected from local medical societies
and bar associations. Use of a panel is voluntary, and if the patient
agrees to appear before it he must furnish all of his medical records
to the panel. After examining the record and holding an informal
hearing, the panel decides either that the patient was injured as
the result of the physician's negligence or that no negligence or
injury occurred. If the panel decides that injury resulted from
negligence, an expert witness will be made available to the patient
for trial. If no negligence or injury is found, then under some plans
the attorney for the patient agrees that he will refrain from bringing
suit unless overriding reasons require such action. No matter which
decision is reached, the patient and physician are not bound by
the results, although past indications are that patients do not bring
suit after a panel finding for the physician, and that physicians are
more inclined to settle after a finding for a patient.[110] Generally
these panels find for a claimant as frequently as courts do.[111]

There are many variations in the procedures outlined above. Under

---

[108]Mich. Stat. Ann., sec. 14.542(5) (Supp. 1976).
[109]Miike, *supra* n. 104, at 26.
[110]Holder, "Joint Screening Panels," 212 *J.A.M.A.* 1715 (1971).
[111]HEW, *supra* n. 4, App. at 215.

some plans the panel is composed of physicians, and the purpose of the review is to advise a physician whether to defend or settle the claim. A New Jersey plan differs from most in that the patient may agree in writing to a binding option, whereby he waives his right to sue if the panel decides against him. If he agrees to the option and the panel decides in his favor, he will be given the names of three expert witnesses. No arrangements for expert witnesses will be made for a patient who has not agreed to the option, if the panel decides in his favor; and if the panel decides against him and he brings suit he may not use the same attorney.[112]

Still another, more recent, variation is to require the use of screening panels in all malpractice disputes. In Indiana, claims are investigated by a review panel composed of three doctors and a nonvoting attorney. The panel, after reviewing written evidence, renders one of the following opinions:

> (a) The evidence supports the conclusion that defendant or defendants failed to comply with the appropriate standard of care as charged in the complaint.
> (b) The evidence does not support the conclusion that the defendant or defendants failed to meet the applicable standard of care as charged in the complaint.
> (c) That there is a material issue of fact, not requiring expert opinion, bearing on liability for consideration by the court or jury.
> (d) The conduct complained of was or was not a factor of the resultant damages. If so, whether the plaintiff suffered: (1) any disability and the extent and duration of the disability, and (2) any permanent impairment and the percentage of the impairment.[113]

According to this legislation a court action cannot be initiated until the panel issues an opinion; and the panel's findings, while not binding, are admissible as evidence in court.

A common complaint from physicians is that the first notice they receive of a patient's dissatisfaction is often the filing of the malpractice action. The lack of notice is justified in many instances, however, because the statute of limitations requires the patient's attorneys to commence the action within a relatively short time. As an alternative it has been suggested that patients be required to give physicians a written notice of intent to file the malpractice suit. The notice

---

[112]Holder, *supra* n. 110, at 1716.
[113]Ind. Stat. Ann., sec. 16-9.5-9-1 to 16-9.5-9-10 (Burns Supp. 1975).

would extend the statute of limitations for a specified period to give the parties a chance to negotiate before the physician suffers the unwanted publicity of a malpractice suit.[114]

A final change suggested in the prelitigation process is to impose criminal penalties on persons who sell medical information to attorneys. There is a feeling among physicians that lawyers began turning to malpractice cases after the advent of no-fault auto insurance. In the words of one Michigan urologist: "Lawyers have stopped chasing ambulances and are chasing surgeons."[115] In Michigan, legislation directed toward these "surgeon-chasers" provides for a maximum penalty of $500 or six months in prison, or both of these, for any person who sells or offers to sell, or who buys or offers to buy, information concerning the identity or treatment of a patient, including records of a hospital, physician, or insurance company.[116]

PROCEDURAL AND SUBSTANTIVE CHANGES

The second group of reforms is directed toward procedural and substantive aspects of litigation. Two reforms are aimed directly at eliminating the backlog of court cases which can cause long delays between commencement of the suit and trial and can increase not only defense costs but, in inflationary times, the amount of a judgment. One proposal would require courts to give first priority to malpractice claims. The New York legislature, for instance, has requested the courts to establish rules to speed up trials of malpractice actions.[117] Another reform, similar to the prelitigation screening panels discussed above, calls for the use of mediation panels. In New York, pending malpractice suits are submitted to a panel of mediators composed of a judge, an attorney, and a physician. The panel reviews the record and assists the parties in reaching a settlement. Records show that settlement has been achieved under this system in 29 per cent of the cases.[118] If the case reaches trial, recent legislation provides that the panel's decision, if unanimous, may be submitted to a jury.[119] Florida requires all malpractice claims to be submitted to a mediation panel and also provides that the panel's conclusions will be admissible evidence in subsequent trials.[120]

---

[114] HEW, *supra* n. 3, at 37.
[115] Bloom, "Malpractice—The Mess That Must Be Ended," *Reader's Digest*, April, 1975, at 79.
[116] Mich. Stat. Ann., sec. 28.642 (Supp. 1976).
[117] N.Y. Judiciary Law, sec. 213(9) (McKinney Supp. 1975).
[118] Bergen, "Mediation of Liability Claims," 222 *J.A.M.A.* 241 (1972).
[119] N.Y. Judiciary Law, sec. 148 (8) (McKinney Supp. 1975).
[120] Fla. Stat. Ann, sec. 768.133 (Supp. 1975). At this writing, courts in New York and Florida have upheld the constitutionality of review panels: *Halpern v. Gozan*,

Another proposal would eliminate the practice of naming specific dollar amounts in the pleading in what is known as the ad damnum clause. Although these amounts are much higher than the actual recovery which the plaintiff could reasonably expect, the exaggerated claim is the one most often publicized. A survey in California showed that demands were fifty-three times higher than actual awards in malpractice cases.[121] Under legislation recently enacted in Florida, dollar amounts specified in complaints are limited to actual losses (medical expenses, lost wages, and the like) and do not cover pain, suffering, and expected loss of earnings, although these damages can be proved at trial.[122] A few states, including Indiana, have gone further and prohibited the use of ad damnum clauses altogether.[123] Wisconsin allows claimants only to state whether the claim is more or less than $10,000.[124]

As might be expected, reforms in the present interpretation of the statute of limitations have been suggested. Two general types of reform have been enacted into legislation to date. Several states have set an absolute cutoff date for bringing suit. In Indiana suit must be brought within two years, starting from the date of the alleged negligence rather than from the date of discovery.[125] Such statutes may extend the period for minors or, as in Ohio, in cases where foreign objects have been left in the patient.[126] Other states have not set an absolute cutoff date but have shortened the time during which suit must be brought. In Michigan suit may be brought within two years from the last date of treatment or six months after the patient should have discovered the alleged malpractice, whichever occurs last.[127]

A number of proposals relate to the standard of care to which the physician is held and to proof of that standard. "Good Samaritan"

---

381 N.Y.S. 2d 744 (1976), *Carter v. Sparkman*, 335 So. 2d 802 (1976). The Illinois Supreme Court has held that the Illinois review panel legislation is unconstitutional, however, on the grounds that it empowers nonjudicial panel members to exercise judicial functions in violation of the state constitution. *Wright v. DuPage*, 347 N.E. 2d 736 (1976). And a New York trial court has ruled that admitting a panel's conclusions into evidence is unconstitutional. *Comiskey v. Arlen*, 45 L.W. 2019 (1976).
[121] Bernstein, "Law in Brief," 49 *J.A.H.A.* 150 (1975). In a survey of 58 physicians in Connecticut who had been sued for malpractice, 25 physicians reported that their cases were publicized initially by newspaper or radio. In 20 cases there was newspaper publicity regarding the ultimate disposition of the case, although this publicity was slight compared with the original. Wyckoff, "The Effects of a Malpractice Suit upon Physicians in Connecticut," 176 *J.A.M.A.* 1096 (1961).
[122] Fla. Stat. Ann., sec. 768.042 (Supp. 1975).
[123] Ind. Stat. Ann., sec. 16-9.5-1-6 (Burns Supp. 1975).
[124] Wis. Stat. Ann., sec. 655.009 (1).
[125] Ind. Stat. Ann., sec. 16-9.5-3-1 (Burns Supp. 1976).
[126] Ohio Rev. Code Ann., sec. 2305.11.
[127] Mich. Stat. Ann., sec. 27A.5838 (Supp. 1976).

laws, for example, have been broadened to provide physicians with greater immunity from negligence actions. A Michigan statute provides that "in instances where the actual hospital duty of that person did not require a response to that emergency situation, a physician . . . who in good faith responds to a life-threatening emergency . . . within a hospital or other licensed medical care facility, shall not be liable for any civil damages as a result of an act or omission in the rendering of emergency care, except an act or omission amounting to gross negligence or willful or wanton misconduct."[128]

Other states have enacted legislation relating to informed consent. As noted in a later chapter, there is a trend in informed consent cases to reject the idea that a doctor's duty to disclose the risks and hazards of treatment is based upon prevailing customs among practitioners in similar situations. Recent legislation reverses this trend. In Florida, for example, no recovery will be allowed in an action based upon lack of consent where:

> (a) The action of the physician, osteopath, chiropractor, podiatrist, or dentist in obtaining the consent of the patient or another person authorized to give consent for the patient was in accordance with an accepted standard of medical practice among members of the medical profession with similar training and experience in the same or similar medical community; and
> (b) A reasonable individual from the information provided by the physician, osteopath, chiropractor, podiatrist, or dentist under the circumstances, would have a general understanding of the procedure and medically acceptable alternative procedures or treatments and substantial risks and hazards inherent in the proposed treatment or procedures which are recognized among other physicians, osteopaths, chiropractors, podiatrists, or dentists in the same or similar community who perform similar treatments or procedures; or
> (c) The patient would reasonably, under all the surrounding circumstances, have undergone such treatment or procedure had he been advised by the physician, osteopath, chiropractor, podiatrist, or dentist in accordance with the provisions of paragraphs (a) and (b) of this section.

A written consent meeting these requirements is conclusively presumed to be a valid consent unless fraudulent representation in

---

[128]Mich. Stat. Ann., sec. 14.563(12) (Supp. 1976). The prior Good Samaritan law remains in effect. This law provides that when physicians or registered nurses render emergency care in good faith at the scene of an emergency, they will not be held liable for negligent acts. This immunity does not apply in cases where there was a prior physician-patient relationship, or where the acts amounted to gross negligence or willful and wanton misconduct. *Id.*, sec. 14.563 (1976).

obtaining the signature can be proved.[129] In New York the plaintiff must prove his case through the use of medical testimony, and informed consent cases may not be brought after emergency therapy or after procedures that do not invade or disrupt the integrity of the body.[130]

The res ipsa loquitur rule has also been the target of legislative reform. States which have enacted statutes relating to this rule have either eliminated the rule or limited its use to certain circumstances.[131] In a few states the judicial trend to look beyond the same or similar locality in determining the standard of care to which the physician is held has been slowed by state legislatures. In Oregon a recent statute provides that physicians have the duty "to use that degree of care, skill and diligence which is used by ordinarily careful physicians in the same or similar circumstances in his or a similar community."[132]

DAMAGE AWARDS

The final group of reforms relates to the amount of damages awarded patients who have been injured by a negligent physician. Several approaches are illustrated in actions by state legislatures. A few states have limited the size of damage awards. An Idaho statute, for example, limits liability to $150,000 for a single injury and $300,000 for each occurrence.[133] Indiana not only limits damage awards to $500,000 but also provides that the liability of an individual health care provider may not exceed $100,000; any excess liability must be paid from a compensation fund financed by surcharges on malpractice insurance premiums.[134] The constitutionality of such limitations is doubtful. In the only appellate court decision to date, the Illinois Supreme Court decided that a $500,000 limitation on damages was unconstitutional because it amounted to a "special law" in violation of the Illinois constitution.[135] Another approach used by several states is to reduce damage awards by the amount the plaintiff received from collateral sources.[136] Others provide that collateral sources of payment are admissible at trial.[137]

---

[129] Fla. Stat. Ann., sec. 768.132 (Supp. 1975).
[130] N.Y. Pub. Health Law, sec. 2805-d(2) (McKinney Supp. 1975).
[131] Wash. Rev. Code Ann., sec. 4.24.290 (Supp. 1975); Nev. Rev. Stat., sec. 41 A.100 (1975).
[132] Ore. Laws 1975; ch. 796, sec. 10d.
[133] Idaho Code, sec. 39-4204-5 (Supp. 1975).
[134] Ind. Stat. Ann., sec. 16-9.5-2-2 (Burns Supp. 1975).
[135] Wright v. DuPage, 347 N.E. 2d 736 (1976).
[136] Iowa Code Ann., sec. 147.136 (Supp. 1976).
[137] N.Y. Civ. Prac. Law, sec. 4010 (McKinney Supp. 1975). An Ohio trial court has held the collateral source legislation unconstitutional as a denial of equal protection. Graley v. Satayatham, 343 N.E. 2d 832 (1976).

CONTINGENCY FEES

Much controversy has been generated over the use of contingency fees to pay attorneys. While there are inequities in the use of contingency fees, especially when an attorney receives half of a large damage award plus expenses, the HEW report concluded that such fees were not unconscionably large. This conclusion was based on a study which showed that plaintiffs' attorneys who used the contingency fee were paid what amounted to an average hourly fee of $63, while defense attorneys billing on an hourly basis charged an average hourly fee of $50.

Despite these findings several states have taken steps to limit the contingency fee. Under a Michigan court rule adopted in 1975 maximum fees for attorneys were set at: 40 percent of the first $5,000 received, 35 percent of the next $20,000, 25 percent of the next $225,000, 20 percent of the next $250,000, and 10 percent of any amount over $500,000.[138] Alternatively an attorney and client can agree to a maximum fee of one-third of a recovery amounting to no more than $250,000, 20 percent of the next $250,000, and 10 percent of any amount over $500,000. In either case the recovery is based on the net sum recovered, after deducting expenses; and all contingency fee agreements must be in writing. The attorney must also advise the client that he may hire an attorney under other fee arrangements, such as on an hourly basis.

Other states have used different approaches. Indiana limits attorneys' fees to 15 percent of awards from the state compensation fund.[139] Iowa, on the other hand, allows the court to determine whether the fees in a malpractice action are reasonable.[140]

There is some question whether such contingency fee limitations place an unconstitutional limit on the freedom of contract. A recent decision of the New Jersey Supreme Court, however, has upheld New Jersey's contingency fee schedule on the basis of the state's right to regulate the practice of law.[141] One issue raised by attorneys challenging contingency fee limitations is whether such limitations constitute a denial of equal protection. A physician and his insurance company, the argument runs, have the financial resources to hire the best counsel available; but patients need a contingency fee arrangement if they are to hire competent counsel. This issue was not discussed by the New Jersey court.

---

[138]Mich. Gen. Ct. R. 928.
[139]Ind., Stat. Ann., sec. 16-9.5-5-1 (Burns Supp. 1975).
[140]Iowa Code Ann., sec. 147.38 (Supp. 1976).
[141]*American Trial Lawyers Association, New Jersey Branch v. New Jersey Supreme Court*, 66 N.J. 258, 330 A. 2d 350 (1974).

Proposed Replacements for the Tort System

Two major proposals which have been seriously considered call for replacing the present tort system with alternative mechanisms for resolving disputes. One proposes arbitration, the other a no-fault program for malpractice claims.

ARBITRATION

Arbitration bypasses the court system, and disputes are resolved at a hearing before an impartial referee. Among the advantages cited for the use of arbitration are these: (1) Arbitration is speedier than the court system. (2) Once the dispute is aired, arbitration saves the time of all parties. (3) Matters under arbitration may be decided by an expert in the field. (4) The formalities and complex evidence rules of a court proceeding are relaxed with arbitration.[142] (5) Arbitration costs much less than a jury trial. (6) Arbitration proceedings are conducted with greater privacy than court proceedings.[143]

Two major types of arbitration are relevant to malpractice disputes. First, arbitration may be imposed on the parties to the dispute by statute or court rule. For several years courts in Allegheny County and Philadelphia County, Pennsylvania, have required arbitration for tort disputes under $10,000. After arbitration the losing party may appeal the decision and have a trial de novo, but he must pay certain costs before doing so. Less than 5 percent of the cases have been appealed.[144] Pennsylvania has also led the way in imposing arbitration upon the parties to a malpractice dispute. Under recently enacted legislation all claims for damages brought by patients must go to an arbitration panel composed of two health care providers, two attorneys, and three laymen. Appeals from the decision of the arbitration panel are by trial de novo, although the decision and findings of fact of the panel are admissible as evidence before the trial court.[145]

The second type of arbitration is voluntary, agreed to by the parties either when they initially enter into a contractual relationship or after the dispute becomes known. A typical example of a contractual provision is the uninsured motorist clause of an automobile insurance policy which provides that if the insured and the insurance company

---

[142] HEW, *supra* n. 3 at 94.
[143] Bergen, "Arbitration of Medical Liability," 211 *J.A.M.A.* 176 (1970).
[144] *Id.* at 176.
[145] Pub. A. 111. Similar legislation was determined to be constitutional in *Application of Smith*, 381 Pa. 223, 112 A. 2d 625 (1955), *appeal dismissed sub nom. Smith v. Wissler*, 350 U.S. 858 (1955).

cannot agree on the amount of a loss, the dispute shall be settled by arbitration in accordance with the rules of the American Arbitration Association. Although a few states do not recognize the enforceability of agreements entered into before a dispute arises, most states allow the use of such agreements.[146]

In medical malpractice cases, voluntary arbitration is not a recent development. Two plans in California illustrate the possibilities for resolving malpractice disputes by arbitration. One frequently cited plan is used by the Ross-Loos Medical Group in Los Angeles, a closed-panel medical plan primarily serving groups who purchase health insurance. The insuring agreement contains the following provision:[147]

> ARBITRATION: In the event of any controversy between a Member (whether a minor or an adult), or the heirs-at-law or personal representatives of a Member, as the case may be, and Ross-Loos (including its agents, employed physicians or employees), whether involving a claim in tort, contract, or otherwise, the same shall be submitted to binding arbitration. Within fifteen (15) days after any of the above named parties shall give written notice to the other of demand for arbitration of said controversy, the parties to the controversy shall each appoint an arbitrator and give notice of such appointment to the other. Within a reasonable time after such notices have been given the two arbitrators so selected shall select a neutral arbitrator and give notice of the selection thereof to the parties. The arbitrators shall hold a hearing within a reasonable time from the date of notice of selection of the neutral arbitrator. All notices or other papers required to be served shall be served by United States mail. Except as herein provided, the arbitration shall be conducted and governed by the provisions of the California Code of Civil Procedure.

Of the thirty-five files closed since 1964, when records were first available, three Ross-Loos cases reached arbitration and the remaining thirty-two were settled. Typical of the settlements was a case where a Ross-Loos physician failed to notice a straight pin in the patient's stomach wall when he reviewed the x-ray. The pin was later removed and the patient recovered. The claim was settled for $6,750.[148]

Among the three cases to reach arbitration, one resulted in an award of $70,000 to the claimant. The medical group won the other

---

[146] HEW, *supra* n. 4 at 94.
[147] *Id.*, App. at 445.
[148] *Id.*, App. at 434.

two, one of which involved a three-year-old patient being treated at a Ross-Loos office for recurrent vomiting. Thorazine suppositories were prescribed, and later the child developed a skin eruption on the abdomen which lasted three or four days. A month later the child was admitted to a hospital where physicians made diagnostic guesses of encephalitis or brain tumor. Although the patient later recovered, she was left with slurred speech and ataxia, and it was suspected that she might have suffered a toxic reaction to Thorazine. On the basis of these facts, the arbitrator decided in favor of Ross-Loos.[149]

One of the major legal problems with arbitration provisions is that a court might consider them to be unenforceable since they might constitute a contract of adhesion, that is, a contract entered into by a person who is in a weak bargaining position because he must have the services provided by the other party to the contract. An obvious example would be an arbitration clause forced on a patient urgently needing medical services. Despite the possibility of adhesion problems, the California Supreme Court has held that the Ross-Loos arbitration clause was valid in the leading case of *Doyle v. Guiliucci,* which contested the arbitrator's decision in favor of Ross-Loos in the case involving the three-year-old patient. The court decided that "the arbitration provision in such contracts is a reasonable restriction, for it does no more than specify a forum for the settlement of disputes."[150] However, a court may not order arbitration if a hospital or clinic has not manifested an intention to arbitrate the dispute. In one instance a clinic lost its chance to take a patient's claim to arbitration because it failed to demand arbitration immediately after suit was commenced, and because even after making the demand it continued actively to litigate the case.[151]

In another arbitration plan accepted by ten hospitals in southern California, great care has been taken to avoid adhesion problems. Although the arbitration provision is a part of the "Conditions of Admission" signed by the patient upon admission, the arbitration clause clearly gives a patient the choice of deleting the option or revoking it within thirty days after his discharge from the hospital:

> Arbitration Option: Any legal claim or civil action in connection with this hospitalization, by or against the hospital or its employees or any doctor of medicine agreeing in writing

[149] *Id.,* App. at 430.
[150] 62 Cal. 2d 606, 610, 43 Cal. Rptr. 697, 699, 401 P. 2d 1, 3 (1965).
[151] *Gunderson v. Superior Court,* 46 Cal. App. 3d 138, 120 Cal. Rptr. 35 (1975).

> to be bound by this provision, shall be settled by arbitration
> at the option of any party bound by this document . . .
> unless the admitting physician has not agreed in writing to
> be bound by this provision, or unless patient or undersigned
> initials below or sends written notification to the contrary
> to the hospital within thirty (30) days of the date of patient
> discharge.
>   If patient, or undersigned, does not agree to the "Arbitra-
> tion Option," then he will initial here. [152]

Furthermore a patient who refuses the option may not be denied
admission to the hospital because of such a refusal.

Even if no adhesion problems exist, however, a number of other
arguments have been raised by patients in an attempt to avoid
arbitration. In *Burton v. Mt. Helix General Hospital* the court considered
and rejected several objections of a patient who had signed an
arbitration agreement. First, the court decided that the patient's failure
to read or understand the agreement was no defense to enforceability
of the agreement. A person who has the capacity to read and
understand a contract which he signs is bound by its terms. Furthermore the terms of the arbitration agreement were "clear and unmistakable." Second, the court found no evidence that the hospital
defrauded the patient or exercised undue influence. Third, the court
noted that arbitration is beneficial in that it provides an alternative
to court litigation and thus saves both time and expense. Finally,
the court decided that the arbitration agreement in question was
not an adhesion contract; the court distinguished an earlier California
case where an agreement which relieved the hospital of all liability
and was offered as a condition of admission was held to violate
public policy.[153]

The southern California plan has proved attractive to state legisla-
tors. A Michigan statute, for instance, provides that a hospital and
substantially all of the independent hospital staff must offer arbitration
to patients. A physician treating patients in his office, however, is
not required to offer arbitration. The arbitration agreement may
not be offered as a prerequisite to treatment; and patients may revoke
the agreement within sixty days after execution (or if it was signed
on admittance to a hospital, within sixty days after the patient's
discharge). Arbitration in Michigan is conducted by three arbitrators:

---

[152] HEW, *supra* n. 3, at 95.
[153] Cal. Ct. App. 4th Dist., Div. 1 (Feb. 24, 1976). This case, originally certified for
publication, was later decertified and thus does not stand as precedent. *Burton* and
related cases are discussed in greater detail in Chapter VI.

an attorney, a physician, and a layman, although a hospital administrator may be substituted for the physician if the claim is solely
against a hospital.[154] The Michigan statute has not yet been tested
in court, but its constitutionality is doubtful. It might be argued,
for example, that requiring hospitals to offer arbitration agreements
to patients denies these institutions equal protection and a right
to a jury trial.

No-Fault

The other alternative to the present system, no-fault, has already
existed in the United States for a number of years in relation to
other injuries. One form of no-fault, workmen's compensation, was
originally enacted into law in the early 1900s. More recently many
states have adopted no-fault to replace to some extent the tort system
in automobile accident cases. In its most simple terms no-fault coverage
is purchased by the owner of an automobile. If a person riding
in the automobile is injured, the owner's insurance pays for the
loss regardless of who caused the accident.

No-fault concepts are fairly adaptable to automobile accidents,
where it is usually clear that an injury was the result of the accident.
The concepts are theoretically more difficult to apply to medical
injuries when the patient was to some degree ill or injured before
receiving treatment. The co-authors of the famous Keeton-O'Connell
no-fault automobile insurance proposal have separately analyzed this
problem. Robert E. Keeton notes that in medical injuries a major
problem with a true no-fault system is in proving that the physician
caused the harm. The HEW malpractice commission also recognized
this difficulty:

> But what is a "medical accident"? A medical injury compen-
> sation system which is not fault-oriented presumably would
> authorize compensation for an injury which may be termed
> a "medical accident," an "untoward result," "a therapeutic
> misadventure" or some similar concept. All these phrases
> in substance describe an unanticipated event or result and
> while they may be intelligible in the abstract, one is still faced
> in particular cases with the requirement to discover the causes
> of the compensable event.[155]

---

[154]Mich. Comp. Laws Ann., sec. 500.3053–.3061, 600.5041–.5044. See also: Desenberg,
"Medical Malpractice Arbitration: The New Michigan Statute," 54 *Mich. S.B.J.* 536
(1976).
[155]HEW, *supra* n. 3, at 101.

To Keeton, one alternative would be a private social security system with broader criteria for determining who is entitled to compensation.[156]

The other pioneer in no-fault proposals for automobile users, Jeffrey O'Connell, has suggested that health care providers be able to elect which risks are covered by a no-fault policy. Once the choice is made, the patient can recover for actual wage losses and expenses; but no recovery would be allowed for punitive damages or for pain and suffering. If a provider does not elect a certain coverage, the patient can sue in tort as in the past.[157] On the surface O'Connell's proposal does not solve the basic question posed by the malpractice commission. Furthermore it seems to give some patients more rights than others, according to the option of the health care provider.

Despite the theoretical problems of applying no-fault to medical injuries, specific proposals have been made regarding the implementation of a no-fault system. Senators Kennedy and Inouye offer a national insurance program of compensation for medical injuries, under which coverage would be purchased from the federal government. Patients would use either an administrative process or jury procedure to determine their compensation from a benefits schedule, and lawyers would be compensated in accordance with a set schedule. In order to qualify for the plan a physician's work would be reviewed by a professional standards review organization. Under an AMA proposal, on the other hand, administrative tribunals would be established which would use schedules similar to those used in workmen's compensation to determine awards.[158] Such systems still leave the problem of proving what constitutes a medical accident, as one can see in the system adopted by New Zealand in 1974, the most comprehensive accident compensation plan in the world. As an attorney working for the Accident Compensation Commission of New Zealand remarked in discussing medical malpractice, "Obvious cases like leaving something in the wound are covered, but the difficult area is misdiagnosis or failure to follow standard medical practice."[159]

---

[156] Keeton, "Compensation for Medical Accidents," 121 *U.Pa.L.Rev.* 590 (1973).
[157] O'Connell, *Ending Insult to Injury: No-Fault Insurance for Products and Services* (1975). For other no-fault proposals see Havighurst and Tancredi, "Medical Adversity Insurance—A No-Fault Approach to Medical Malpractice and Quality Assurance," *Insurance L. J.* 69 (Feb., 1974); Carlson, "Conceptualization of a No-Fault Compensation System for Medical Injuries," 7 *Law and Society Rev.* 329 (1973); Switzer and Reynolds, "Medical Malpractice Compensation—A Proposal," 13 *Am.Bus.L.J.* 65 (1975). See also: 21 *Loyola L.R.* 194, 211 (1975) for an analysis of recent proposals.
[158] Peterson, "Malpractice," *The National Observer*, Feb. 15, 1975, at 10.
[159] Hartley, "Helping the Hurt," *Wall Street Journal*, Sept. 16, 1975, at 1.

PART FOUR

The Hospital-Patient
Relationship

VI

Admission and Discharge

The relatively narrow yet important question to be considered initially in this chapter is whether or not a patient has a legal right to be formally admitted to a hospital. Admission policies for each institution must necessarily be developed according to a number of different factors because the legal aspects of admitting and discharge may depend upon the facts of the particular situation.

Formal Voluntary Admission

In the first place, it is convenient to distinguish between medical emergency patients and others. The right of patients to be treated or formally admitted and the corresponding duties of the hospital may depend upon whether or not their condition is identifiable as an emergency, and in turn whether the hospital in fact has the facilities and staff to render emergency care. The rights of the patient and duties of the hospital with respect to formal admission may also depend upon whether the patient has previously received any treatment or service from the institution. Care of emergency patients is discussed in the next chapter.

Secondly, ownership of the hospital may be relevant to the rights of the patient to be admitted. A governmental hospital may be subject to different standards of conduct from those legally imposed on a private hospital, since local statutory law may apply to particular governmental institutions in some states.

Finally, federal funding of the voluntary hospital sector through the Hill-Burton Act casts a duty on institutions benefited under this legislation to provide service for the indigent to an extent which will be noted.

161

It is a general common law maxim that a nonemergency patient
has no legal right to be admitted to any voluntary or proprietary
hospital or to most governmental hospitals.[1] Thus most institutions
can generally accept or refuse nonemergency cases with impunity
as long as admission policies are not racially discriminatory, and
as long as the relevant Hill-Burton Act regulations are followed.
Refusal to admit would therefore not ordinarily give the patient
a cause of action in damages, or entitle him to a court order changing
hospital policies.

An exception to the general assertion that a patient has no legal
right to be admitted to a voluntary or proprietary hospital could
be created by special contract. A hospital could enter into a contract
with a particular class or group of patients, or with another party
(such as an employer) for the benefit of a class or group of employees,
thereby undertaking a legal obligation to admit group members for
care and treatment whenever the need arose. Breach of the voluntarily
assumed contractual obligation would give the other party to the
contract, or the intended beneficiary of the contract, a right to sue
for damages.[2]

Legal risks arise, however, when a hospital asserts too vigorously
the general rule that a patient has no right to be admitted. These
will be more apparent in the cases, discussed in the next chapter,
where patients present themselves at the emergency room requesting
or demanding treatment. It has already been mentioned in several
contexts throughout this book that admission policies based on such
discriminatory criteria as race or inability to pay raise serious legal
issues.

The governing board and the administration of a hospital, rather
than being concerned with the presence or absence of a patient's
legal right to be formally admitted, should be more concerned with
the hospital's purpose and role in the community. Having defined
this purpose and role, with proper reference to statutes in the case
of governmental hospitals and relevant state licensure regulations,
the board's task is then to provide adequate facilities, equipment,
and staff to fulfill the purpose and carry out the role. If such policies
are adhered to, the narrow legal question of the patient's right to
be admitted does not generally arise.

Governmental hospitals are created by statutory enactments; stat-

---

[1] *Hill v. Ohio County*, 468 S.W. 2d 306 (Ky. 1971), *cert. denied*, 404 U.S. 1041 (1972):
(A pregnant patient had no right to be admitted to a hospital when no emergency
was apparent); *Fabian v. Matzko*, 236 Pa. Super. 267, 344 A. 2d 569 (1975).
[2] *Norwood Hospital v. Howton*, 32 Ala. App. 375, 26 So. 2d 427 (1946).

utes specify the purpose of the hospital. Many state statutes refer to and define the people intended to be served by the hospital, classified according to their particular diseases, their financial status, or their place of residence.[3] From such statutes a patient's legal right to be admitted to the hospital if he falls within the class may at least be inferred, although actual court cases on the matter are lacking. It would appear, however, that even if such a legal right exists it is not absolute; hence not every patient who is refused has a cause of action in damages. For instance, any legal right created by the statutes would still be subject to the ability of the hospital to care for the particular patient and the availability of bed space at the particular time of the patient's request for admission. Furthermore admissions would still be subject to the rules and regulations of the governing board, so long as these rules were within the statutorily delegated authority of the board. For example, the board might properly require proof of inability to pay when the hospital is statutorily set up to serve those who cannot pay for private care. On the other hand, even when a state statute indicates that the hospital's purpose is to care for those unable to pay, there is generally nothing to prevent a governmental hospital from admitting patients who are able to pay if facilities are available.

Residency requirements are found in many statutes pertaining to governmental hospitals. Sometimes the statutory definition is very broad and would include all persons who fall ill within a particularly defined geographical area, even though they do not reside within the area. Other statutes appear to require actual residence within a specified area, but there are no cases which construe the meaning of this concept. Even so, the governing board may promulgate the rules and regulations which permit the admission of nonresidents.

Like a private general hospital a governmental institution functioning as a general hospital may usually exclude persons suffering from illnesses which it is not equipped to treat adequately. For example, a general hospital may ordinarily deny formal admission to a mental patient, or to one afflicted with a contagious disease, when facilities and staff are not available to care for such individuals; and such a patient would have no cause of action in damages, particularly if his admission would endanger other patients.

---

[3]For example, a Colorado statute applicable to certain governmental hospitals provides in effect that the institution shall be primarily conducted for the legal residents of Colorado who are unable to pay for care. Colo. Rev. Stat., sec. 23–21–103 (1973). For other statutory references see, generally, "Admitting and Discharge," *Hospital Law Manual*, Aspen Systems Corp., Rockville, Md., 5–10.

Governmental hospitals, which are liable in tort law and not
protected by the still important doctrine of governmental immunity
(in some jurisdictions), owe the same duty of exercising reasonable
care with respect to patients who appear at the emergency room
seeking treatment, even though such persons are not among those
statutorily defined as the primary beneficiaries of the institution.
In other words, a refusal of service, or a failure to exercise reasonable
care once service is undertaken, cannot be justified on the basis
that the patient did not reside within the service area of the hospital
or was not indigent—thus being outside the classes of persons to
be served by the hospital.

Once a patient has been voluntarily admitted to the hospital, a
duty to exercise reasonable care for his treatment under all the
facts and circumstances is of course created, unless some relevant
doctrine of immunity for tort liability is present. Moreover admission
can occur and the duty to exercise reasonable care can arise without
formal admission procedures, as the case of *LeJeune Road Hospital,
Inc. v. Watson* illustrates.[4] In this case the hospital refused a bed
to a minor suffering from appendicitis, because his mother had not
paid the required cash advance deposit, although staff members
had already put a hospital gown on the patient and examined him.
Surgery on the youth was delayed until his parents could locate
an institution that would care for him. In a suit for damages, the
defendant hospital contended that formal admission had not occurred, and accordingly that no duty to exercise reasonable care
had been created. This argument was rejected. The court held that,
even though the hospital had no positive duty to admit, admission
had in fact occurred.

Once a decision is made to admit a nonemergency patient, certain
formalities should be accomplished. In general the patient or his
authorized representative should be asked to sign a form containing
a number of different items. Admissions personnel should not suggest
by act or language that this is a formal contract, since the patient
might then think that he could bring suit against the hospital alleging
breach of contract if he suffered injury while hospitalized. Rather
the form should simply provide evidence of an understanding between
the hospital and the patient with respect to certain matters.

For example, the admissions form should expressly identify the
person responsible for payment of the hospital bill and should contain
language legally sufficient to establish this express obligation or

---

[4] 171 So. 2d 202 (Florida Dist. Ct. App. 1965).

otherwise identify the expected source of reimbursement. The person responsible will usually be the patient himself, but a third person could be responsible. If the patient is a minor, for example, the party responsible for payment would normally be the father, or in his absence the mother. Although a legal obligation to pay for services rendered an unemancipated minor does not require the parent's signature, it is wise and practical to obtain it. In cases where a third party who is not legally responsible for supporting the patient undertakes to guarantee payment of the account, most states require that this party's promise to pay must be in writing to satisfy the statute of frauds. The legal aspects of hospital credit and collections are beyond the scope of this discussion, but the major point is that it is always better, even if not legally necessary, to obtain an express, written promise from the person who will be responsible for the hospital bill, or the balance of the bill in excess of insurance coverage, at the time of the patient's admission to the hospital.

Another matter to clarify at the same time is the patient's consent for routine medical treatment and diagnostic procedures.[5] Again, the patient or his authorized representative should be asked by an employee of the admitting office to sign a generalized consent statement. Although oral consent to treatment is legally effective if proved, a written consent, filed as a part of the patient's record, provides far better protection to the hospital in the event of later misunderstanding. It should be particularly emphasized, however, that this statement of consent is not sufficient to provide proof of informed consent for surgical procedures or many of the more sophisticated diagnostic tests. For surgery and for extraordinary diagnostic procedures, a special consent form is strongly advised, as will be emphasized in the chapter on consent for treatment. The signature on such a special consent form should be obtained by the physician undertaking the procedure—not by admissions personnel.

The admitting form should also give notice to the patients that the hospital has an organized system for the safekeeping of any valuables that they may bring with them. The patient should be invited to deposit these with the hospital and should be advised that the institution cannot normally assume responsibility for loss of money or personal property kept by a patient's bedside. The

---

[5] *Parr v. Palmyra Hospital*, 228 S.E. 2d 596 (Ga. App. 1976). (A Georgia statute requiring consent to medical and surgical treatment applies to hospitals as well as physicians. If the consent is in writing it is "conclusively presumed" to be valid in the absence of fraudulent misrepresentations of material facts.)

particular language employed in the admitting form must, of course, be consistent with local state law regarding hospital liability for loss or theft of patients' property.

At the time of admission it is also wise to obtain the patient's consent to release medical information to legitimately interested third parties such as insurance carriers or governmental agencies paying for services rendered to the patient. It is now a fact that hospitals often receive multiple requests for medical information regarding a particular patient. The hospital need not ask the patient for a separate release form for each request. A better understanding is achieved and administrative procedure simplified if consent for releasing information is obtained at the time of admission to cover the most frequent situations. Special requests for medical information—certainly those from parties whose interests are adverse to the patient's—should be handled separately as they are received.

Still other matters might be covered in the written admission form, depending upon the advice of local legal counsel. Counsel might advise, for instance, a statement that the hospital does not routinely provide special duty nursing and that patients requiring or wishing such care must arrange for the special duty nurses, perhaps from a roster maintained by the hospital of persons available for such service.

In a recent development in the Los Angeles area, selected hospitals are asking at the time of patients' admission that they agree to submit voluntarily to binding arbitration any claims for negligence or malpractice which may arise as a result of the hospitalization. This plan, if deemed effective to alleviate malpractice claims and if legally enforceable, may well be adopted by hospitals and physicians in other parts of the country and will have the effect of removing claims of liability from the normal process of court litigation.

The plan for voluntary binding arbitration of medical malpractice claims has been the subject of litigation, and to date cases are inconclusive. California and many states have statutes which recognize and legalize agreements to arbitrate if statutory criteria are met. Regardless of statutory approval of arbitration as a substitute for court litigation, however, a primary legal issue is whether the agreement was truly voluntary. By definition a contract of adhesion is thrust upon a person contrary to his free will or without his full understanding on a take-it-or-leave-it basis; accordingly it is unenforceable.

In *Burton v. Mt. Helix General Hospital* the California Court of Appeals upheld an agreement to arbitrate, finding that the language was clear enough for lay persons to understand and that the hospital had committed no fraud in obtaining the patient's signature.[6] After certifying the opinion for publication, however, the court decertified it, thus nullifying the case as precedent. Later, in another court of appeals case in the same district, the court refused to uphold an alleged agreement to arbitrate. At the time of admission to the hospital the patient failed to indicate in the manner provided for by the "Conditions of Admissions" form that he refused to agree to the arbitration option. He also failed to revoke the presumed agreement to arbitrate within thirty days of discharge from the hospital, as was his right under the terms of the agreement. Hence the hospital claimed that his signature on the admissions form constituted a voluntary agreement to arbitrate. The court found, however, that the arbitration option had not been brought to his attention by hospital personnel. He had therefore assumed that the form contained only matters relating to hospital procedures and an agreement to pay for services, being unaware of the arbitration provision.[7]

In contrast, a provision for arbitration contained in a group health plan for state employees was found legally enforceable.[8] The contract for the group health insurance had been entered into between the board of administration of the California State Employees Retirement System and Kaiser Foundation Hospitals. It was not a contract of adhesion, since the board of administration, as the patient's agent, was in a position of relatively equal bargaining power with Kaiser. It has also been held that a parent can bind a minor to arbitrate a malpractice claim, when such is a condition to voluntary membership in a group practice health plan.[9] There will surely be further litigation in California and elsewhere with respect to agreements between hospitals, physicians, and patients to arbitrate malpractice disputes.

Legislation Guaranteeing Equal Protection

In developing admission policies and practices, hospital administration must take cognizance of legislation by Congress, administrative regulations of federal agencies, state statutes and regulations, and local governmental ordinances which are designed to prohibit discrimination on the basis of race, color, creed, national origin, or other

[6]Cal. Ct. App. 4th Dist., Div. 1 (Feb. 24, 1976).
[7]*Wheeler v. St. Joseph Hospital,* 63 Cal. Ct. App. 3d 345, 133 Cal. Rptr. 775 (1976).
[8]*Madden v. Kaiser Foundation Hospitals,* 17 Cal. 3d 699, 131 Cal. Rptr. 882, 552 P. 2d 1178 (1976).
[9]*Doyle v. Guiliucci,* 62 Cal. 2d 606, 43 Cal. Rptr. 697, 401 P. 2d 1 (1965).

arbitrary criteria. Aside from these various legislative enactments, straightforward court decisions interpreting the Fourteenth Amendment prohibit discriminatory policies in admitting patients, furnishing services and facilities, and appointing hospital medical staff. All of this statutory and judicial law developed rapidly during the 1960s and unequivocally committed the United States to the concept that all persons are entitled to equal protection of law. This extremely significant body of law does not grant an affirmative right to the patient to be admitted to a hospital, but simply proscribes discriminatory practices and policies.

Before noting the primary sources of federal and state law prohibiting discriminatory policies, it is of historical interest that some states formerly had statutes that actually required certain hospitals to segregate patients on the basis of race or color. Some of these enactments were applicable only to governmental institutions; others applied to both governmental and voluntary hospitals. In either case, such state laws were clearly and patently unconstitutional and hence of no force and effect, on the basis of the *Brown* case and others. In *Brown* the Supreme Court of the United States held in 1954 that public school segregation on the basis of equal but separate facilities was a denial of the equal protection clause of the Fourteenth Amendment.[10] The scope and breadth of this amendment are more thoroughly explained in a later chapter.

The major antidiscriminatory legislation is the federal Civil Rights Act of 1964. One section of this act (Title II) prohibits racial but not sexual discrimination in designated places of "public accommodation"; another applies to publicly owned facilities including governmental hospitals; a third (Title VII) relates to racial and sexual discrimination in employment opportunities and embraces private hospitals as well as public; most significantly, Title VI of the act prohibits discrimination on the basis of race, color, or national origin by an institution receiving federal financial assistance.[11]

In turn, every federal agency or department administering a financial program is authorized by Congress to promulgate administrative rules and regulations to effectuate the purpose of the primary legislation.[12] This has been done by the Department of Health, Education, and Welfare specifically with reference to hospitals.[13] A

---

[10] *Brown v. Board of Education of Topeka*, 347 U.S. 483, 98 L. Ed. 873, 74 S. Ct. 686, 38 A.L.R. 2d 1180 (1954).
[11] 42 U.S.C. sec. 2000 a–e (1964).
[12] 42 U.S.C. sec. 2000 d–1 (1964).
[13] 45 C.F.R. 80 (1973).

major illustration of the impact of the 1964 act is provided by the Medicare program effective July 1, 1966. To be eligible for participation a hospital must comply with Title VI of the Civil Rights Act. Accordingly a hospital receiving Medicare funds must not discriminate on racial or ethnic grounds in its admission policies, room assignments (although the patient's medical condition, age, and similar factors can be considered in assigning rooms), and the availability of hospital facilities and services.

The constitutional basis of the Federal Civil Rights Act is the power of Congress to regulate interstate commerce. Presumably matters of intrastate commerce are beyond the power of congressional action. However, as a result of numerous Supreme Court decisions dating back to the 1930s, nearly all economic relationships can be legally classified as interstate commerce; and in any event the constitutionality of the sections of the act relating to public accommodations and federal financing as defined in the legislation and applicable to private enterprise have been specifically upheld.

Another very important federal statute pertaining to antidiscriminatory practices is the Hospital Survey and Construction Act, known more simply as the Hill-Burton Act.[14] When first enacted in 1944, the legislation was interpreted as permitting hospitals to provide separate but equal facilities for persons of different races in accordance with the then existing constitutional law relative to public school facilities. As is now well known, this doctrine was struck down as unconstitutional in the *Brown* case; and hence the administrative regulations promulgated to carry out the purposes of the Hill-Burton Act were changed to make it perfectly clear that if hospitals received planning and construction funds they should not discriminate on the basis of race, color, or creed in the use of their facilities.

In addition to federal legislative and administrative regulation articulating forceful policies against racial and sexual discrimination, there are state statutes and local city ordinances to the same effect. Hence hospital administration must consult state and local, as well as federal, law in developing policies relating to the admission and discharge of patients. Considerably more than half the states and many major cities have enacted statutory law forbidding discrimination on racial or ethnic grounds by business and institutions serving the public. The applicability of such laws to a particular hospital and the criteria for defining prohibited forms of discrimination are determined, of course, by the precise wording or interpretation of

[14] 42 U.S.C. sec. 291–291n (1944).

the particular statute in question. Generally, however, these laws are made applicable to all types of hospitals.

Some of these local civil rights statutes or ordinances may specifically mention hospitals. Most, however, speak simply in terms of public accommodations, which in turn may be broadly defined as a place which offers goods, services, or facilities to the general public.[15] Such a concept embraces hospitals, even proprietary institutions, unless a specific exemption is provided. Extended care facilities and nursing homes may be subject to these state laws as well as federal law, although local law must be carefully interpreted.[16]

Antidiscrimination provisions may also be found in state hospital licensure laws, as contrasted to civil rights statutes.[17] The Michigan statute on licensure reads that "all phases of the hospital's operation shall be without discrimination against individuals or groups of individuals on the basis of race, creed, color, or national origin." Statutes or regulations pertaining to tax-exempt status, such as those in Oklahoma, may also proscribe discriminatory practices.[18]

In developing admission policies, hospital administrators must consult local law prohibiting forms of discrimination other than racial. Such statutes are not yet frequent or commonplace; but Montana, for instance, has a statute to the effect that a voluntary hospital may not discriminate between patients of licensed staff physicians and those of licensed doctors not on the staff.[19]

Quite aside from federal and state statutory law designed to guarantee against discriminatory practices, the Fourteenth Amendment assures equal protection of the laws and due process of law. Specifically, the relevant language reads: "Nor shall any State deprive any person of life, liberty, or property without due process of law, nor deny to any person within its jurisdiction the equal protection of the laws." The amendment therefore applies to state or governmental action but not to purely private action. In other words, it is "state action" denying equal protection or due process that is unconstitutional—not "private action." Hence, racial and other types of discrimination by private individuals or private business are not, in theory, prohibited by the Fourteenth Amendment, although local

---

[15] For example: New Mexico Stat. Ann, sec. 4–33–7F (1953).
[16] For example: Michigan's Civil Rights Law, Mich. State Ann., sec. 28.343–.344 (1962) applies to places of "public accommodation." The Attorney General has ruled that this does not include private nursing homes. (1957–58) Mich. Att'y Gen. Biennial Rep. vol. I, at 349.
[17] Michigan Stat. Ann, sec. 14.1179 (11) (1969).
[18] Okla. Stat. Ann., sec. 68–2405 (j) (1966).
[19] Mont. Rev. Codes Ann., sec. 69–5217, 69–5221 (1947).

statutes or ordinances may properly regulate private conduct to attain justifiable social policies. State constitutions may also contain equal protection and due process clauses similar to those of the federal constitution.

As a matter of federal constitutional law the issue becomes one of defining state action, and through a series of court decisions the concept has been greatly expanded in recent years. Clearly ownership by government is not necessary to bring the Fourteenth Amendment into play. Under various facts and circumstances a private voluntary hospital may be so closely allied or associated with government that it becomes subject to the mandates of the Fourteenth Amendment with respect to a number of different issues: admission policies, the availability of facilities and services to all patients on a nondiscriminatory basis, and medical staff appointments and privileges—to name only three major areas of concern. Neither acceptance of governmental financial aid nor tax-exempt status converts per se a voluntary hospital into a public hospital, and many cases have so held. Nevertheless such support and reliance on government may make the Fourteenth Amendment applicable in several contexts.

Illustrating this point is a leading case decided in 1963, *Simkins v. Moses H. Cone Memorial Hospital.*[20] This litigation concerned two private nonprofit hospitals which were participating in the Hill-Burton program, thus cooperating in the planning function with state and federal governments and also receiving public funds. Accordingly the action of the hospitals was deemed to be state action, and the court held that the Fourteenth Amendment prohibited racial discrimination with respect to both admission of patients and appointments of medical staff.[21] The contact with government can be even less direct than in *Simkins*. In *Eaton v. Grubbs* the voluntary hospital was located on land which, by terms of the deed, was to revert to government if the corporation dissolved. Furthermore the hospital had received financial aid from the local municipal government. These factors were sufficient to make the Fourteenth Amendment applicable to hospital admission policies.[22]

---

[20] 323 F. 2d 959 (4th Cir. 1963), *cert. denied,* 376 U.S. 938 (1964).

[21] Similarly, in *Flagler Hospital, Inc. v. Hayling,* 344 F. 2d 950 (5th Cir. 1965), the court enjoined the hospital, which had received a Hill-Burton grant, from denying patient admissions on the basis of race, and it retained jurisdiction for such further orders as might be shown necessary by actual experience or sound medical reasons with respect to separate rooms and other facilities.

[22] 329 F. 2d 710 (4th Cir. 1974), the *Simkins* and *Eaton* cases do not of course create a constitutional right in the patient to be admitted. They simply prohibit discriminatory conduct. See: *Stanturf v. Sipes,* 355 F. 2d 224 (8th Cir, 1964), *cert. denied,* 379 U.S. 977 (1965).

Thus there are several sources of law that require nondiscriminatory policies with respect to admission of patients and availability of facilities and services: local city ordinances, state statutes, federal legislation, state and federal administrative regulation pursuant to delegated legislative authority, and finally and simply, judicial interpretation of constitutional law.

The last-named source is sometimes the least visible and the least publicized, but it is probably the most significant and important. A point deserving major emphasis is that specific legislation is frequently not needed to accomplish change in the conduct of individuals or institutions. Hospital managements are well advised to keep their eyes on the trend of court decisions. Today this trend is clearly toward viewing a voluntary hospital as performing a public and hence a quasi-governmental function—and hence subject to many of the same rules governing institutions actually owned by government, at least with respect to relations between patients and the hospital and between physicians and the hospital.

Hill-Burton Act and Mandated Free Care

The Hospital Survey and Construction Act, commonly known as the Hill-Burton Act, provided that applicants for financial grants under the act must assure that a "reasonable volume" of services be available to persons unable to pay, although the act allowed exceptions for institutions financially unable to provide such services to the indigent.[23]

Nevertheless for many years hospitals were allowed to neglect the apparent intent of this statutory requirement; at least it was not effectively implemented. Early in the 1970s, however, it became the basis for several class action lawsuits contending that institutions which required cash deposits or evidence of adequate hospitalization insurance before admission of patients and those which automatically billed patients without regard for ability to pay were in violation of the Hill-Burton Act. The initial legal issue presented for court decision in these suits was whether or not the plaintiffs had standing to sue to enforce the provisions of the act and regulations, in other words, whether a private cause of action existed to require hospitals receiving Hill-Burton funds to provide a given volume of free care or care below cost. This issue was answered in the affirmative by the leading and most authoritative case on the matter, which held

---

[23] 42 U.S.C. sec. 291 (c) (e) (1944).

that a private cause of action did exist.[24]

Following these court decisions the Department of Health, Education, and Welfare promulgated new regulations. An institution which receives Hill-Burton financing can presumptively meet the requirements of free care or care below cost by budgeting for such care 3 percent of its operating costs less Medicare and Medicaid reimbursement for a fiscal year, or by budgeting 10 percent of the federal Hill-Burton assistance for such care, whichever is less. If they choose, however, they can simply certify that they do not refuse admission solely on the ground of inability to pay. The latter option for compliance is sometimes referred to as the open-door policy. The writing off of uncollectible debts will not qualify as a way of meeting these requirements. Under the original regulations a hospital was permitted to determine a patient's eligibility for free care after his discharge from the hospital, rather than at the time of admission, as long as it did not give a routine invoicing of an account to a collection agency or an attorney prior to determination of eligibility.[25]

These regulations permitting routine invoicing and deferring the determination of eligibility for free care until the patient had been discharged were held to be invalid by a federal district court.[26] Amended regulations were then issued and made applicable to hospitals and other institutions that had received Hill-Burton grants within the previous twenty years, or those that had outstanding loans assisted by Hill-Burton funds. The new rules require a written determination of a patient's eligibility for charity before services are rendered, except in an emergency. Further, an eligibility can be determined after the services whenever there are "changed circumstances"; for example, the patient's financial condition may have changed because his illness resulted in a loss of wages, or insurance coverage might be less than expected, or the cost of care greater. Such a determination must precede any collection effort other than a routine billing to the patient. Eligibility may also be determined at any time if the original efforts were hindered or delayed because the information furnished by the patient was erroneous or incomplete.

The amended regulations require hospitals and other facilities

---

[24] Cook, et al. v. Ochsner Foundation Hospital, et al., 319 F. Supp. 603, 11 A.L.R. 3d 677 (E.D. La. 1970). Cook relied on the earlier case of Gomez v. Florida Employment Services, 417 F. 2d 569 (5th Cir. 1969), which had held that migrant workers had standing to enforce certain provisions of the Wagner-Peyser Act. To the same effect as Cook was Organized Migrants in Community Action, Inc. v. James Archer Smith Hospital, 325 F. Supp. 268 (S.C. Florida 1971).
[25] 42 C.F.R. sec. 53.111 (d) and (f) (1974).
[26] Corum v. Beth Israel Medical Center, 373 F. Supp. 557 (S.D.N.Y. 1974).

receiving Hill-Burton funds to post a notice in appropriate areas—the admissions office, emergency department, and business office—informing patients that a reasonable amount of charity care is available and advising that criteria for eligibility will be furnished upon request. If the hospital's presumptive obligation has been satisfied (as noted above and as distinguished from compliance with the open-door option) for the current period, the notice must state this fact and also say when additional uncompensated services will again be available. An invoice rendered for emergency care must contain substantially the same information as the posted notice.[27]

The criteria for determining the eligibility of persons unable to pay for services are established by the Hill-Burton agency in each state, with the approval of the Secretary of Health, Education, and Welfare. Factors to be considered are: insurance coverage, family income, size of family, state standards for Aid to Families with Dependent Children, and federal poverty income guidelines. The state agency will also determine the reasonable level of uncompensated services for each health care institution, not to exceed the presumptive compliance guidelines noted previously, after considering the institution's adopted budget, annual statement, the nature and quantity of its health services, the need within the geographical area, and the ability of other nearby health care organizations to provide uncompensated services.

The amount of uncompensated service is determined by the "reasonable cost" of the services, if no charge is made to the patient, or the excess of cost over charges. Reasonable cost is to be determined by the same principles applicable to Medicare reimbursement. Excluded from the computation of uncompensated services are services for which the institution has received, or is entitled to receive, reimbursement from a third-party insurer or from a governmental program such as Medicare or Medicaid.

Each institution must elect the presumptive guideline that it wishes to be applicable. If no choice is made, the first presumptive compliance guideline—the lesser of 3 percent of operating costs or 10 percent of the Hill-Burton assistance—will apply. Even if this presumptive compliance guideline is made applicable, however, a given institution may budget a lower level of uncompensated services and then request approval from the state agency for the deviation.

Under the regulations the period of obligation to furnish uncompensated services is twenty years after completion of the construc-

[27] 42 C.F.R. sec. 53.111 (f) and (i) (1975).

tion for which the grant was furnished. If the Hill-Burton assistance was subsidy for a loan and interest, rather than a grant, the period of obligation is the term of the loan. The state Hill-Burton plan provides for methods of enforcing the regulations. Sanctions such as termination of state assistance, revocation of the hospital's license, and court action are available.

A point to be especially noted is that the regulations do not expressly state how a hospital which elects to meet its obligations by budgeting 3 percent of operating costs for charity care shall actually allocate these funds. An issue in recent litigation has been whether a hospital must provide such care on a strictly first-come-first-served basis, or whether it may group patients as emergency, urgent, or elective, and then allocate Hill-Burton obligations according to these priorities. In the latter case it could ensure that means were on hand for treating those charity patients in greatest need of medical care, whereas available funds might be exhausted relatively early in a fiscal year under a first-come–first-served policy.

Forsyth County Hospital Authority in North Carolina adopted the priority method of allocation. When the practice was challenged, the federal district court first ruled that primary jurisdiction with respect to implementation of the free care obligations resides in the state and federal agencies administering the program. Following plaintiff's acquisition of approval of the hospital's priority system of allocation and continuing challenge, the court ruled that the policy did not violate the Hill-Burton Act or regulations, since the law does not mandate any particular method of allocation of funds.[28] The decision was affirmed by the Fourth Circuit Court of Appeals.[29] Thus each hospital may determine its method of compliance, although the adopted policy will be subject to review by administrative agencies and thereafter by the courts.

Admission of Unwilling or Incompetent Patients

The legal rights of an incompetent patient to be admitted to a hospital or other institution for care are most commonly determined by state statutory law concerning the care and treatment of the mentally ill as interpreted by judicial decision. Hospital managements therefore need competent advice concerning local law regarding the admission, voluntary or involuntary, of mentally ill patients. Constitutional law as developed by recent cases has also articulated certain

---

[28] *Gordon v. Forsyth County Hospital Authority*, 409 F. Supp. 708 (M.D.N.C. 1976).
[29] *Gordon v. Forsyth County Hospital Authority*, 544 F. 2d 748 (4th Cir. 1976).

defined rights to treatment following admission. A detailed survey of the substantive and procedural rights of incompetent patients would be beyond the scope of this work.

It is possible, however, to consider briefly the question sometimes encountered by general hospitals: should an unwilling, incompetent patient be formally admitted, for example at the urgent request of relatives? The family of such a patient has no absolute right to have him admitted to a general hospital, especially if the institution's facilities are inadequate and its staff cannot furnish proper care and at the same time protect other patients from the risks associated with such patients. Ordinarily a refusal to admit an incompetent person will not lead to hospital liability. On the other hand, a hospital may decide temporarily to admit an unwilling, incompetent patient for his own safety or for the protection of others. Admission procedures must then carefully follow local statutes as ascertained by the hospital attorney and communicated to hospital personnel. Otherwise the hospital risks liability to the unwilling patient for the common law torts of false imprisonment as well as assault and battery. False imprisonment can be generally defined as unreasonable restriction of another's freedom of mobility accompanied by the use of force or the threat of force. Assault and battery, briefly, is an unconsented touching of the person.

Minimum precautions against risks of liability for one or both of these torts are first, to follow local statutory requirements regarding involuntary hospitalization; second, to make certain that only such force as is reasonable under all the facts and circumstances is used to detain the patient, that detention continues only for a reasonable length of time, that the detention has the legitimate purpose of protecting the patient or the public, and that the express consent or authorization of the nearest relative is obtained whenever involuntary hospitalization is requested by such a relative.[30] (Requests for involuntary hospitalization may of course come from persons or agencies other than relatives—for example, the police—in which case the hospital should still protect itself from liability by following these guidelines.) Finally, admission and detention should never take place except upon the order of a licensed physician exercising his professional judgment in good faith.

---

[30] Hospitals need not investigate the apparent good faith of relatives requesting hospitalization unless circumstances suggest an ulterior motive. *Maben v. Rankin,* 55 Cal. 2d 139, 10 Cal. Rptr. 353, 358 P. 2d 681 (1961).

Discharge from Hospital

The discharge of most patients from the hospital presents no significant legal problems. Most discharged patients are of sound mind and do not suffer from a contagious disease; hence they respresent no risk of harm to themselves or others. Most are medically ready for discharge and wish to be at home or at another institution better suited to their need for further care.[31]

It is elementary that patients should not be discharged without a written order from a licensed physician. It is also fundamental that unless the institution is protected by the doctrine of governmental immunity under local state law a hospital, like a physician, can be held liable for abandoning or discharging a patient who is in need of further medical care. The legal test is whether or not the hospital acted reasonably under all the facts and circumstances of the particular case. The standard for what is reasonable is whether the patient's condition is likely to be aggravated by his discharge or transfer to another hospital. If an unreasonable risk was taken, it does not matter why the hospital discharged the patient despite his need of further attention. Failure by a patient to pay his bill is certainly no justification for discharge or transfer to another institution. If transfer to a less costly institution is contemplated or seemingly mandated by standards of utilization review, the attending physician must be certain in his professional judgment that the receiving institution is adequately equipped and staffed to care properly for the patient in the light of his physical and mental condition.

Several reported cases illustrate the prospect of tort liability when a hospital discharges a patient in need of further care. For example, in *Meiselman v. Crown Heights Hospital* there was liability when the defendant hospital discharged a minor while his legs were in casts and open wounds in the legs were draining.[32] Further professional care at home was known to be necessary, and this was to be arranged and supervised by the chief of the hospital's surgical staff. The home care proved to be inadequate, however, and the patient had to be sent to another hospital. Since the probable need for further care was foreseeable, the discharge was held to be unreasonable under the facts and circumstances. There was also some evidence that the motive for discharging the patient was financial.

[31] Discharges and transfers to other hospitals of patients who are brought to the emergency room entail particular legal hazards, however. See the following chapter.
[32] 285 N.Y. 389, 34 N.E. 2d 367 (1941).

If a patient represents a threat of harm to third persons, and the hospital and attending physician know or ought to know of the danger, they can be liable to any person injured by the patient. In a New York case, a patient released from Pilgrim State Mental Hospital assaulted two women on the day of his release. The attending psychiatrist had convened a commission of three physicians to approve the patient's discharge. After evaluating his condition the commission declared that he could be discharged; but he was not actually released for more than forty days, since housing and out-patient care had to be arranged for him. During the interval, several incidents of violent behavior required him to be placed under restraint. Nevertheless he was discharged without further medical evaluation. Since the hospital and the attending physician were on notice that the patient's condition had apparently deteriorated after the commission's approval of his release, the failure to conduct a further evaluation of his condition constituted negligence that was the proximate cause of the injuries suffered by the plaintiffs.[33] Note especially, however, that liability is not imposed simply because of an erroneous medical judgment. Rather, the known facts of violent and uncontrollable behavior immediately prior to discharge were the basis for the finding of negligence.

In *Semler v. Psychiatric Institute of Washington, D.C.*, a man who plead guilty to the criminal charge of abducting a young girl received a suspended prison sentence contingent upon continued in-patient treatment at a psychiatric institution. On the later recommendations of his physician and probation officer, the court approved his transfer to day care, permitting him to live at home and commute daily to the hospital with his parents. Soon, however, he began living alone and working as a bricklayer's helper, all with the knowledge of his attending physician and the court probation officer, but without approval of the court. He then murdered a girl. In a civil suit for damages, the Psychiatric Institute, the physician, and the probation officer all were liable in damages for transferring the patient to full out-patient status without obtaining the court's approval. Since the court had not authorized the probation officer to approve the transfer, the institution was not protected from liability on the basis of the officer's approval. Further, the officer's unauthorized act constituted a ministerial decision, not discretionary, thus rendering him also personally liable in damages.[34]

---

[33] *Homere v. State of New York*, 370 N.Y.S. 2d 246 (App. Div. 1975).
[34] 538 F. 2d 121 (4th Cir. 1976), *cert. denied*, 97 S. Ct. 83 (1976).

The development and implementation of home and ambulatory care programs require that each patient's medical and mental condition must be properly evaluated and continually monitored in accordance with his individual needs. The interest and protection of the community must not be overlooked. If his care and treatment are rendered under the jurisdiction of a court, the orders of the court must be strictly followed.

A difficult problem is presented when a patient of sound mind and in full control of his faculties insists upon leaving the hospital when he is still in need of immediate care. He cannot be held in the hospital against his will because that would constitute the tort of false imprisonment regardless of the medical urgency of the case. The only thing the attending physician can do is to give the patient medical advice and encourage him to remain hospitalized. If he still refuses, he must be discharged. In that event the hospital should try to obtain an appropriately worded release form which can then be filed in the medical record. This form should state that a full explanation of his medical condition was given the patient; that he was advised not to leave the hospital; that his discharge is solely at his own responsibility; and that he is acting of his own free will and volition. It is entirely possible, of course, that the patient of sound mind who insists on leaving the hospital against medical advice will refuse to sign the release form. If so, he cannot be forced to sign, but the situation should be thoroughly explained in the medical record by the attending physician, who should affix his signature to the explanation. The entries should be witnessed by other competent medical personnel familiar with the situation.

Patients of unsound mind may be reasonably restrained from leaving if they insist on doing so against medical advice, one justification being that departure would endanger their health or life. A further justification in such situations is that the lives or property of others may be endangered if mentally unstable patients are discharged too soon. The same can be said of the patient of sound mind who is suffering from a contagious disease. Not only is reasonable restraint permitted in these circumstances; there is an affirmative duty on the part of the hospital to the community to refuse to discharge such patients. Restraint in preventing them from leaving the hospital must be reasonable under all the facts and circumstances of each particular case; and competent medical evidence of the contagious disease or the mental instability of the patient, whichever the case may be, is essential.

A patient must never be held in the hospital for failure to pay his bill or held until arrangements are completed for the payment of the bill. Such action, at least where force or the threat of force is used, constitutes false imprisonment and gives the aggrieved patient a cause of action in damages against the hospital.[35]

An unemancipated minor should be discharged only to his parents, or in their absence those the hospital knows to be legally entitled to custody. When the whereabouts of the parents is unknown and there is no court-appointed guardian, steps should be taken to procure a guardian. Social welfare agencies should be of help to the hospital in these situations. If the whereabouts of the parents, or the parent entitled to custody, is known, but for some reason the parent cannot come to the hospital for the child, discharge to another should take place only if the person produces a written order from the parent.

Emancipated minors—that is, minors who are earning their own living and are permitted by their parents to retain these earnings for their own use—can be discharged from the hospital in the same manner as adults. Emancipation is a matter of agreement between the parent and child; it is a question of fact in each case and does not depend on whether the youth is or is not living at home. In some states emancipation results when a minor marries.

Generally it is legally sound to discharge the infant child of an unmarried mother to the custody of the mother. The hospital cannot prevent the mother from claiming her child, at least when she intends to retain custody and responsibility for raising the infant. Further, even if she intends to place the child for private adoption, most states would recognize her legal right to do so in accordance with local limitations and restrictions. Some jurisdictions, however, prohibit all private and independent adoption. Thus, if an unmarried mother claims her child and the hospital personnel knows that she intends to place the infant for private independent adoption, hospital administrators should consult legal counsel for advice consistent with local law. If the unmarried mother does not herself claim the child but requests his discharge, then the child should in no case be discharged except on the recommendations of an approved and legally recognized social service adoption agency.

Utilization review committees do not and certainly should not order the discharge of individual patients. As previously stressed, only the patient's attending physician can authorize his discharge or transfer to another health care institution. If a review committee should insist

---

[35] *Gadsden v. Hamilton,* 212 Ala. 531, 103 So. 553 (1925); *Bedard v. Notre Dame,* 89 R.I. 194, 151 A. 2d 690 (1959).

upon discharge contrary to the professional judgment of the attending physician, and if the patient later suffers harm or injury as the proximate cause of premature release, then the hospital would probably be liable in damages, since the organized utilization review committee would have acted as the agent of the hospital. If the attending physician properly documented his exercise of reasonable care in resisting the committee's order of discharge, he of course would not be personally liable to his patient for the premature discharge. On the other hand, if the attending doctor acquiesces in the discharge contrary to professional standards, then his personal liability would be established.

The role and function of the utilization review committee is thus simply to make recommendations with respect to the need and appropriateness of continued hospitalization of individual patients. Moreover, and most significantly, the impact of the committee's recommendations is solely financial: when the committee finds that a patient's medical condition no longer warrants continued hospitalization, the third party paying for the care—the federal Medicare program or Blue Cross–Blue Shield—will no longer reimburse the hospital for in-patient care. As is well known, utilization review is mandated by governmental programs financing hospital-medical care, and it is also required by many private third-party agencies, especially Blue Cross–Blue Shield. This mandated review has resulted, of course, from the ever-increasing cost of care, and it is only one of several techniques for reducing the cost of health care.

When the review committee refuses to find a need for continued hospitalization and recommends discharge or transfer to a less expensive place, the patient must assume responsibility for payment of costs if he remains at the institution. All of this must be carefully explained by the attending physician to his patient and the family, and together they must then decide on the future course and place of care. As long as the committee functions within its defined role and exercises good faith, individual members of the committee run no significant risk of legal liability for rendering a decision adverse to the patient. In many states local statutes specifically provide that the members of a utilization review committee shall not be personally liable for damages when they conduct their review in good faith within the confines of the committee's proper functions.

VII

Legal Aspects of Emergency Hospital Care

Ordinarily a patient does not have a legal right to be admitted formally to a hospital, whether private and voluntary or governmental, or to be seen and treated in an out-patient clinic. That is, as a general rule the hospital has no common law or statutory duty to admit or even serve all who apply for accommodation or service.

With respect to some hospitals owned and operated by government in some jurisdictions, however, the local statutes may be construed as creating a right among some classes of individuals to be both served and admitted to the hospital. Statutes creating certain governmental hospitals and specifying the purposes to be accomplished by the hospital may define or designate groups, or classes, of persons to be served: for example, the population of a given county or patients suffering from a particular disease. From such statutes a duty to serve emergency patients might well be implied. (A review of these statutes and an interpretation of the extent to which particular patients have the legal right to be admitted in particular circumstances appear in the preceding chapter.)

The general rule denying the patient a legal right to be admitted may be changed if the hospital has voluntarily undertaken to serve a defined population by entering into an express contract. Such a contract could be between the hospital and an identifiable class or group of patients, or between the hospital and, for example, an employer, the latter's employees being designated beneficiaries of the undertaking.[1] Naturally, and understandably, an obligation

---

[1] *Norwood Hospital v. Howton*, 32 Ala. App. 375, 26 So. 2d 427 (1946).

182

created by an express contract must be performed, and a duty to serve emergency patients would normally be included among such obligations.

One route of attack on the rule that there is no duty to serve comes through, or arises from, the maintenance and operation of the hospital's emergency room, the subject of the present chapter. It is perfectly evident that the American public expects service from the nation's hospitals and their medical staffs. Primarily through the mechanism of the private lawsuit, judicial decision is establishing that the hospital's emergency facility has a duty to see and treat, or at least refer, all patients who apply for service. Hospitals and their staffs must thus be organized and prepared to meet the expectations of the public as expressed in the judicial decisions to be reviewed here. The most recent decisions of influential courts appear to be consistent with the newly developed and frequently articulated philosophy that health care is a right and not a privilege.

Considered below are situations where a patient presents himself at the hospital, usually at the emergency room or unit, requesting examination and treatment. Many such persons appear without benefit of a private physician who is a member of the hospital's medical staff, or they will appear at times when their private physicians are unavailable. The hospital's legal responsibilities to the patient may depend, first, on whether the situation is governed by statutory or common law; secondly, whether the institution in fact has an emergency room; and, finally, upon the apparent condition of the patient at the time he presents himself for diagnosis, advice, and treatment.

Initially the question is whether or not a hospital must maintain a facility for emergency care. If it must, or if it voluntarily maintains such a facility, the issue is then the extent of the institution's duty to the patient.

Necessity for Maintaining Emergency Care Facilities

The common law does not impose a duty upon a general community hospital to provide treatment and care for emergency patients. This means that a hospital, whether governmental or private, need not generally have any special room, equipment, or personnel for the care of those who suddenly fall ill or who are the victims of accident.

Approximately half the states, however, have statutory laws that either directly or indirectly require certain categories of hospitals to maintain emergency care facilities. These requirements may be found in some states in rules and regulations of hospital licensure statutes. Wisconsin, for example, has a statute requiring that county hospitals in counties having a population of 250,000 or more "establish and maintain . . . an emergency unit or department for the treatment . . . of persons in said county who may meet with accidents or be suddenly afflicted with illness not contagious."[2] Not only is there a duty to maintain an emergency facility, there is a duty to treat emergency patients, although the statute authorizes "safe removal" of the patient to another hospital or to his home and thus does not require formal admission of all such patients. Moreover, the statute permits the county to provide this emergency care by contract with a private hospital. The point is that the statute casts upon local county government the obligation to provide emergency care facilities either directly or by contract with some other capable agent.

In Illinois a statute, applicable to both private and governmental hospitals where surgical operations are performed, requires the hospital to extend emergency care.[3] Pennsylvania requires all hospitals receiving payments from the Department of Public Welfare to have at least one licensed doctor or resident intern on call at all times.[4] New York provides that operating certificates can be revoked for any general hospital refusing to provide emergency care.[5] In practical effect such statutes and the rules and regulations of hospital licensure which attempt to assure that emergency care will be available require the establishment and maintenance of an emergency room. Violation will be penalized as provided for in the particular statute, perhaps by a criminal sanction, revocation of license, or both of these. Moreover, and this is more significant perhaps than the usual criminal sanction, violation of such a statute could be the basis of a private civil lawsuit for damages.

These statutes apparently represent a trend toward requiring hospitals to establish and maintain emergency care facilities and staff. The public expects community general hospitals to be so equipped, but the trend will have to be monitored and coordinated with sound public policy pertaining to area-wide planning of hospital facilities and services. Granted that every community and every population group should have ready and convenient access to a hospital emer-

---

[2]Wisconsin Stat. Ann., sec. 46.21(8)(b) (1957), as amended (Supp. 1973).
[3]Illinois Stat. Ann., Title 111 $\frac{1}{2}$, sec. 86 and 87 as amended (Smith-Hurd 1977).
[4]Pa. Stat. Ann, Title 35, sec. 435 (1977).
[5]N.Y. Publ. Health Law, sec. 2806(1)(b) (McKinney 1971). Tennessee also requires all general hospitals to provide emergency service. Tenn. Code Ann., sec. 53.5201 (1977).

gency department, it does not follow that all general hospitals should be legally required to maintain relatively expensive emergency care capabilities.[6]

Duty to Treat and Aid

At common law there is no duty to aid another in peril. This doctrine, even though contrary to the morals and the ethics of the medical profession, has been applied to physicians and to hospitals as well as to lay persons. Hence a physician has no common law responsibility to respond to a call for help from one not already his patient, or from a person acting on behalf of one not his patient.

Illustrative is the case of *Childs v. Weis.*[7] A pregnant patient presented herself at the hospital emergency room at 2:00 a.m. apparently suffering from bleeding and thinking herself to be in labor. The nurse on duty conducted an examination and telephoned the staff physician on call. The doctor, who was a private practitioner, told the nurse to have the patient telephone her private physician for advice. The hospital as a matter of policy did not require the physician on call to see and examine all emergency room patients. The nurse apparently mistook the message and told the patient to go to her private doctor, located some miles away. After leaving the hospital and while en route, she gave birth to the baby, which lived only twelve hours.

In a suit against the physician, the court held that a dismissal of the action was proper on the basis that the doctor's duty to exercise reasonable care was dependent upon a contract with the patient and that there was no such contract here and hence no duty to treat. In other words, no doctor-patient relationship had been established, and accordingly the physician was not liable for even an arbitrary refusal to respond to the call. Moreover, he was not liable for the negligence of the nurse, if any, since she was not his employee. The possible liability of the hospital and the nurse in this factual setting is another question and will be discussed later in the chapter.

The only common law exception to the rule that there is no duty to aid another in peril is when the person failing to give aid was responsible for the victim's being in peril. In such circumstances,

---

[6]In 1970 the Illinois State Hospital Licensing Board approved regulations, consistent with the statute previously cited, allowing hospitals to pool their emergency care facilities and staff. The regulations recognize levels of service: "comprehensive," "basic," and "standby." Sec. 7–1.1 (1972).
[7]440 S.W. 2d 104 (Texas Ct. Civ. App. 1969).

his failure to aid could result in liability. Some cases, however, have restricted liability to negligent conduct which placed the plaintiff in peril. In short, the plaintiff had to show first that *negligent* conduct of the defendant placed him in peril, and second that the defendant then failed in his duty to aid. Other cases have found liability for failure to aid whenever any conduct by the defendant put the plaintiff in peril.

Similarly a hospital need not, by application of the early common law, employ its facilities and staff to aid the person who presents himself for treatment. Recent court cases and some statutes, however, suggest that this attitude has changed, at least with respect to hospitals which maintain emergency care facilities. The public expects aid, and sound moral doctrine dictates that hospitals extend aid which they are capable of rendering.

Such changes occur in the first place because statutory law in particular jurisdictions directly or by inference changes the common law. As mentioned above, statutes in Wisconsin, Illinois, New York, and Pennsylvania, for example, require the provision of emergency care in certain hospitals. Also to be noted is a Florida statute pertaining to certain governmental hospitals which are declared to be for the benefit of those who fall ill or are the victims of accidents within the governmental boundaries.[8] From statutory language mandating the maintenance of emergency care facilities it is reasonable to infer a duty to aid victims of an emergency. An affirmative duty to aid follows logically from a duty to maintain emergency care facilities.

Bearing more expressly and directly on the issue of a duty to aid is a relatively new statute in California. The act, first passed in 1970, requires that health centers having "appropriate facilities and qualified personnel" extend emergency care in cases of serious injury or illness. The law further provides that the health center, its personnel, and the physician are not liable in damages for refusal to render emergency care if good faith and reasonable care were exercised in determining whether the available facilities and personnel could care for the patient.[9]

Certainly a public hospital, or a private hospital receiving Hill-Burton funds or other governmental support, may not refuse emergency care or hospital admission on the basis of race, color, creed, or national origin. To do so would clearly violate the Fourteenth

[8]Florida Stat. Ann., sec. 155.16 (1972).
[9]West Cal. Health and Safety Code, sec. 1317 (West Supp. 1974). Florida also prohibits denial of emergency care in hospitals maintaining emergency departments. Florida Stat. Ann., sec. 401.45 (1973).

Amendment to the federal Constitution.[10] Such discriminatory practices would also violate the public accommodations section of the
federal Civil Rights Act of 1964 and the regulations governing the
Medicare-Medicaid program.

Judicial law, moreover, is developing a duty to aid under certain
circumstances without benefit of statute; and hence the traditional
common law rule that there was no duty to aid one in peril is no
longer a reliable guide for hospitals. In the recent case of *Williams
v. Hospital Authority of Hall County* the Georgia Appellate Court held
that a governmental hospital which had an emergency care department must extend aid to the victim of an accident who had presented
himself at the hospital for treatment of a fracture.[11] The court stressed
that the defendant hospital was tax supported and a public institution,
and it expressly rejected the argument that the hospital had an
absolute right to refuse emergency services. The judge described
as "repugnant" a refusal to serve where an emergency care facility
was available. Although the decision was carefully limited in applicability to a governmental hospital, it would be a short step indeed
to extend this same philosophy to a voluntary hospital which maintains
an emergency department.

The Missouri Supreme Court has apparently already taken this
step. In *Stanturf v. Sipes*, a patient with frozen feet was refused
treatment and admission to a private hospital. The reason initially
was that he was not able to pay an advance cash deposit; but the
hospital maintained its refusal even after friends offered the deposit,
the hospital apparently being doubtful that further payment could
be assured. The delay in care necessitated the amputation of both
feet. The court's opinion was that a hospital which has an emergency
service holds itself out as providing care and may not then refuse.[12]
Hence, even if it is legally justifiable to require a preadmission cash
deposit from ordinary patients, it is not justifiable with respect to
the patient who presents himself in need of immediate care. Most
observers believe that the holding of this court should now be accepted
as the rule governing hospital emergency room policies.

---

[10]*Simkins v. Moses H. Cone Memorial Hospital*, 323 F. 2d 959 (4th Cir. 1963); *Flagler
Hospital v. Hayling*, 344 F. 2d 950 (5th Cir. 1964); *Eaton v. Grubbs*, 329 F. 2d 710
(4th Cir. 1964). See also: *Penn v. San Juan Hospital*, 528 F. 2d 1181 (10th Cir.
1975). (A class action alleged that Navajo Indians were denied emergency medical
care solely because they were Indians. District court denied temporary and permanent
injunctions following only preliminary hearings. Circuit court remanded for further
proceedings, holding that plaintiffs were entitled to an adequate opportunity to show
the merits of the case.)
[11]119 Ga. App. 626; 168 S.E. 2d 336 (1969).
[12]447 S.W. 2d 558, 35 A.L.R. 3d 834 (Mo. 1969).

Even before the *Williams* and *Sipes* cases the Delaware Supreme
Court had issued a landmark decision in *Wilmington General Hospital
v. Manlove.*[13] In this case an infant was suffering from acute diarrhea
and a high temperature. The mother, unable to locate the family
pediatrician, took the child to a private hospital's emergency room.
The nurse on duty refused to examine the baby or call another
doctor, however, because the patient was already under the care
of a private physician. The nurse did try to call the private doctor
but was also unsuccessful. She then suggested that the mother return
with the infant to the hospital clinic the next day if she were still
unable to reach her doctor. The mother then returned home, where
the baby died four hours later.

In a suit for damages the hospital was held liable on the basis
that the nurse had at least a duty to determine whether an "unmistakable" emergency existed and to extend aid if it did. Hence, as a
minimum, a nurse in an emergency room must exercise reasonable
care to ascertain the patient's condition and then act accordingly.
A professional judgment, made with reasonable care in the light
of all the facts and circumstances, leading to the conclusion that
the patient was not in need of immediate medical care and treatment
would not result in liability under the *Manlove* reasoning. Nevertheless,
since a medical diagnosis is normally beyond the scope of nursing
practice, it is difficult to see how a nurse can adequately perform
her duty and protect the hospital from possible liability unless she
calls a licensed physician to examine the patient and recommend
treatment.

On the basis of these judicial decisions, a hospital policy is strongly
recommended which would require that all patients presenting
themselves at the emergency room be seen, examined, and advised
by a licensed physician. The physician, in the exercise of his professional judgment, would then order formal admission, transfer to
another institution, or return to home. Diagnosis and advice by
telephone is not recommended, since a legally valid physician-patient
or hospital-patient relationship can be established by telephone, thus
creating a duty to exercise reasonable care and skill under all the
circumstances. A doctor may risk breach of this duty when he relies

[13] 54 Del 15, 174 A. 2d 135 (Sup. Ct. 1961). *Accord: Guerrero v. Copper Queen Hospital,*
22 Ariz. App. 611, 529 P. 2d 1205 (1974), *aff'd,* 537 P. 2d 1329 (1975). (A licensed
private hospital with an emergency room must extend care.) See also: *Carr v. St.
Paul Fire and Marine Insurance Co.,* 384 F. Supp. 821 (D.C. Ark. 1974). (Where a
patient's readily apparent condition indicated a medical emergency, and hospital
personnel failed to summon a physician, a jury verdict against the hospital was justified.)

upon diagnosis by telephone, especially when he is not personally acquainted with the patient and his condition.[14]

Beginning of Aid—Duty to Exercise Reasonable Care

The foregoing recommendation is also based upon the long-standing and well-accepted common law rule that the voluntary beginning of aid creates a duty to exercise reasonable care under all the facts and circumstances. The rule clearly applies to both physicians and hospitals. The slightest act of aid or exercise of control over the patient may be legally the starting of aid, thereby bringing into play this judicial doctrine. To illustrate, in *Bourgeois v. Dade County* the police brought an unconscious patient to the hospital. The physician on emergency call conducted only a cursory examination without benefit of x-rays, decided that the patient was intoxicated, and approved his removal to jail, where he died. It was then established that he had been suffering from broken ribs which had punctured the chest. The issue of negligence was one for jury determination.[15]

Many other cases have involved the same principles and resulted in the finding of liability for negligence. There is no need to call attention to all these decisions here, but a hospital administrator should be familiar with such other important cases as *New Biloxi Hospital v. Frazier,*[16] *Jones v. City of New York,*[17] *Methodist Hospital v. Ball,*[18] and *O'Neill v. Montefiore Hospital.*[19] In *Frazier, Jones,* and *Ball* the facts were fundamentally the same. In all instances the victims of violence or accident were accepted into the emergency room, and the hospital staff failed to exercise reasonable care in diagnosis, treatment, and disposition of the case.

In the *Jones* case, an intern of a voluntary hospital cleaned and dressed stab wounds and without further care ordered the patient transferred to a city hospital, the delay causing death. In both *Frazier* and *Ball,* the patients were unattended for a considerable time (forty-five minutes in the *Ball* case, an hour or more in *Frazier*),

---

[14] Compare the case of *Childs v. Weis,* 440 S.W. 2d 104 (Texas Ct. Civ. App. 1969), discussed above, where the suit was against the physician on hospital emergency call duty, the hospital's policy did not require him personally to see patients at the emergency room, and the doctor gave no advice to the patient or nurse other than apparently telling the nurse to have the patient telephone her private physician.

[15] 99 So. 2d 575, 72 A.L.R. 2d 391 (Florida 1957).

[16] 245 Miss. 185, 146 So. 2d 882 (1962).

[17] 134 N.Y.S. 2d 779 (Sup. Ct. 1954), *modified,* 286 App. Div. 825, 143 N.Y.S. 2d 628 (1955).

[18] 50 Tenn. App. 460, 362 S.W. 2d 475 (1961).

[19] 11 App. Div. 2d 132, 202 N.Y.S. 2d 436 (1960).

given minimal attention and diagnosis from hospital nursing and medical staff, and then transferred to other institutions with adverse results.

These litigated cases emphasize the legal and humane necessity of exercising reasonable care in making a diagnosis and deciding the course (and place) of treatment.[20] They also show the necessity for hospital personnel to determine which patients need immediate attention. Delay cannot be excused on the basis that others are being treated. To collect damages, of course, the plaintiff must prove, usually by expert witness testimony, that the delay in diagnosis and treatment, or the delay occasioned by the transfer to another institution, was the proximate cause of death or of a worsened condition.[21]

The *O'Neill* case in New York is one of the most instructive of all. A man and his wife arrived at the hospital emergency room in the early morning hours and told the nurse on duty that they believed the husband was experiencing a heart attack. Upon inquiry, he said he was a participant in the Health Insurance Plan (H.I.P.) of New York. The nurse thereupon informed the couple that the hospital did not serve such individuals and that it would be necessary for the patient to see his H.I.P. physician. She did, however, telephone the H.I.P. physician. Speaking directly with Mr. O'Neill, the physician apparently told him to return home, and that he could see the doctor at the H.I.P. clinic later in the day. The hospital nurse thereupon refused the couple's further request that a staff member at the defendant hospital examine Mr. O'Neill. They returned home, where Mr. O'Neill died before he could see his physician.

The court held that there were two issues to be resolved by a jury: Did the nurse's action in telephoning the H.I.P. physician constitute the beginning of aid, thus creating the duty to exercise reasonable care? If so, did the nurse exercise the proper standard of care? In response to the first question, juries would not normally be expected to be sympathetic to the hospital. In other words, even in a jurisdiction which nominally recognizes the historical common

---

[20] For still another case involving an inadequate examination and a decision by a hospital intern in the emergency room to send the patient home before the results of a throat culture were known, see *Barcia v. Society of N.Y. Hospital*, 241 N.Y.S. 2d 373, 39 Misc. 2d 526 (Sup. Ct. 1963).

[21] *Ruvio v. North Broward Hospital District*, 186 So. 2d 45, (Fla. Dist. Ct. App. 1966), *cert. denied*, 195 So. 2d 567 (Fla. 1966). *Cooper v. Sisters of Charity of Cincinnati*, 27 Ohio St. 2d 242, 56 Ohio Op. 2d 146, 272 N.E. 2d 97 (1971): (Although the physician was negligent in failing to conduct adequate examination of a minor who had been struck by a truck, there was no proof that the patient would have survived had an appropriate examination been conducted. Hence neither the physician nor the hospital was liable). *Accord: Rosen v. Parkview Hospital*, 265 So.2d 93 (Florida Dist. Ct. App. 1972).

law rule that there is no duty to aid one who presents himself at the hospital, the slightest act by emergency room personnel on behalf of the patient is likely to be interpreted as the exercise of control, thus creating a duty to act reasonably.

Logically, the issues emphasized in the *O'Neill* and similar cases that were decided in the early 1960s and before are now moot in the light of the *Manlove, Williams, Sipes,* and *Guerrero* cases. In other words, if a hospital having an emergency department has a positive duty to recognize a medical emergency, or simply to extend aid to all who present themselves, it is not necessary to argue or determine whether aid was, in fact, started or control over the patient exercised. By either process of reasoning, however, the proper conduct is clear—all patients who present themselves should be seen, examined, and treated as their condition requires.[22]

The recent Maryland case of *Thomas v. Corso* dramatically illustrates the legal duty of all parties to exercise reasonable care under all the facts and circumstances.[23] It further illustrates the substantial risk of liability that hospitals incur when they rely upon a system of on-call rosters for physicians covering the emergency room, and when the hospital nurse and doctor confer by telephone. In *Corso* the patient had been struck by an automobile and was taken to the hospital at approximately 11:30 p.m.; the emergency room nurse conferred by telephone with the on-call physician, who ordered the patient admitted for observation and for x-rays to be taken in the morning. The patient was permitted by the hospital personnel to remain in the corridor outside the nurses' station, although they knew him to be in shock with low blood pressure. Moreover, the nurses failed to telephone the physician immediately upon discovery of shock as indicated by a change in vital signs. Later a further report was made to the physician, and he came to the hospital to attend to the case personally, but the patient had already died.

The opinion held that the physician had clearly established a patient-physician relationship over the telephone by making a diagnosis and undertaking care. Although there was a dispute of fact concerning the extent and content of the nurse's initial telephoned reports to the physician, he knew enough about the patient's accident and his condition to realize that his personal attendance was required. Hence he was personally liable for his negligence in failing to come at once to the hospital; and expert testimony was not necessary to

---

[22] See generally: Powers, "Hospital Emergency Service and the Open Door," 66 *Michigan Law Review* 1455, no. 7, May, 1968.
[23] 265 Md. 84, 288 A. 2d 379 (1972).

establish this negligence, since lay persons of the jury were capable of determining that the failure to attend the patient was the proximate cause of death. The hospital nurses and their employer were likewise negligent in permitting the patient to remain in the corridor, where it was more difficult to carry out the constant observation of the patient that the circumstances required, and in failing to report promptly to the doctor a significant change of the patient's vital signs.

Also dramatic and tragic is the 1973 case of *Niles v. City of San Rafael*, in which the jury's judgment in favor of a thirteen-year-old boy and his father exceeded $4 million.[24] The youth had suffered a head injury during a summer recreational program sponsored by the city of San Rafael and the local school district. At the emergency room of Mount Zion Hospital in San Francisco, where he was taken, an intern determined that admission to the hospital was indicated. The admitting office, however, mistakenly advised him that unless the patient was in the care of a private physician he could not be admitted.

Just at this time Dr. David Haskin, a private board-certified pediatrician, who was also an employee of the hospital on salary as director of the pediatric out-patient clinic, appeared in the emergency room, and the house officer asked Dr. Haskin to examine the patient, explaining the difficulties involved in arranging formal admission. Dr. Haskin advised that the patient be sent home with his father, having arrived at this judgment without examining the injured youth or looking at his chart. Moreover, not all of the patient's vital signs had been promptly recorded on the chart by the hospital's house staff and nurses.

At this point, again contrary to hospital policy, the father was not given a written list of instructions and symptoms to observe in cases of head injuries. These were prepared standing instructions, one of which was that the patient should return immediately to the hospital if certain described symptoms appeared. No reason was given why neither Dr. Haskin nor the house staff furnished this information to the father of the patient. Within less than two hours, the boy's condition had so greatly deteriorated that he was returned to the hospital, where another physician immediately recognized an epidural hematoma. By the time a neurosurgeon could be summoned, it was too late to save the patient from nearly total paralysis.

Another recent case similar to *Thomas* and *Niles* is *Citizens Hospital*

---

[24] 42 Cal. App. 3d 230, 116 Cal. Rptr. 733 (1974).

Association v. Schoulin, where there was liability when the nurse on duty at the hospital failed to communicate effectively with the on-call physician. In this case it was not discovered that the patient's back had been fractured.[25]

Obviously not all emergency room patients need to be formally admitted to the hospital. Transfer to another hospital is justified when no negligence occurs in diagnosis or treatment in the emergency room, and when the exercise of reasonable professional judgment indicates that the transfer will not aggravate or worsen the patient's condition. Such was the situation in the recent case of *Joyner v. Alton Ochsner Medical Foundation.* An accident victim was properly cared for on an emergency, first aid basis according to his condition and in conformance with recognized standards of medical care. He was then transferred to another hospital with the approval of his wife, since they were unable to pay the required deposit for admission.[26] The case is clearly distinguishable from the *Sipes* litigation in the Missouri Court, previously discussed, because there all care was refused, even after third parties agreed to pay the deposit.

Similarly, the rendering of emergency care does not obligate a hospital to violate its legitimate rules regarding formal admission; nor does it commit the hospital to admit patients when it is not adequately equipped to give them continuing treatment. In *Birmingham Baptist Hospital v. Crews,* a relatively old case, the hospital had a rule that patients with contagious disease could not be admitted. A victim of diphtheria was seen and treated in the emergency room. She died soon after being sent home. The court held that the hospital could not be held liable, saying that there was no legal right to formal admission. Requiring the hospital in this instance to violate its rule regarding contagious disease would encourage the hospital, it was said, to refuse even emergency aid in the future, and requiring admission might endanger the health of other patients.[27] Indeed, a hospital is under a positive duty to transfer a patient to another institution if it does not have the appropriate facilities and staff to care properly for the patient and if the circumstances thus indicate a need for such a transfer.[28] The transferring institution also has

---

[25] 48 Ala. App. 100, 262 So. 2d 303 (1972). Compare: *Falcher v. St. Luke's Medical Center,* 19 Ariz. App. 2d 247, 506 P. 2d 287 (1973). (Leaving an emergency room patient for a short time was not negligence, since expert witness for the defendant testified that under the particular circumstances of the case there had been no violation of standards of care.)
[26] 230 So. 2d 913 (La. Ct. App. 1970). See also: *Murray v. United States,* 329 F. 2d 270 (4th Cir. 1964).
[27] 229 Ala. 398, 157 So. 224 (1934).
[28] *Carrasco v. Bankoff,* 220 Cal. App. 2d 230, 33 Cal. Rptr. 673, 97 A.L.R. 464 (1963).

a duty to forward with the patient the diagnosis and other appropriate medical information, and the receiving hospital has a duty to obtain this information.[29]

As these cases demonstrate, in summary, patients who present themselves at the hospital emergency room should never be turned away until they have been seen and examined by a licensed physician, who thus determines the seriousness of the illness or injury and then orders admission, return home, or referral to another facility, depending upon the facts and circumstances of each particular case. Undue delays should not be tolerated. These policies should be expressed in clearly understood written rules which can be readily carried out by hospital personnel and emergency room physicians. Because written rules which are ignored or violated can be evidence of negligence, it is extremely important to follow established hospital policies meticulously, once they are expressed in written form.

It is also important to follow in full the standards of emergency care promulgated by public and private agencies as well as by professional groups. Among the former are the rules and regulations issued by the state department or agency responsible under law for hospital licensure. If the particular state has a licensure law, and if there are regulations pertaining to emergency care, a violation of these regulations could be evidence of negligence in a civil suit by the patient for damages. Most important is the further fact that standards established by such private agencies as the Joint Commission on Accreditation of Hospitals and the American College of Surgeons have the same legal implications. Both groups have published standards relative to emergency room equipment, staffing, and care. For example, the Joint Commission's "Principle for Emergency Services" states: "Adequate appraisal and advice or initial treatment shall be rendered to any ill or injured person who presents himself at the hospital."[30] Under this principle, Standard I requires a well-defined plan for providing care consistent with community need and the capability of the hospital. According to the published interpretations, this does not mean that all hospitals must actually maintain a full-service emergency department. Rather, the plan for emergency care may recognize limited capabilities, or even call for all emergency patients to be transferred to other institutions. The point is that a plan for emergency care must exist, and if the hospital is, in fact, capable of caring for the patient he should not be arbitrarily

[29] *Mulligan v. Wetchler,* 39 App. Div. 2d 102, 332 N.Y.S. 2d 68 (1972).
[30] *Accreditation Manual for Hospitals,* Joint Commission on Accreditation of Hospitals, Chicago (1976), 69, and *Second Supplement to Manual* (1977), 69.

sent elsewhere. For institutions which do maintain an emergency department, further standards relate to organization, direction, staffing, facilities, written policies, and medical records. The Medicare "Conditions of Participation" contain standards for emergency care similar to those promulgated by the Joint Commission on Accreditation.

The chief legal point to be emphasized here is that regulations of public or governmental agencies and standards of private agencies—together with hospital rules often expressed in medical staff bylaws—may be introduced into evidence for jury consideration in a liability suit for damages.[31]

Also to be stressed is the necessity to maintain written medical records for each person seen in the emergency room, even if that person is not formally admitted to the hospital. Not only are such records mandatory in the interests of adequate medical care, but the hospital may be called upon later to document in the courtroom the standards of care rendered to a particular patient, in which event a medical chart is indispensable. Moreover, records are required by various hospital licensing regulations and by the Joint Commission on Accreditation of Hospitals. These should include the instructions given the patient for continuing care when he is sent home, as well as information furnished an institution or physician to whom he is referred.

All of the foregoing cases and discussion of hospital liability arising out of emergency care must be qualified by the doctrine of governmental immunity from tort liability in any case involving a state or local governmental hospital. Immunity of the state and its agencies from suit is a matter of individual state law. In one or two states which still retain the remnants of charitable immunity, the outcome of a suit for damages against a charitable hospital would be controlled by that doctrine. But a hospital's immunity for tort never protects the individual emergency room nurse, technician, or physician from individual liability. Moreover, by virtue of the Federal Tort Claims Act, a hospital owned and operated by the federal government is fully liable in tort to the same extent as a private hospital.[32]

In *Childs v. Greenville Hospital Authority*, a companion case to *Childs v. Weis* arising from the same facts discussed earlier in this chapter, the hospital was not liable for the nurse's negligence, if any, since the institution was a county hospital performing a governmental

[31] *Darling v. Charleston Community Memorial Hospital*, 33 Ill. 2d 326, 211 N.E. 2d 253, 14 A.L.R. 3d 860 (1965).
[32] *McBride v. United States*, 462 F. 2d 72 (9th Cir. 1972).

function in Texas, which follows the doctrine of governmental immunity. As was noted in the opinion, however, the emergency room nurse could be found negligent in relaying the wrong message from the physician to the patient. On this issue there was a factual question for the jury to decide.[33]

Staffing the Emergency Department

All of the foregoing suggests that the legal duty of reasonable care owed to patients who present themselves at the emergency room mandates a well-organized department, staffed with qualified personnel, and possessed of the equipment and facilities necessary to assure prompt diagnosis and treatment on referral. Not only is this true according to general common law of judicial decisions previously discussed, at least for those general hospitals that maintain emergency departments, but a number of states require competent personnel, and some also specify certain equipment, through rules and regulations relevant to hospital licensure. For example, some states provide by regulation that there must be a physician covering the emergency room at all times. Standards promulgated by private accreditation agencies or professional groups may contain similar provisions relative to the staffing and the facilities of an emergency department.

Organizationally those in charge of the department must be an integral part of the medical staff and accountable to relevant staff committees for the quality of care. Ultimately the governing body of the hospital is responsible for the professional standards of the emergency department, just as the board is responsible for other clinical standards of the institution.[34] Medical staff privileges in the emergency room should be delineated for each individual physician staffing the facility, as is done in other hospital departments.

For moderately sized and larger hospitals, staffing the emergency room with nurses and interns, supported only by medical staff on a rotating on-call basis, no longer meets the expectations of the public or satisfies the legal responsibilities required in malpractice cases. When physicians serve only on call, there is too much opportunity for error in diagnosis and delay in treatment, both of which lead to unfortunate situations and increase such liability problems as those illustrated in the cases reviewed above. Liability may, perhaps ironically, be made more likely by the modern specialization in medical

---

[33] 479 S.W. 2d 399 (Texas Ct. Civ. App. 1972).
[34] *Darling v. Charleston Community Hospital,* 33 Ill. 2d 326, 211 N.E. 2d 253, 14 A.L.R. 3d 860 (1965).

practice. That is, some specialists may not be professionally competent to deal with certain emergency cases and hence should not be on emergency duty. Nor should interns, physicians' assistants, and foreign medical school graduates without a local license to practice medicine be employed for primary care of emergency room patients. On the other hand, as a general legal proposition a nurse, an intern, or even a layman is authorized, so far as the medical licensure laws are concerned, to do anything that is reasonably calculated to save life in a genuine life-or-death emergency. However, this general rule does not help the hospital avoid liability in the factual situations previously noted, since it pertains in the final analysis only to the issue of illegal practice. Substantial efforts must yet be made in many hospitals to correct what is probably the weakest link in standards of medical care provided to the community.

Consequently hospitals called upon in their respective communities to furnish full-scale emergency services should have a department with a full-time staff of locally licensed, experienced physicians competent to handle cases of trauma. Making emergency medicine a recognized specialty might well facilitate and encourage further development of full-time arrangements. Emergency room nurses of course should be adequately trained in life-saving techniques.

Hospitals have several alternatives in arranging full-time coverage of the emergency department by a physician. In most states nonprofit institutions may employ physicians directly on salary; that is, the judicial rule prohibiting a corporation from practicing medicine will not inhibit or prevent salaried arrangements. Years ago the prohibition was announced as a means of discouraging commercialization and exploitation of the professional person and to emphasize that the physician owes his individual loyalties to his patient. It was developed, however, in the context of the private, profit-making corporation and is believed to have little or no relevance to the modern voluntary hospital. In those few states which do prohibit the payment of a salary, or when an alternative to salary is desired, a fee-for-service arrangement could of course be used.

More typical than direct employment of salaried or fee-for-service physicians for emergency department staff is a contractual arrangement with a corporation of physicians, or a partnership, whereby the physicians undertake to provide full-time coverage. Nearly all states now permit professional individuals to incorporate their practice under authority granted by special statute. Such a contract must be carefully drafted to make sure that the corporation or partnership is obligated to provide the services contemplated by the hospital and that the hospital retains adequate control with respect to the privileges of the physicians in the emergency department and the standards of their practice. By entering into such an arrangement the hospital must not abdicate its ultimate responsibility for the quality of health care. The contract, among other provisions, must provide guidelines for the following responsibilities: full-time coverage; the supervision of hospital nurses and house staff as well as equipment and facilities; fees and billing; and referral of patients. The document must also provide for the term of the arrangement and contain provisions for renewal. Above all, the medical staff of the hospital must be involved in monitoring the standards of practice in the emergency service and delineating clinical privileges, even when service is contracted to an independent group of physicians. This medical staff function must be clearly articulated in the contract with the physicians' group. The emergency room group should also be required to carry adequate malpractice insurance and agree to indemnify the hospital if judgments of malpractice arise from the negligence of any physician or employee of the corporation or partnership.

The financial arrangements between the hospital and the group of physicians may legally consist of two charges to the patient—one for hospital services and another for the physician's service. The group may bill directly to the patient or may assign the account to the hospital for collection. The hospital may legally guarantee the physicians an agreed annual or periodic minimum income.

Contracts for emergency department coverage between a hospital and a corporation, or partnership, of physicians give rise to legal questions involving the hospital's liability for the malpractice or negligence of any of the doctors. The contract will normally recite that the physicians are "independent contractors," and at common law under the doctrine of respondeat superior an employer is not legally liable for the negligence or other tort of an independent contractor. The reason given for this long-established rule is that an employer has no right to control the means and methods of the independent contractor's work, although the employer does control ultimately the overall specifications and quality of the contractor's performance.

The Georgia Appellate Court, adhering to this traditional legal concept, held in 1969 that the hospital was not liable for the negligence of a physician who was staffing the emergency department as a member of a medical partnership under contract with the hospital. The court observed that the hospital retained no control over individual professional decisions of the physicians, and that the contract in this case expressly said the doctors were considered independent contractors. Identification of the partnership's general responsibilities and surveillance of standards of practice by the medical staff were not sufficient "control" to deny the hospital the defense of independent contractor. Accordingly, dismissal of the action was proper.[35]

A contrary result has been reached by the Supreme Court of Delaware. Even if a physician is an independent contractor vis-a-vis the hospital, the hospital can be held liable for the negligence of the doctor if the institution has "held out" or "represented" to the patient that the doctor is its agent or employee. This is the doctrine of apparent agency that, when applicable, justifies the imposition of liability on the hospital for the wrong of one who is not in fact an employee of the hospital. In *Vanaman v. Milford Memorial Hospital, Inc.*, the patient had twisted her ankle and appeared at the emergency room for treatment. The family physician was not available. Since the patient and her mother indicated no preference with respect to physicians, the staff doctor on call was summoned. His treatment resulted in further injury to the patient. The trial court dismissed the suit against the hospital on the general basis that the institution had not held itself out as a "provider of medical care." On appeal, however, the state's supreme court reversed, saying that the jury must decide whether the doctor was acting in his private capacity or staffing the emergency room as agent of the hospital.[36] The fact that the physician was not paid directly by the hospital is relevant, but not conclusive.

Subsequent to *Vanaman* the same court held that a hospital could be liable for the negligence of a physician who was a partner of a medical partnership under contract to provide coverage of the emergency room. Again, the Delaware court denied the hospital's defense of independent contractor on the basis of the "holding out" or apparent agency doctrine. It was improper, the court said, to grant a summary judgment for the hospital, and a new trial must

[35] *Pogue v. Hospital Authority of DeKalb County*, 120 Ga. App. 230, 170 S.E. 2d 53 (1969). See also: *Dumer v. St. Michael's Hospital*, 69 Wis. 2d 766, 233 N.W. 2d 372 (1975). (A hospital was not liable for alleged negligence of a physician who was a member of Physicians Emergency Service Corporation, under contract with the hospital.) Compare: *Newton County Hospital v. Nickolson*, 132 Ga. App. 164, 207 S.E. 2d 659 (1974). (The hospital was liable for an emergency room physician's negligence when he was paid an hourly wage and his schedule was controlled by the hospital.)
[36] 272 A. 2d 718 (Delaware 1970). Cases with similar reasoning are *Lundberg v. Bay View Hospital*, 175 Ohio St. 133, 191 N.E. 2d 821 (1963), involving a pathologist, and *Kober v. Stewart*, 148 Mont. 117, 417 P. 2d 476 (1966), involving radiologists.

be held to determine, in effect, whether the patient relied upon the hospital to provide medical service.[37] The decision is directly contrary to the *Pogue* case in Georgia, since in Delaware a contractual clause reciting that the emergency room physicians are to be considered independent contractors would clearly not be regarded as a bar to the plaintiff's action against the hospital.

It is evident, of course, that not all hospitals are able to provide physicians in the emergency room at all times or even have them available on call around the clock. From a legal point of view, hospitals providing such limited emergency service should make their limitations clear, in a tactful manner, to their respective communities. The institution should not give the impression of full-service capabilities when these are lacking.

In metropolitan and suburban areas having several hospitals with overlapping services, not all of these institutions should undertake, or represent that they undertake, full emergency service. Regional planning and rationalization of facilities and services are needed, accomplished either through voluntary action that is truly effective or by statutory laws for the planning of health facilities. Perhaps some hospitals should have no emergency facility, others limited capabilities, and still others full service and permanent staffing. After the development and implementation of such regional plans, the public in general and police agencies and ambulance companies in particular should be made aware of each hospital's capability for emergency care. Not only is such regional planning necessary as a matter of the economics of health care, it is necessary to the quality of care. Improvement of care in the whole community will help to alleviate the legal problems currently facing hospital emergency departments. Such "categorization" of emergency care facilities is legally permissible as long as there is no misrepresentation to the public regarding the capabilities of a given hospital and the quality of care available at any given institution. Categorization is best accomplished, legally, through appropriate rules and regulations of a governmental agency responsible for hospital licensure. As noted earlier in this chapter, this has been done in Illinois.

---

[37] *Schagrin v. Wilmington Medical Center*, 304 A. 2d 61 (Delaware 1973). See also: *Mduba v. Benedictine Hospital*, 384 N.Y.S. 2d 527, 52 A.D. 2d 450 (1976). (A physician operating the emergency room was an employee of the hospital despite contractual language to the contrary, since the hospital controlled the means or manner of achieving emergency care through rules and regulations. Even if the physician was not an employee, the hospital was liable for his negligence, since it held itself out to the public as furnishing emergency care.)

The Good Samaritan Statutes

Most states have enacted statutes typically known as Good Samaritan laws. From the point of view of public policy the purpose of the statutes is to encourage physicians and other professional persons to extend aid at the scene of an emergency even though no physician-patient relationship already exists. Legally, the essence of the legislation is to provide that a physician, registered nurse, or other professional person as designated by each particular statute is not to be held liable for ordinary negligence or malpractice when extending aid at the scene of an emergency, as long as the aid is extended in good faith and without gross negligence or willful and wanton misconduct. Although the applicability of each statute to designated professional personnel and to particular factual situations depends upon the precise statutory language of each state, several general observations can be useful.

The statutes were really unnecessary as a matter of law and legal liability and can be further criticized on the basis that their coverage is limited only to certain persons who aid in an emergency. None of the statutes are applicable to laymen or professional persons not specifically designated in the relevant local statute, and such individuals are still held to the well-recognized common law rule that the beginning of aid raises the duty to exercise reasonable care under all the facts and circumstances. Further, very few, if any, actual lawsuits are on record against a defendant physician, nurse, or ambulance attendant alleging negligence in rendering aid to a victim of a medical emergency on a highway or at the scene of an out-of-hospital emergency. The fear of suit and liability which prompted the enactment of the Good Samaritan legislation was accordingly unfounded. Moreover, "reasonable care" at the scene of an out-of-hospital emergency would be a rather minimal requirement, inasmuch as the common law would not expect a physician, for instance, to possess life-saving equipment or drugs when he gives aid at the scene of a highway accident or treats the victim of sudden illness. Finally, even though most of these statutes, as enacted at present, are not clear on the matter, it is generally believed that they would not be applicable to an emergency in a hospital or to care being rendered in a hospital emergency room.[38] Hence, in none of the cases discussed and cited in this chapter was the Good Samaritan statute an issue.

---

[38] See: *Guerrero v. Copper Queen Hospital*, 537 P. 2d 1329 (Ariz. 1975).

In some states, however, there is currently an effort to extend immunity for ordinary negligence to the hospital emergency, at least in circumstances where medical persons attending the stricken patient have not previously established a doctor-patient relationship or otherwise have a duty to aid. Such attempts to enact legislation of this nature represent one of several approaches to alleviate the current costs and burdens of malpractice litigation. In the judgment of this writer, however, such legislation, which grants immunity to individual physicians and nurses from liability for malpractice, and which may reestablish institutional immunity for the negligent acts of professional personnel, is not the proper approach—from the viewpoint of public policy—to the malpractice situation.

VIII

Consent for Treatment

In Anglo-American law it is a fundamental principle that the consent of the patient, or of someone authorized to act for a legally incompetent patient, must be obtained before any medical or surgical treatment is undertaken, unless an emergency justifies treatment without consent. The reason for this is that any unpermitted, intentional touching of the patient's person constitutes the tort of assault and battery.

Any unpermitted touching constitutes an assault and battery even if the person touched is not harmed or injured in any way. Indeed, the wrong exists even when the person touched has benefited; the good faith of the one committing the wrong is immaterial and not relevant. Assault and battery is one of the intentional torts, or personal wrongs, as distinguished from negligence or malpractice. The requisite of intent, however, is fulfilled simply by showing that the defendant intended to touch; it is not necessary to show that he possessed an evil intent, or intended to harm or injure the patient.

Once the wrong has been established, the patient has a cause of action and may sue for damages. If he has, in fact, been physically injured by the assault and battery or has suffered pain and disability, the damages are compensatory in nature and could be substantial. If he has not been injured, the patient's recovery is limited to a nominal sum. Upon proper proof, loss of wages could be an element in the calculation of damages.

In certain situations an assault and battery may be a criminal act as well as a civil wrong. The wrongdoer could then be prosecuted by the state in addition to being subjected to a civil lawsuit. Indeed, even if consent is obtained for a given touching, a crime may have been committed—for example, in the performance of an unlawful abortion—and a civil cause of action might also be brought in spite of consent granted.

Furthermore, in most states if a battery is committed on a married woman, her husband probably has the right to bring his own cause of action for damages for loss of consortium and loss of his wife's services. Similarly, an increasing number of states are now recognizing a wife's right to bring action for loss of her husband's consortium. This does not mean, however, that a spouse's consent is necessary for treatment of the patient. As explained elsewhere, if an adult, mentally competent patient gives an effective consent, the consent of the spouse is generally not required.

The law of assault and battery emphasizes, of course, that a mentally competent adult is the master of his own person. Generally, medical or surgical treatment cannot be forced on a patient against his will, regardless of the urgency of the situation, unless some especially strong social policy is called into play to protect the interests of others.[1] It can therefore be said that a competent adult has the right to die if he wishes; as will be seen, however, courts have sometimes ordered that care be rendered even when a competent adult has expressly refused it. Regarding minors or the mentally incompetent, the same generalization applies. Medical treatment cannot be rendered over the objection of the parents or guardian, although the courts often protect the patient in such situations. When the patient cannot speak for himself because of incompetency, the law demands that someone in the proper position of authority speak for him.

The classic judicial statement supporting the foregoing general principles is by Justice Cardozo in *Schloendorff v. Society of New York Hospital:*

> Every human being of adult years and sound mind has a right to determine what shall be done with his own body; and a surgeon who performs an operation without his patient's consent commits an assault for which he is liable in damages. This is true except in cases of emergency, where the patient is unconscious and where it is necessary to operate before consent can be obtained.[2]

---

[1] *Jacobson v. Massachusetts,* 197 U.S. 11, 49 L. Ed. 643, 25 S. Ct. 358 (1905): (Compulsory smallpox vaccination was held not in violation of a patient's constitutional rights). *Buck v. Bell,* 274 U.S. 200, 71 L. Ed. 1000, 47 S. Ct. 584 (1927): (A compulsory eugenic sterilization statute was held to be constitutional).
[2] 211 N.Y. 125, 129, 105 N.E. 92, 93 (1914).

The tort of assault and battery must be carefully distinguished from malpractice. Malpractice is professional negligence, or the failure to adhere to legally imposed professional standards. Liability is based upon deviation from the standards of medical practice as determined by reasonably prudent practitioners of the art of medicine in the same or similar communities under similar facts and circumstances; or sometimes it is based simply on lack of reasonable care. In contrast, assault and battery is an intentional tort, as distinguished from negligence, and the wrong can occur even if all established professional standards have been followed in a given case. Lack of care is not relevant to a determination of whether or not an assault and battery has occurred. Both the torts of assault and battery and of malpractice may result, however, from a failure to obtain proper consent.

Court decisions have emphasized, as a legal necessity, that an effective consent must be an "informed consent." To grant an informed consent the patient must possess reasonably complete information about the advised medical treatment or surgery. The courts have said that if a doctor fails to warn the patient adequately regarding the risks accompanying the contemplated treatment or surgical procedure, the acceptable alternate methods of treatment, and the contemplated benefits of the proposed course, the consent given is not "informed" and is hence ineffective. Thus such a failure by the physician would result in liability for damages.

Several leading decisions stressing this doctrine of informed consent have focused on negligence or malpractice in evaluating how far a physician must go in explaining the risks of surgery or care, the alternative methods of treatment, and the probable results of each alternative. Some overlapping and legal confusion have hence arisen between the historically separate and distinct torts of battery and negligence.

It is, of course, not unusual or contradictory for the plaintiff's attorney to bring two separate allegations against a physician or a hospital in the same lawsuit. One allegation would be based upon a cause of action founded in negligence and the other upon assault and battery. In such situations the court must make clear the essential legal requirements of each alleged wrong when it gives instructions to the jury. Not only do the substantive rules of law differ with respect to these different causes of action, but the statute of limitations may also differ.

Perhaps the clearest factual example of the overlap between a cause of action based on assault and battery and one based on negligence occurs when the patient's identity is mistaken in surgery or in administering medication. When the wrong patient undergoes surgery or receives medication, the tort of assault and battery has clearly occurred. Another example is surgery applied to a properly identified patient but to the wrong part of the body, for instance, amputation of the patient's left leg when the right leg required the surgery.[3] Here again, a case of battery could be clearly established as long as the patient had consented only to surgery on the right leg. In such cases there would be no legal necessity for the aggrieved patient to prove lack of reasonable care, or malpractice, on the part of the physician or hospital personnel through the use of expert medical witnesses or application of the doctrine res ipsa loquitur. Many of these cases do proceed in the courts on a theory of negligence, however, simply because negligence is relatively easy to prove whenever there has been mistaken identity or a mistake regarding the part of the body requiring surgery.[4]

Types of Consent and Recommended Procedure

Legally sufficient consent can be classified as either express or implied in fact. The latter is often referred to as voluntary submission. The difference between an express consent and an implied consent lies in the method by which the patient, or the one authorized to consent for him, manifests his consent. Express consent is manifested by words, oral or written, while implied consent is manifested by acts on the part of the patient and by all the circumstances surrounding the rendering of medical or surgical treatment. Both types of consent, to be sufficient, require that the patient, or the one authorized to consent for him, be conscious, be legally capable of giving consent and competent to do so, and possess knowledge and understanding regarding the medical or surgical treatment that is about to occur. Lack of knowledge and understanding regarding the nature and extent of the medical care that is purportedly consented to can overcome either express or implied consent presumably given.

Legally, therefore, consent need not be in writing. Oral express consent, if proved, is adequate. Moreover a completely evident situation of voluntary submission is clearly adequate to protect the

[3] *Moos v. United States*, 225 F. 2d 705 (8th Cir. 1955).
[4] Moreover there is some authority for the proposition that any unauthorized surgery, although clearly an assault and battery, also amounts to malpractice, thereby granting to plaintiff the benefit of the statute of limitations pertaining to malpractice, which may be longer than the statute pertaining to battery. *Physicians and Dentists Business Bureau v. Dray*, 8 Wash. 2d 38, 111 P. 2d 568 (1941).

physician, nurse, or hospital from allegations of nonconsensual touching. To illustrate, a routine physical examination of a mentally competent, adult patient in a physician's office, or of a minor accompanied by a parent, need not be fortified by an express oral or written consent. A further illustration of a voluntary submission, or consent implied in fact, is a patient in labor presenting herself at the maternity department of a hospital.

When physicians or hospitals rely upon an oral consent or upon implied-in-fact consent, however, at least two very real related problems of proof arise. First is the question of whether the patient, or the one authorized to consent for him, in fact consented to any treatment at all. Consent may be difficult to prove if reliance must be placed upon an alleged oral consent or upon implication from the facts of the particular case. Secondly, even if consent of some sort is established, a further question is whether the one consenting had full understanding and knowledge regarding the nature and the extent of the treatment that was in fact rendered.

Even when a written consent is obtained, subsequent proof by the patient that he or she lacked knowledge and understanding of what in fact took place will negate the written consent. Hence one should never use a written consent purporting in very general language to authorize the surgeon or physician to do any procedure that he deems necessary in his professional judgment for the welfare of the patient. Such vague, general consent forms are no better protection for the physician and the hospital than simple reliance upon voluntary submission. To illustrate, in *Rogers v. Lumberman's Mutual Casualty Company*, the patient signed such a general consent form. The defendant surgeon successfully performed a hysterectomy. Subsequently the patient established that she thought she was consenting to an appendectomy, and she had not understood that the operation was to be a hysterectomy. No evidence existed of an emergency demanding immediate action by the surgeon to preserve life or health, hence the written, generalized consent was worthless to the physician. The fact that the surgery was skillfully performed and the fact that a hysterectomy was medically advisable were immaterial, since these reasons do not justify proceeding without consent.[5]

---

[5] 119 So. 2d 649 (La. Ct. App. 1960). See also: *Pegram v. Sisco*, 406 F. Supp. 776 (D. Ark. 1976). (A signed consent form in generalized language does not relieve a surgeon from explaining the nature of the diagnosis, the material elements and the risks of a recommended treatment utilizing radium implants, as well as alternative methods of treatment.)

Physicians and hospitals are therefore strongly advised to utilize two different written consent forms. The first should be obtained at the time of the patient's admission to the hospital, perhaps by the person processing the admission. It should recite simply that the patient, or the one authorized to act for him, consents to routine hospital care, nursing service, and diagnostic procedures. The form should name the attending physician, and the wording should recognize that others—nurses and laboratory technicians, for instance—will touch the patient during his hospitalization. The form should recite that no guarantees of cure have been made to the patient and that he fully understands the nature of the medical care to which he is consenting.

In addition to the consent form obtained at the time of admission, the hospital should insist upon obtaining a separate, special consent form whenever any surgery is undertaken, any anesthesia is used, any radium or x-ray therapy is employed, or any special diagnostic procedures are indicated. Other situations may arise where the special consent form should be employed. The guiding principle should be to use a special form whenever the in-hospital procedure or treatment is classified as something more than routine hospital care.

The signature on the special consent form should be obtained by the attending physician, or by an intern or resident physician associated with the case, not by a nurse or some member of the hospital's administrative staff. The reason is that the patient must fully understand the nature and extent of the surgical or medical procedure about to be undertaken if his consent is to be effective. Only a physician can properly convey the required knowledge and understanding.

The form should name the physician or surgeon, authorize him to select assistants, list the procedures to be undertaken, recite that the patient understands the procedures, recite consent to the administration of anesthesia under the supervision of a named physician or nurse, and state that the patient has received an explanation of the contemplated procedures. In addition, the language should recognize that unforeseen conditions arising during the surgery may dictate additional or different procedures from those contemplated, and that the patient realizes this and consents to such additional or different procedures as may in the professional judgment of the surgeon or physician be advisable.

It is elementary, of course, that any consent obtained by fraudulent misrepresentation is no consent at all. Moreover, signatures obtained after the partial administration of anesthesia or while the patient is under the influence of drugs may be worthless in proving valid consent, if the patient is able to show that his condition at the time of signing prevented him from fully understanding the consequences of his purported consent.[6]

Sometimes it is thought that the coordinated use of two written consent forms is unnecessary "paperwork" for physicians and hospital personnel. It is also sometimes argued that the procurement of written forms represents undue interference with sound medical practice and patient-physician relationships. One hears that patients as well as medical practitioners resent the use of consent forms and that such forms may make a patient even more apprehensive about his condition.

Experience indicates that the tactful, professional use of consent forms should have opposite effects. Certainly for the hospital and for the medical profession the use of the recommended consent forms ensures inexpensive protection from claims, perhaps unjust claims, of nonconsensual surgery or medical treatment. From the viewpoint of the patient-physician relationship, the use of the forms should increase, not decrease, the patient's understanding and should improve communication between the parties. Tactful application of techniques that make for better communication between doctor and patient should be encouraged. For that reason these consent procedures are recommended here, not solely as a matter of legalistic formality.

Consent in Emergencies

In a medical emergency no consent at all is required. The law, in effect, presumes that consent has been given, and the lack of an express or implied-in-fact consent will not justify an action based upon assault and battery or negligence against a physician or hospital. This rule applies to all patients regardless of age and is sometimes called consent implied by law.

It is not always easy, however, to define a medical emergency. To justify medical treatment without consent, the defendant must show, first, that it was not possible at the time treatment was undertaken to obtain the consent of the patient or the consent of the person authorized to act for him. One must always remember

---

[6]An example is found in a recent case, *Demers v. Gerety*, 85 N.M. 641, 515 P. 2d 645 (Ct. App. 1973). (A consent form signed when the patient was under the influence of nembutal was not effective.) There are many other cases involving similar factual situations. *Rev'd and remanded on procedural grounds, Gerety v. Demers*, 86 N.M. 141, 520 P. 2d 869 (1974).

that a conscious, competent adult is generally entitled to refuse medical aid, even if failure to receive immediate care is likely to result in death. Hence treatment without consent is permissible only when the patient or the one authorized to act for him is unable to express his wishes. The medical need for a prompt operation or treatment is not tantamount to an emergency.

Secondly, the traditional legal concept of a medical emergency demands a situation where there is an immediate threat to life, or a threat of permanent impairment of health. According to some judicial decisions, if delaying treatment while consent is obtained would not increase the hazards to the patient, the "emergency" is not sufficient to justify treatment without consent.[7] Some cases, however, appear to have liberalized the traditional legal definition of an emergency by permitting treatment without consent whenever immediate action is necessary to alleviate pain and suffering, even though no threat of irreparable harm is present.[8]

The doctor who treats without consent always has the burden of proof. That is, he must establish by the preponderance of the evidence that an emergency existed. Physicians and other medical personnel who treat without consent should thus make every reasonable effort to document the circumstances in such a situation. Adequate notes should be included in the medical record explaining the immediate threat to life or health. Consultation with other physicians, if they are available and time permits, is most wise and helpful in justifying the attending physician's action.

Akin to the medical emergency, where treatment can proceed without consent, is the discovery of unanticipated conditions during surgery. The legal question is whether the surgeon is justified in extending the surgery to correct the unanticipated or undiagnosed conditions. Certainly, if the patient consented to a given procedure at a time when he was competent and rational, and if he specifically prohibited any extension of the procedure, then the surgeon must not perform any extension, even if life depends upon such extension. Normally, however, there will not be any specific instructions from the patient prohibiting extensions of surgery. The traditional and older legal rule is that the surgeon must not engage in any extension

---

[7] An example is *Zoski v. Gaines*, 271 Mich. 1, 260 N.W. 99 (1935). (A surgeon was held liable for removal of a minor's tonsils without parental consent. Although the tonsils were infected, there was no immediate threat to life or health.) For a contrasting situation involving an immediate threat to life or health see *Luka v. Lowrie*, 171 Mich. 122, 136 N.W. 1106 (1912), discussed in the section on consent for treatment of minors.

[8] *Sullivan v. Montgomery*, 155 Misc. 448, 279 N.Y.S. 575 (New York City Ct. 1935).

of the contemplated procedure unless he encounters an unanticipated condition during surgery which must be corrected at once to obviate an immediate threat to life or a permanent impairment of health.[9]

Some cases, however, have developed a more liberal legal rule: a surgeon may extend the originally contemplated surgery whenever an unanticipated condition becomes evident during surgery and makes it medically advisable in his professional judgment to correct the condition immediately.[10] This liberalized approach, however, is not legal sanction to the surgeon to proceed without consent whenever he thinks it advisable. The courts will still insist that medical and surgical treatment is a matter for the patient to decide. The more liberal legal approach is rather based upon the undoubtedly justified assumption that, perhaps to avoid a second operation at a later time, the patient would have consented if the extension had been foreseeable, or that he would consent during surgery if he were not under anesthesia. These assumptions become a limitation upon the surgeon's right to proceed with the extension, in the sense that he must justify the probability that express consent would have been granted if it had been possible. Moreover, such a liberal approach is undoubtedly limited to surgical extensions involving the same incision as the primary procedure, and also to situations not entailing substantially different risks from those originally contemplated.

A relatively recent American case illustrating the more liberal approach to the question of surgical extensions is *Kennedy v. Parrott*.[11] In this litigation it was shown that the patient had expressly consented to an appendectomy. During the operation the surgeon discovered follicular cysts on the ovaries and punctured the cysts. The court held that this action was justified and that a battery had not been committed.

To sum up, it would appear wise to include in the surgical consent form a statement that the surgeon and his assistants may, in the exercise of their professional judgment, extend the originally contemplated procedure to correct or alleviate unanticipated conditions discovered during the course of the operation. Such language in the consent form and the liberalized attitude of the courts are both consistent with common sense and good surgical technique. Physicians realize and patients should also realize that a precise diagnosis is

---

[9] *Mohr v. Williams*, 95 Minn. 261, 104 N.W. 12 (1905). See also: *Tabor v. Scobee*, 254 S.W. 2d 474, (Ky. Ct. App. 1951). (During surgery a surgeon discovered infected fallopian tubes; it was ruled that he might not extend the operation and remove the tubes without consent unless an immediate threat to life or health existed.)
[10] *Bennan v. Parsonnet*, 83 N.J.L. 20, 83 A. 948 (Sup. Ct. 1912).
[11] 243 N.C. 355, 90 S.E. 2d 754, 56 A.L.R. 2d 686 (1956).

frequently difficult if not impossible prior to surgery. Physicians should adequately explain to the patient the frequent advisability of surgical extensions. With proper explanations of this kind before the surgery is undertaken, the surgeon has no need to fear that a medically justified extension will produce a claim by the patient that he was treated without consent.

The Hospital's Role in Consent Cases

Most lawsuits alleging lack of consent are brought against the individual who allegedly committed the wrong, the most likely individual being the attending physician or surgeon. Any professional or nonprofessional person, however, could be the alleged wrongdoer, and hence all individuals having responsibility for patients must be familiar with the law protecting the patient from nonconsensual touchings.

Further, attorneys for the plaintiff show an increasing tendency to bring assault and battery or negligence actions against the hospital, either as a sole defendant or as one of several defendants. It is not unusual for a suit to be brought against the hospital as well as against all the individuals who by reason of one legal theory or another are supposedly responsible for the alleged wrong.

In actions arising out of an assault and battery or negligence, the hospital can be liable on either one of two theories. First, it is liable vicariously for the torts of its employees committed within the scope of their employment. This is the doctrine of respondeat superior, which is translated as "Let the master answer." The theory rests upon the principle that an employer should be liable for the personal wrongs his employees commit while they are furthering his business.

The second theory, in contrast to the doctrine of respondeat superior, is based upon the hospital's own corporate neglect or fault in failing to see that treatment without proper consent does not take place upon its premises. If a hospital knows, or if in the exercise of reasonable care it should know, that a battery or negligence is about to be committed upon its premises and does nothing to prevent the event, the hospital is quite likely to be liable in damages to the aggrieved patient. This theory is actually a theory in corporate or institutional negligence: the hospital has failed to perform a duty it owes to the patient.

When the patient who is the victim of a tort proceeds against the hospital upon the theory of respondeat superior he must establish, first, that the individual committing the wrong was an employee of the hospital. Legally, an "employee" is an agent or a servant of the hospital and should be distinguished from an independent contractor. An individual is an agent or a servant whenever the hospital has the right to control the means and the methods of the employee's work. This is in contrast to the relation between an employer and an independent contractor, in which the employer has the right to specify or control the final results of the contractor's work but has surrendered the right to control the means and the methods of accomplishing the final results. An agent differs from a servant in that the former is employed, subject to the employer's control, to negotiate contracts with third parties on behalf of the employer-principal, while a servant is employed to perform mechanical tasks for the employer-master.

Respondeat superior holds the master liable for the torts of his servant and the principal liable for the torts of his agent; but, since the employer has no right to control the activities of independent contractors, he is not liable as a rule to third parties for their torts. In the hospital setting, it can generally be said that all nonprofessional people, as well as nurses, x-ray technicians, physiotherapists, interns, and resident physicians are either agents or servants. As a result, the hospital would normally be liable for torts committed by these individuals.[12] In some states a staff physician is considered to be in the employ of the hospital in some circumstances, thus rendering the hospital liable for his torts under the theory of respondeat superior. Having established that the individual committing the wrong was an agent or a servant, the patient must further establish that the wrong was committed within the scope of employment. This is done simply by showing that the tort was committed while furthering the employer's business. As we shall see, the doctrine of respondeat superior comes into play in other questions of hospitals' liability. Here it is mentioned to emphasize that it is applicable to cases alleging treatment without proper consent.

Staff physicians are generally not agents or servants of the hospital but independent contractors. Normally therefore the hospital would not be liable for treatment by a staff physician without the patient's consent so far as the doctrine of respondeat superior is concerned,

---

[12]For example: *Inderbitzen v. Lane Hospital*, 124 Cal. App. 462, 12 P. 2d 744 (Dist. Ct. App. 1932). (A hospital was held liable for permitting medical students, who were under hospital control and hence employees, to examine a patient without her consent.)

at least when the doctor had been privately employed by the patient. In some states, however, the payment of a salary is considered sufficient to invoke this doctrine and thus to hold the hospital liable for the battery or negligence of the physician. Moreover some courts have developed the theory of "ostensible" or "apparent" agency to justify holding the hospital liable for the tort of one who in fact is an independent contractor. This theory rests upon the notion that the hospital has acted to "hold out" to the patient, or represent to him, that a given physician is in its employ. In the cases to date, the hospital procured the physician for the patient, in contrast to a situation where the patient expressly employed his own doctor.

Exceptions to the general result that a hospital is liable under the doctrine of respondeat superior for the torts of an agent or a servant would be created for governmental hospitals in some jurisdictions by the governmental immunity doctrine, and in a very few states for the voluntary hospital by the charitable immunity doctrine. Aside from possible immunity, the only other exception would be the borrowed- or loaned-servant rule.

The borrowed-servant rule has the effect of insulating the usual and general employer, the hospital, from liability for the torts of an agent or servant if the tort was committed while the agent or servant was temporarily working under the control of someone not an employee of the hospital. To illustrate, a registered nurse is generally an agent or a servant of the hospital while performing her usual and customary nursing functions. However, she may on occasion be called upon to work under the direct control of a staff physician or surgeon who is not himself in the employ of the hospital, and thereupon she would temporarily leave the employ of the hospital. If she should treat a patient without proper consent while under the direct control of a staff physician or surgeon, the hospital would not be liable under respondeat superior for her act. The physician, as her new and temporary employer, would be liable vicariously for her wrong.

The performance by a nurse of routine nursing care and treatment, including the administration of drugs pursuant to the order of a staff physician, is not enough to invoke the borrowed-servant rule. The right of a physician who is not an employee to control her acts must be more immediate and direct to justify a finding that a nurse, intern, resident, or other hospital employee has temporarily left the employ of the hospital and entered into an employment relationship with another. Accordingly the borrowed-servant rule has been frequently applied when the nurse, intern, or resident physician is assisting in surgery or in the delivery room of a maternity department. These principles of judicial law are more thoroughly discussed in the chapter on hospital liability.

When the patient proceeds against the hospital on the theory that the institution has violated its direct duty to use reasonable care in ascertaining that batteries do not occur on the hospital premises, he need not establish that the alleged wrongdoer was an employee of the hospital. It is only necessary, after establishing that a nonconsensual touching did occur, to show that the hospital knew or in the exercise of reasonable care should have known that a battery or negligence was about to occur and did nothing to prevent the act.

Previous discussion has emphasized that consent must be an "informed consent" and that hospitals and their medical staffs should use two separate written consent forms. The first would be obtained at the time of admission to the hospital and would cover routine hospital care; the second would pertain to surgical procedures and extraordinary or high-risk diagnostic procedures. Also stressed was the principle that the patient's signature on the second consent form should be obtained by the attending physician and not by the hospital's administrative or nursing personnel, since only a doctor is professionally qualified to see that the consent is "informed."

The issue that then arises is this: how far must a hospital go in making certain that its medical staff physicians are in fact obtaining the informed consent of their patients? If a hospital is to protect itself from liability for treatment or surgery without consent, the hospital must as a minimum have administrative rules and regulations regarding the procurement of a properly drafted written consent. Having adopted rules and regulations, it must then devise procedures to ensure enforcement of the rules. Operating room supervisors or the chief surgical nurse should be assigned the responsibility of checking on the patient's identity and of making certain that no surgery is undertaken before proper consent is obtained. Do hospital personnel need to go even further and inquire whether the private attending physician or surgeon has explained the contemplated treatment or procedure well enough to meet the legal tests of informed consent? A New York court said no in *Fiorentino v. Wenger*.[13]

---

[13]*Fiorentino v. Wenger*, 280 N.Y. Supp. 2d 373, 19 N.Y. 2d 407, 227 N.E. 2d 296 (1967). *Cf.: Parr v. Palmyra Hospital*, 228 S.E. 2d 596 (Ga. App. 1976). (A Georgia statute providing that a written consent to medical and surgical treatment shall be conclusively presumed valid in the absence of fraudulent misrepresentations of material facts applies to hospitals as well as physicians.)

In this case the hospital personnel had no reason to know that the doctor's explanation was inadequate when he asked the father of a minor patient to sign the written consent form for surgery. Nor was the hospital aware that the surgery itself constituted malpractice, the surgery on the spine of the patient not being generally recognized in the medical profession as acceptable. The defendant surgeon himself had developed the particular procedure and was at the time the only surgeon utilizing the particular techniques. In the absence of proof that the hospital knew or should have known that the surgeon failed to furnish adequate information to the father of the patient, or that conduct of the surgery would be malpractice, the hospital was not held to be responsible.

In conclusion, so far as the doctrine of informed consent is concerned, the hospital appears to perform its duty to the patient by making private staff physicians aware that they must properly inform the patient and by insisting that adequate written consent forms be obtained and placed in the patient's medical chart. The hospital, in other words, need not be an actual party or participant in the privately employed physician's discussions with the patient or with the person legally authorized to consent for the patient. However, if nursing or administrative staff of the hospital know or ought to have known that a private physician has not obtained a legally sufficient consent, then the hospital has a duty to prevent the unauthorized surgery or treatment; liability could follow from a breach of this duty.

The Doctrine of Informed Consent

Since the patient is the master of his or her person, unless the facts and circumstances of the particular situation indicate an overriding social policy to the contrary, consent granted for medical care or surgery must be an informed consent, as emphasized throughout this chapter. But how far must a physician go in explaining to the patient the status of the diagnosis, the nature of the recommended treatment or procedure, the alternatives available, the possible or probable risks involved, and the expected benefits or outcome of the contemplated care?

The judicial cases on this question can be classified into three types. In the first, the issue is whether the physician has either affirmatively or by silence misrepresented the nature or character of the treatment or surgery. Illustrative of this type is *Rogers v. Lumberman's Mutual Casualty Company,* a case already mentioned, in which the patient understood that she was to undergo an appendectomy when in fact a hysterectomy was performed. The consent form, written in very general language and failing to name the surgical procedure to be performed, did not protect the doctor from liability.[14] This charge can be, in a sense, characterized as misrepresentation by silence, since the physician failed to explain the nature of the contemplated surgery and the medical indications of the patient's condition. The fiduciary duty that exists between the doctor and the patient certainly requires, as a minimum, full disclosure of the nature of the diagnosed condition, all material or significant facts concerning the condition, and an explanation of the more probable consequences and difficulties inherent in the situation.

The relatively old case of *Corn v. French* illustrates a doctor's affirmative misrepresentation of the surgery to be undertaken.[15] After examining the patient, the physician recommended that she submit to a "test" for a possible malignancy. The patient then asked her doctor if he intended to remove her breast. He apparently replied in the negative. She signed a written consent form indicating that a "mastectomy" was to be performed, but received no explanation of this medical term and did not, in fact, know what the word mastectomy meant. Clearly there was liability for an unauthorized operation, even without allegation or proof of medical malpractice in departing from acceptable professional treatment.

The second type of cases involving informed consent is based on the rule that the patient is entitled to know the inevitable risks or results of the contemplated surgery. To illustrate, in *Bang v. Charles T. Miller Hospital*, a Minnesota case decided in 1958, an elderly male patient expressly consented to a transurethral prostatic resection. He was not told that because of the particular circumstances, including his age, and the possibility of infection, the professionally acceptable surgical technique would inevitably render him sterile. Accordingly there was liability.[16] This case can also be cited as authority for the proposition that a patient is entitled to an explanation of the alternatives to treatment or surgical techniques. In this situation the surgeon should have explained to the patient that protecting his ability to father children might entail a substantial risk of infection.

The third type of case—and clearly the most difficult for both

---

[14] 119 So. 2d 649 (La. Ct. App. 1960). See also the case of *Darrah v. Kite*, 301 N.Y.S. 2d 286, 32 App. Div. 2d 208 (1969). (The father of a minor patient was told that "routine brain tests" and a "general work-up" was necessary. In fact, the surgeon opened the patient's skull and penetrated the brain itself. Whether informed consent had been obtained was a question for the jury.)
[15] 71 Nevada 280, 289 P. 2d 173 (1955).
[16] 251 Minn. 427, 88 N.W. 2d 186 (1958).

physicians and the courts—involves the duty to disclose the foreseeable collateral risks and hazards of the proposed treatment or surgery. These cases in turn break down into subcategories, or at least express differing legal theories or underlying philosophies, depending upon the particular facts and the particular jurisdictions in which they are decided.

Both of the leading cases of *Natanson v. Kline* in Kansas and *Mitchell v. Robinson* in Missouri seem to speak in terms of liability based upon negligence or malpractice for failure to disclose possibly serious collateral risks. In *Natanson* the physician recommended cobalt radiation therapy following removal of the patient's breast for cancer. The therapy was skillfully performed. The patient was not, however, informed that such therapy involved substantial risk of tissue damage. The Kansas Supreme Court held that the patient was entitled to be told in advance of probable consequences or hazards known to the doctor, and the physician was obligated to make "reasonable disclosures" as determined by what a reasonable medical practitioner would make under the same or similar circumstances.[17] Similarly, in *Mitchell* the Missouri Supreme Court said that plaintiff, who was given electroshock and insulin therapy, had the right to be informed that from 18 to 25 percent of such patients suffered convulsions as a result of the treatment. In this particular litigation a convulsion caused fractured vertebrae. Although there was no allegation or evidence of negligence or malpractice in the diagnosis or the recommendation for treatment by electroshock and insulin, the court held that a jury must decide the factual question of whether the defendant was negligent in failing to apprise the patient of the risks.[18] The duty owed was to make reasonable disclosure of significant facts and probable consequences.

When such liability is based upon the legal theory or cause of action involving negligence or malpractice, the plaintiff must generally establish by expert testimony what disclosures of risks and hazards a reasonable medical practitioner would make under the particular circumstances. The answer may in turn depend upon the custom or generally accepted professional standards of practice in the local

---

[17] 186 Kansas 393, 350 P. 2d 1093 (1960), *second opinion*, 187 Kansas 186, 354 P. 2d 670 (1960).

[18] 334 S.W. 2d 11, 79 A.L.R. 2d 1017 (Missouri 1960). (A retrial in this litigation resulted in a verdict for defendants as they satisfactorily proved that they had adequately informed the patient. 360 S.W. 2d 673 [Missouri 1962].) See also: *Shack v. Holland*, 389 N.Y.S. 2d 988 (Sup. Ct. 1976). (The absence of informed consent from a mother with respect to risks, hazards, and alternative delivery procedures is malpractice and gives to a child born permanently deformed a derivative cause of action; the statute of limitations begins to run when the child is twenty-one years old.)

medical community. For example, according to expert evidence, a risk of untoward damage to the voice existed in only 2 percent of the competently performed thyroidectomy operations, and it was not the custom of the medical profession in the area to warn patients of this risk. The court ruled that the defendant physician had no legal duty to disclose the risk.[19]

The plaintiff in a negligence action need not always present expert medical testimony to establish liability, since the court may rule as a matter of law that the physician had a duty to disclose. The Kansas court did so in *Natanson*, where the evidence is clear that there had been no explanation of risks at all. Nevertheless the usual malpractice action does require expert witness testimony to establish deviation from recognized professional standards or custom among practitioners, as was held in the *DiFilippo* case and others.[20]

By this line of decisions, if no expert witness testimony whatever is presented by the plaintiff to show the prevailing standards of disclosure in the medical community relevant to the particular case, then the court will rule as a matter of law for the defendant. On the other hand, if there is conflicting expert testimony, the matter usually becomes a question for the jury.

In *Collins v. Itoh*, a Montana decision, the court held that there must be expert testimony to establish negligence in a malpractice action, and that the duty of the physician was to disclose "known risks" which a "reasonable medical practitioner would disclose." This case arose from the performance of a thyroidectomy, to which the patient had consented. During the operation the surgeon removed a parathyroid gland, allegedly by mistake, thus causing a condition known as hypoparathyroidism, which required the administration of large amounts of calcium for the remainder of the patient's life to prevent severe cramps in the limbs. Testimony established that such a result from the removal of parathyroid tissue would be a

---

[19] *DiFilippo v. Preston*, 53 Del. 539, 173 A. 2d 333 (Sup. Ct. 1961).
[20] Also see: *Haggerty v. McCarthy*, 344 Mass 136, 181 N.E. 2d 562, 94 A.L.R. 2d 998 (1962). *Petterson v. Lynch*, 299 N.Y.S. 2d 244, 59 Misc. 2d 469 (Sup. Ct. 1969). *Govia v. Hunter*, 2 Wyo. 1, 374 P. 2d 421 (1962): (Plaintiff contended that she was not informed that a vein-stripping operation would disfigure her leg. Her case failed because of lack of proof that the defendant surgeon had deviated from the accepted practice of other competent surgeons). *Williams v. Menehan*, 191 Kansas 6, 379 P. 2d 292 (1963): (Custom among practitioners is the guide to how much information is to be given and how it is to be transmitted to the patient). *Bowers v. Talmage*, 159 So. 2d 888 (Florida Dist. Ct. App. 1964): (It was a question for the jury whether the neurologist fulfilled his duty of disclosing the risks of an arteriogram to the parents of a nine-year-old patient. According to expert testimony by a neurosurgeon, it was the custom of practitioners to disclose a 3 percent risk of paralysis). *Kaplan v. Haines*, 96 N.J. Super. 242, 232 A. 2d 840 (App. Div. 1967): (Expert testimony was required, and then the issue was one for the jury).

risk in only .5 to 3 percent of all thyroid surgery. Under such
circumstances the court held as a matter of law that the physician
had not breached any duty owed to the patient, and that there
was no issue to be submitted to the jury for decision.[21] The sole
fact that the patient incurred an injury does not justify an award
of damages, and the rare occurrence of removal of parathyroid tissue
does not in itself indicate any negligence by the defendant. Moreover,
testimony at the trial which attempted to establish the custom and
practice of a reasonable practitioner was inconclusive, failing to
determine general practice.

On the other hand, informed consent cases like *Corn v. French*
and *Bang v. Charles T. Miller Hospital*, which proceed on an assault
and battery cause of action, do not require expert testimony to support
a verdict for the plaintiff, since the facts can be established by credible
lay testimony. Further, punitive damages might be available to a
plaintiff in a battery action if he could establish an evil or malicious
intent on the part of the defendant, whereas only compensatory
damages for actual harm or injury are normally available in a cause
of action based upon negligence or malpractice.

Even when it may not be entirely clear whether the action is based
upon assault and battery or negligence, the holding of some recent
cases involving informed consent rejects the idea that the doctor's
duty to disclose is based upon the prevailing custom among similarly
situated practitioners, and hence that the plaintiff must produce
expert testimony to prove his case. A Florida court held that no
expert testimony was required to establish departure from customary
professional practice in a case where the patient was not informed
that orthopedic surgery on the hip was likely to leave one leg shorter
than the other.[22] All the patient had to do was convince the jury
that she would have withheld consent for the surgery had she been
so informed. California has also ruled that the plaintiff need not
establish deviation from the usual community standards of disclosure
in a suit alleging the absence of informed consent.[23] In sum, it would
seem that the fiduciary duty of the physician requires full disclosure
of all facts and risks which are relevant to the patient's granting
of an informed consent, regardless of what other physicians custom-

[21] 160 Mont. 461, 503 P. 2d 36 (1972).
[22] *Russell v. Harwick*, 166 So. 2d 904 (Fla. Dist. Ct. App. 1964).
[23] *Berkey v. Anderson*, 82 Cal. Rptr. 67, 1 Cal. App. 3d 790 (1969). See also: *Salgo v. Leland Stanford, Jr. University*, 154 Cal. App. 2d 560, 317 P. 2d 170 (1957). (The duty of a doctor is to disclose all facts necessary for a patient to form a basis for granting consent.)

arily disclose. The issue may still be one for the jury to decide, but it will rest on lay testimony rather than expert evidence.

The view that the nature and extent of a doctor's disclosure of collateral risks and hazards are to be measured by the prevailing standards of practice among similarly situated practitioners, thus normally requiring the patient to present expert medical testimony to prove a departure from standards, is of course highly favorable to the medical profession. It permits physicians to establish their own standards of extent of disclosure, and it burdens the plaintiff with the difficulty of obtaining expert witnesses in support of his case. Accordingly the trend of the cases, as noted above, is twofold: to adopt some other criteria of disclosure than those of prevailing professional standards of practice when the court or jury determines the duty of the physician; and to eliminate the evidentiary requirement of expert witness testimony.

Illustrating departures from the rule that the physician's duty to disclose is measured by generally accepted and prevailing medical standards are the *Berkey* case decided by the intermediate appellate court in California and the Pennsylvania decision in *Cooper v. Roberts*.[24] The first has already been cited. In the second, before undergoing a gastroscopic examination the patient signed a "blanket" consent form without being told of the risk of a perforated stomach. Actually the risk of such a perforation was minimal—one occurrence in 2,500 cases, according to scientific evidence at the trial. The plaintiff presented no expert medical testimony establishing the prevailing standards of practice relative to disclosure. Nevertheless a trial court's ruling for the defendant was reversed for a new trial, the appellate court ruling that the patient was entitled to know all facts, risks, and alternatives that a reasonable layman would consider material to his or her decision. In other words, the patient's right to know cannot be made dependent upon self-imposed standards of the medical profession as evidenced by expert witnesses. Such a rule only encourages physicians to remain silent or to provide minimal explanations to the patient.[25]

Also rejecting the concept that a physician must disclose to the extent that his peers disclose are three major 1972 decisions in Rhode

---

[24] 220 Pa. Super. 260, 286 A. 2d 647 (1971).
[25] Essentially the same ruling was made in a Washington appellate court decision, *Hunter v. Brown*, 4 Wash. App. 899, 484 P. 2d 1162 (1971), *aff'd*, Washington Supreme Court, 81 Wash. 2d 465, 502 P. 2d 1194 (1972). (The patient was an Oriental. Risks of adverse results of a dermabrasion procedure are greater for Orientals than for others, and she was entitled to know the risks relating to her situation.)

Island, California, and the Circuit Court of Appeals for the District of Columbia. All three were based on the theory of negligence and not battery. In the Rhode Island case, *Wilkinson v. Vesey*, the patient experienced pains in her limbs; the tentative diagnosis was "lymphoma of the mediastinum or possibly a substernal thyroid." Radiation therapy reduced the size of the shadow shown in the x-ray examination, and a diagnosis of malignancy was made although no biopsy was conducted. Further treatments by radiation resulted in severe radiation burns, which required eight subsequent operations, and it was eventually determined that the patient had never suffered from cancer.

In a suit based upon the absence of an informed consent along with other allegations, the Rhode Island Supreme Court reversed the trial court's directed verdict in favor of the defendant radiologists, ruling that the patient was entitled to be informed of all known material information and risks and need not present expert testimony pertaining to prevailing practices of other practitioners and the extent to which they customarily disclose.[26] The question of what the medical profession "knows" about risks in the particular treatment would require expert testimony, but the point here is that a lay jury can decide if sufficient disclosure was made of material hazards and risks to enable the patient to make an intelligent choice. "Materiality" was defined by the court in terms of both the "dangerousness" of the treatment or surgery and any other matters that would be significant to a reasonable person. The statistical remoteness of a risk does not determine its materiality, since even a very small hazard or chance of untoward result could well be significant to a reasonable person.

Similarly, the California Supreme Court in *Cobbs v. Grant* held that the extent and scope of disclosure is not to be measured by generally acceptable professional practices.[27] Rather, disclosure of known hazards, inherent risks, and untoward results must be based upon matters that are material to the individual patient's needs and decisional process, although to assert a successful claim the patient must apparently prove to the satisfaction of the jury that he as a reasonably prudent person would have refused consent for the treatment or surgery if he had been informed. This proof would then establish that insufficient information relative to the surgery

[26] 110 R.I. 606, 295 A. 2d 676 (1972).
[27] 104 Cal. Rptr. 505, 8 Cal. 3d 229, 502 P. 2d 1 (1972). *Accord: Trogun v. Fruchtman*, 58 Wisc. 2d 569, 207 N.W. 2d 297 (1973); *Riedinger v. Colburn*, 361 F. Supp. 1073 (D. Idaho 1973).

was the proximate cause of the injuries suffered. The physician need not disclose minor risks of common knowledge to the lay patient, nor must he disclose if the patient exhibits a desire not to be informed. Finally, disclosure is unnecessary if, in the physician's documented opinion, full revelation of material information would adversely affect the patient's rational decision about consenting to the recommended treatment.

In *Cobbs* the patient underwent surgery for a duodenal ulcer in the course of which an artery at the base of the spleen was severed. As a result that organ had to be removed. Still later a gastric ulcer required removal of 50 percent of the patient's stomach. Although the patient had consented to the initial surgery, he was not informed that injuries to the spleen occur in approximately 5 percent of such operations. At the trial court level the plaintiff made allegations against the hospital and the surgeon charging both malpractice and negligence: malpractice in the conduct of the surgery and subsequent care, and negligence in the failure to obtain an informed consent. The jury returned a verdict for plaintiff against the hospital for $45,000 and against the surgeon for $23,800.

When the surgeon appealed the verdict against him, the Supreme Court of California returned the matter for a new trial, saying that it could not determine whether the verdict against the surgeon was based on the theory of malpractice in the conduct of the surgery and care or the theory of negligence in failing to obtain an informed consent. If the former, the verdict was not justified because there was inadequate evidence to support a finding of malpractice in the conduct of the surgery. If, on the other hand, the judgment was based on an inadequate explanation to the patient of collateral risks and hazards, then the decision in favor of the plaintiff was proper, as long as it was consistent with the judicial guidelines noted in the case. In addition to the criteria for disclosure outlined above, the case emphasizes once again that the primary responsibility for obtaining an informed consent rests on the attending physician or surgeon who is to treat the patient.

As in *Cobbs v. Grant,* the Circuit Court of Appeals for the District of Columbia has stressed the right of the individual patient to decide what medical care or surgery he agrees to, as long as he is legally and mentally competent. In *Canterbury v. Spence,* the court stated the rule that the physician must disclose all material inherent and potential hazards of the proposed care or surgery, the anticipated benefits, any acceptable alternative methods of treatment, the severity and the degree of incidence of the risk, and the anticipated results if the patient should refuse consent.[28] Note especially these points: the extent and scope of the physician's duty to disclose is not to be determined by the custom of other like practitioners of medicine or surgery; there is an affirmative duty of disclosure whether or not the patient requests full information; and even a remote, statistically rare risk must be explained, because such a risk may nevertheless be material and significant to the patient in his decision-making process.

This, then, is the duty of the physician to exercise "reasonable care under the circumstances," unless he knows that the patient is already aware of the risk or that a given risk would not have any apparent materiality to the patient's decision, or unless he can establish that disclosure would adversely affect the rationality of a patient's decision. All such matters are to be submitted to the jury for decision without requiring plaintiff to provide expert testimony showing materiality of the nondisclosure, although experts must of course be used to establish medical facts—for example, to show that the patient's current condition is a result of the surgery or care rendered.

In the *Canterbury* case, a nineteen-year-old patient suffered partial paralysis and other untoward results following the performance of a laminectomy. Such paralysis was a remote risk of this particular surgery, present in approximately 1 percent of the cases. In the court's opinion, the plaintiff must convince the jury that he, a reasonably prudent person—as measured objectively and *not* subjectively—would not have consented to the surgery had he been informed of the risk of paralysis. This is to say that a patient as an individual may not rely on hindsight in denying that a reasonably prudent person in similar circumstances would have consented. Finally, to be noted in *Canterbury* is the court's ruling that the District of Columbia's three-year statute of limitations applicable to negligence causes of action controls the bringing of the action, not the one-year statute pertaining to assault and battery actions.

In summary, these three major 1972 cases treating the informed consent doctrine as a cause of action in negligence have removed the need for plaintiff to present expert medical testimony with respect to the required extent and scope of disclosure, and they have created judicial rules or criteria for disclosure in place of professional custom and practices. Truly the patient does seem to be the master of his own body and destiny, as Justice Cardozo asserted in *Schloendorff*

---

[28] 464 F. 2d 772 (D. C. Cir. 1972), *cert. denied*, 409 U.S. 1064 (1972).

v. Society of New York Hospital as long ago as 1914.[29]

In response, however, to the malpractice "crisis" which was widely publicized in 1974 and 1975 some courts have specifically rejected the holding of *Canterbury v. Spence*[30] and similar decisions. For example, the highest court of Virginia, although acknowledging that in certain circumstances ordinary human knowledge and experience would indicate that disclosure of risks was so obviously required that expert testimony should not be mandated, and further agreeing that in some situations lay testimony might be competent to show adverse consequences following treatment, has recently held the general rule to be that the patient must show by qualified medical experts whether and to what extent information should be disclosed by the physician.[31] *Canterbury,* in the view of the Virginia court, has the effect of permitting lay witnesses to express medical opinion, and such an effect is not desirable in factual situations, as alleged in *Bly.* In *Bly* plaintiff-patient had undergone a hysterectomy and exploratory surgery followed by complications requiring further surgery, and her suit was based in part upon allegations that the defendant physician had failed to inform her adequately of the risks of the surgery. Since the plaintiff presented no expert testimony with respect to the extent of disclosure required, the trial court granted a summary judgment for the defendant and this was affirmed on appeal.

Moreover, legislation has recently been enacted in several states modifying substantially. the liberalized "modern trend" of judicial decisions. For example, the Ohio statute provides a specific form of written consent containing precise language with respect to certain known risks associated with particular surgical or medical procedures. If the patient or his authorized representative is provided with and signs this statutory consent form, or if the written form utilized by the physician and the hospital meets certain statutory requirements, the form is presumed to be valid and effective, and no evidence shall be admissible in a subsequent lawsuit to impeach, modify, or limit the patient's authorization to perform the treatment or surgery, except where a preponderance of evidence proves that the person who obtained the consent was not acting in good faith, or that the signing of the consent form was induced by fraudulent misrepresentation of material facts, or that the person signing the form was

[29] 211 N.Y. 125, 129; 105 N.E. 92, 93 (1914).
[30] 464 F. 2d 772, (D. C. Cir. 1972), *cert. denied,* 409 U.S. 1064 (1972).
[31] *Bly v. Rhoads,* 222 S.E. 2d 783 (Va. 1976).

226 The Hospital-Patient Relation

unable to understand the language in which the form was written.[32]
Legislation in Hawaii authorizes the board of medical examiners
to establish reasonable standards, applicable to specific surgical and
treatment procedures, for information given to the patient in order
to make him reasonably aware of probable risks. The measure also
provides that these standards shall be prima facie evidence of the
standards of care required.[33] In sum, with respect to the doctrine
of informed consent, the new statutes establish statutory criteria for
written consent forms and the extent of disclosure required. If these
criteria are adhered to by the provider of medical care, the patient
may not later overcome the written document except upon proper
proof of extraordinary circumstances, as in Ohio or as in Hawaii,
unless the patient is able to prove by a preponderance of the evidence
that an informed consent, as contemplated by the statute, was not
obtained.[34]

The courts have recognized that the physician is privileged to
limit or withhold information from the patient for sound therapeutic
reasons.[35] For example, full disclosure might well complicate or hinder
treatment of the patient, depending upon his emotional state or
personal traits. Hence, in the interests of the patient's welfare the
physician may in his professional judgment provide a less than full
explanation of collateral risks and hazards in the proposed treatment
or surgery. The physician should of course document his reasons
for limiting or withholding information by appropriate notations
in the medical record. The privilege could not be successfully asserted
if the facts indicated that a competent and rational patient would
have declined treatment had he been informed.

As should be evident, it is especially important to obtain an informed
consent for any novel or "experimental" procedure or surgery (or
for the administration of experimental drugs) and to evidence the
obtaining of such consent with a specially drafted, written consent
form. In methods of treatment not yet accepted by the medical
profession generally, where the contemplated therapeutic benefits

---

[32]Ohio Revised Code, sec. 2317.54.
[33]Hawaii, H.B. 2700–76 (April 1976), sec. 3 of new chapter of Hawaii Revised Statutes
entitled "Medical Torts."
[34]Proposed legislation in Washington itemizes the necessary elements of proof in
a cause of action based upon the alleged absence of an informed consent and further
provides that a signed consent form meeting specified statutory criteria shall be prima
facie evidence that an informed consent was granted. Sec. 10, 11 S.H.B. 1470 (Feb.
1976).
[35]Roberts v. Woods, 206 F. Supp. 579, (S.D. Alabama 1962); Lester v. Aetna Casualty
Co., 240 F. 2d 676 (5th Cir. 1957); Starnes v. Taylor, 272 N.C. 386, 158 S.E. 2d
339 (1968).

are unknown or speculative, the facts as known and unknown to the physician become of material importance to the patient as he weighs his decision. In a recent case involving the well-known cardiologist and surgeon, Dr. Denton A. Cooley, and his colleague, Dr. Liotta, a soundly prepared consent form, together with actual testimony at trial, resulted in a court directed verdict for the physicians in a malpractice suit by the estate of a deceased surgical patient, alleging that the physicians had failed to obtain an informed consent for ventriculoplasty surgery.[36] The consent form, reproduced here, is an example of a well-drafted document:

> I, Haskell Karp, request and authorize Dr. Denton A. Cooley and such other surgeons as he may designate to perform upon me, in St. Luke's Episcopal Hospital of Houston, Texas, cardiac surgery for advanced cardiac decompensation and myocardial insufficiency as a result of numerous coronary occlusions. The risk of this surgery has been explained to me. In the event cardiac function cannot be restored by excision of destroyed heart muscle and plastic reconstruction of the ventricle and death seems imminent, I authorize Dr. Cooley and his staff to remove my diseased heart and insert a mechanical cardiac substitute. I understand that this mechanical device will not be permanent and ultimately will require a replacement by a heart transplant. I realize that this device has been tested in the laboratory but has not been used to sustain a human being and that no assurance of success can be made. I expect the surgeons to exercise every effort to preserve my life through any of these means. No assurance has been made by anyone as to the results that may be obtained.
>
> I understand that the operating surgeon will be occupied solely with the surgery and that the administration of the anesthetic(s) is an independent function. I hereby request and authorize Dr. Arthur S. Keats, or others he may designate, to administer such anesthetics as he or they may deem advisable.
>
> I hereby consent to the photographing of the operation to be performed, including appropriate portions of my body, for medical, scientific, and educational purposes.[37]

Without doubt the doctrine of informed consent raises significant problems for the physician and surgeon. Many of the fears expressed

---

[36] *Karp v. Cooley*, 349 F. Supp. 827 (S.D. Texas 1972), *aff'd*, 493 F. 2d 408 (5th Cir. 1974), *cert. denied*, 419 U.S. 845 (1974). See also: *Schwartz v. Boston Hospital for Women*, 422 F. Supp. 53 (S.D.N.Y. 1976). (A hospital has responsibility to obtain informed consent when the patient is a participant in a surgical research program.)
[37] *Karp v. Cooley*, 349 F. Supp. at 831.

by the medical community, however, are largely imaginary and unfounded. On balance the courts seem primarily interested in increasing communication between physicians and their patients and in emphasizing the competent individual's freedom of choice. Moreover, from the physician's point of view, a fully informed patient is much less likely to be surprised, disappointed, or angry when unexpected and perhaps unfortunate results do follow medical treatment, diagnostic tests, or surgery. There is every reason to think that a larger number of informed patients will mean a decrease in litigation. Techniques and practices by physicians and hospital personnel which increase communication and foster mutual understanding are the best possible antidotes for misunderstanding and litigation on the part of the patient.

The major criteria for the physician when he is deciding how much to tell the patient should always be the welfare and the needs of the patient. The physician should ask himself such questions as the following: Is the patient likely to be unaware of a known hazard or risk? Would a reasonably prudent patient be likely to withhold consent if he were aware of the risk? Is there any acceptable justification for failing to disclose? Is the risk or hazard, however remote, material to the patient's decision? Above all, the physician should put himself in the place of the patient and discuss all the matters that he would want to know, in language and in a tone that the lay patient would understand and comprehend. Patients do not need to be given a medical school education. But they should be informed and have trust and confidence in those caring for them. There is now a clear-cut judicial attitude that physicians must practice the golden rule and do as they would be done by.

Refusal of Patient to Consent

It will be recalled that an emergency eliminates the need to obtain consent, since the law values the preserving of life and the prevention of permanent impairment to health. This rule, however, applies only when the patient is incapable of expressing his wishes by reason of unconsciousness, mental incompetence, or legal disability. It further applies only when the person legally authorized to consent for the incompetent patient is similarly incompetent or unavailable.

Hence the philosophical and legal situation is quite different when an adult and mentally competent patient expressly refuses consent to medical or surgical treatment, whatever his reason. The logic begins with the point, quite consistent with the need to obtain consent, that the patient's express refusal of treatment or his withdrawal of consent to a continuation of treatment must be honored—since he is the master of his own body—even if death is the likely result. Accordingly one frequently hears that there is a legally recognized "right to die," unless a compelling state interest overrides the rights of the patient.

It follows that there would be civil liability in damages for treatment rendered contrary to the express wishes of the mentally and legally competent patient. It also follows that a court would normally not step in and order treatment for such a patient; his personal right to control his own destiny would outweigh the interest of society in preserving life. There are several leading cases to this effect.[38]

As said by the appellate court in the recent case of *In re Osborne* from the District of Columbia:

> In some cases the patient is comatose and his religious views must be expressed by family members or friends. In other cases, like this one, the patient is fully capable of making the choice. That is one reason why we directed the bedside hearing. Whenever possible it is better for the judge to make a first-hand appraisal of the patient's personal desires and ability for rational choice. In this way the court can always know, to the extent possible, that the judgment is that of the individual concerned and not that of those who believe, however well-intentioned, that they speak for the person whose life is in the balance. Thus, where the patient is comatose or suffering impairment of capacity for choice, it may be better to give weight to the known instinct for survival which can, in a critical situation alter previously held convictions. In such cases it cannot be determined with certainty that a deliberate and intelligent choice has been made.

---

[38] *Erickson v. Dilgard*, 44 Misc. 2d 27, 252 N.Y.S. 2d 705 (Sup. Ct. 1962): (The court refused to order a blood transfusion for a competent adult). *Winters v. Miller*, 446 F. 2d 65 (2d Cir. 1971), *cert. denied*, 404 U.S. 985, (1971): (Medication may not be administered to a mentally ill patient contrary to her wishes when she has not been declared legally incompetent). *In re Estate of Brooks*, 32 Ill. 2d 361, 205 N.E. 2d 435 (1965): (A court may not order administration of blood contrary to a patient's wishes based upon religious convictions). *Palm Springs General Hospital v. Martinez*, case no. 71-12687 (Cir. Ct. Fla. 1971): (*Unreported.* Physicians and hospital would not be civilly liable for complying with a competent, terminally ill patient's wishes to withdraw treatment). *In re Osborne*, 294 A. 2d 372 (D.C. Cir. 1972): (The court would not appoint a guardian and order a blood transfusion to save the life of a 34-year-old male who was competent to express his wishes). *Matter of Melideo*, 390 N.Y.S. 2d 523 (Sup. Ct. 1976): (A competent married adult woman with no children has the right to refuse a blood transfusion in accordance with her religious beliefs, even though transfusion is necessary to save her life; there is no compelling state interest in overriding her decision).

Another circumstance which is often present in cases like this is the existence of children, whose lives, if yet unborn, are also at stake, or whose welfare, as survivors, may be unclear. In those cases, it seems less difficult for courts to find sufficient state interest to intervene and circumvent religious convictions. But even then, it is important to note that courts may be more controlled by the interest of the surviving children when there is lack of clarity respecting first-hand knowledge that the patient's current choice is competently maintained. . . .

. . . Thus Judge Bacon and this court were faced with a man who did not wish to live if to do so required a blood transfusion, who viewed himself as deprived of life everlasting even if he involuntarily received the transfusion, and who had, through material provision and family and spiritual bonds, provided for the future well-being of his two children. . . . Based on this unique record, we have been unable to conclude that judicial intervention respecting the wishes and religious beliefs of the patient was warranted under our law.[39]

The test of mental competence is whether or not the patient understands his condition, the nature of the medical advice rendered, and the consequences of his refusal to consent.

It likewise follows logically that a physician should not be criminally liable for honoring a competent adult's wishes in refusing treatment or in withdrawing from on-going treatment. Although generally the deliberate taking of another's life can be considered criminal homicide, even when done at the conscious request of the victim, the context of the physician-patient relationship would seem to require a recognition that a competent patient has the right to terminate that relationship. Accordingly, the physician's duty to render care (even "ordinary" care) can be considered ended, and thus his "omissions" in the rendition of continuing care should eliminate any possible criminal liability.[40]

Mental competence is, of course, a matter for the physicians to decide in their professional judgment. If it is determined that the patient is incompetent and that his refusal to consent is therefore not based in fact on his free choice, then the matter should be referred to the appropriate court for a legal determination of incompetence and the appointment of a guardian. If there is no time for a court determination, and if the physicians have decided

[39] 294 A. 2d at 374.
[40] See: P. Foreman, "The Physician's Criminal Liability for the Practice of Euthanasia," 27 *Baylor L. Rev.* 54, 57 (1975).

in their professional judgment that the patient is incompetent, then it is better to render treatment in the interest of attempting to protect life, since the legal risk is greater in a malpractice suit based upon inaction than in one based upon alleged treatment contrary to wishes, assuming of course that the doctors have fully documented their determination of incompetence. When a competent adult refuses consent or withdraws consent, the physician or hospital, or both of these, should obtain written acknowledgment of the refusal from the patient and a release of liability. The form should be filed in the patient's medical record. If the patient refuses to sign such a form, then full documentation of his refusal of treatment should be recorded in the chart.

Even when the nonconsenting patient is competent and fully understands the probable consequences of his action, the physicians and hospital may be well advised to take the matter to a court for a ruling, both to protect the physicians and hospital and to serve the interest of the patient, as was done in all the leading cases, noted earlier, dealing with the "right to die."

Sometimes a court will intervene and order treatment of a nonconsenting competent adult, even if refusal of consent is based upon religious convictions. The legal basis for such a ruling may be that society has a "compelling interest in the preservation of life," thus justifying state intervention contrary to individual wishes. There may be interests of minor children to protect, as in the famous case of *In re Application of the President and Directors of Georgetown College, Inc.*, decided in 1964.[41] Further in this opinion the judge justified his order on the basis that the patient was really in no mental condition to make a choice and that her religious convictions would not actually be violated if the court should decide the matter, thus removing responsibility from her shoulders.

The case going the farthest in justifying state intervention is a 1971 New Jersey decision entitled *John F. Kennedy Memorial Hospital v. Heston.*[42] In effect, the court ruled that the state had a "compelling interest" to preserve the life of an adult, a 22-year-old unmarried female. It can therefore be considered as conflicting with other decisions, previously cited, which indicated that a competent individual has a right to die.

---

[41] 331 F. 2d 1000, 9 A.L.R. 3d 1367 (D.C. Cir., 1964). See also: *United States v. George*, 239 F. Supp. 752 (D. Conn. 1965): (The court ordered a blood transfusion for a father of four children). *Raleigh Fitkin–Paul Morgan Memorial Hospital v. Anderson*, 42 N.J. 421, 201 A. 2d 537 (1964), *cert. denied*, 377 U.S. 985 (1964): (The court ordered a transfusion for a female patient who was 32 weeks pregnant).
[42] 58 N.J. 576, 279 A. 2d 670 (1971).

In *Heston*, the New Jersey court ordered that a blood transfusion could be administered to save the life of an accident victim who had refused consent for religious reasons. *Heston* is also inconsistent with a 1972 federal court decision, *Holmes v. Silver Cross Hospital*, which held that physicians and the hospital may have violated constitutional rights of religious freedom and rights under the Civil Rights Act by administering blood despite an express refusal by a twenty-year-old married male, his wife, and his parents, even though the hospital had first obtained an order of probate court declaring the patient to be incompetent. The legal point in *Holmes* is that the Illinois court lacked power to restrict religious freedom, unless the state could show a grave or immediate danger to its interests. Hence the federal court, as a matter of legal procedure, denied a motion to dismiss this action for damages alleging violation of civil rights, and there had to be a trial on the issue of whether or not the Illinois probate court properly found the patient to be incompetent.[43] Thus the struggle to balance individual rights and the interests of society acting through governmental institutions continues unabated.

Consent of Spouse, Relative, or Persons Acting for a Patient

A patient may be unable to grant an effective consent for medical or surgical treatment by reason of mental incompetence or because of legal disability, such as minority. If the incompetence has been recognized by a court through the appointment of a guardian, it is absolutely necessary for the physician and the hospital to obtain the guardian's consent, unless the guardian is unavailable and a medical emergency as previously defined is present.

In the absence of a court-appointed guardian, the extent of incompetence as determined by a qualified physician will govern the question of obtaining consent. Even a patient who is emotionally disturbed and in a sense suffering from "mental illness" may nevertheless be capable of understanding the need for treatment and the significance of his act in granting consent. In this event, the patient's own consent is sufficient, because the legal test of a valid consent is always the knowledge and the understanding of the patient. If the physician doubts the ability of the patient to give his own consent, then a court should be asked to rule on the patient's competence before treatment is undertaken, providing there is time

---

[43]340 F. Supp. 125 (N.D. Ill. 1972).

to obtain a ruling without jeopardizing the patient's physical condition. If time does not allow a court to rule, then presumably a medical emergency exists which would justify treatment without consent.

The consent of the patient's spouse or nearest relative should be obtained in this situation, however, if such a person is readily accessible, both for reasons of law and to maintain the physician-patient relationship. Some states have specific statutes with respect to the mentally incompetent, which place upon a named relative the responsibility of maintaining the incompetent, thereby also establishing the relative's right to consent to treatment of the incompetent person. Even without such a statute, when the patient's condition is such that waiting to obtain a court order would be likely to cause permanent harm to the patient, the spouse or in his absence the nearest relative is probably authorized to give consent.[44]

If the patient is competent to consent for himself, the spouse or other relative is not authorized to render consent. Marriage alone does not make a spouse the agent of his or her partner. Since the spouse's consent is not normally necessary, the only reason for discussing the patient's condition with a spouse or a relative would be to improve relations with the patient's family.[45] In one case, the ruling was to the effect that when it was possible to obtain a patient's consent before administration of sedatives to the patient, and this was not done, the spouse's consent to surgery would not protect the surgeon or the hospital from liability.[46]

In special circumstances a spouse's consent may be advisable as a legal matter, however, even though the patient is competent. This occurs if the treatment to which the patient has consented involves

---

[44]*Farber v. Olkon*, 40 Cal. 2d 503, 254 P. 2d 520, (1953): (A parent can consent for a mentally incompetent adult child). *Anonymous v. State*, 17 App. Div. 2d 495, 236 N.Y.S. 2d 88 (1963). *Steele v. Woods*, 327 S.W. 2d 187 (Mo. 1959). *Lester v. Aetna Casualty Surety Co.*, 240 F. 2d 676 (5th Cir. 1957): (A wife was authorized to consent for electroshock treatments for her husband. It was reasonable under all the facts and circumstances to believe that it would harm the patient to obtain a fully informed consent from him). *Application of Long Island Jewish–Hillside Medical Center*, 73 Misc. 2d 395, 342 N.Y.S. 2d 356 (N.Y. Sup. Ct. 1973): (The court appointed a niece as guardian of an elderly incompetent patient to give consent for amputation of the patient's leg). *Pratt v. Davis*, 224 Ill. 300, 79 N.E. 562 (1906): (A physician was held liable when surgery was performed on an incompetent wife without the husband's consent).

[45]*Jeffcoat v. Phillips*, 417 S.W. 2d 903 (Texas Civ. App. 1967): (A husband's consent was not necessary for surgery on the wife; the jury found as fact that the patient had given effective consent). *Rytkonen v. Lojacona*, 269 Mich. 270, 257 N.W. 703 (1934): (A wife's consent was not necessary for an operation on her husband; he had consented). *Accord: Karp v. Cooley*, 349 F. Supp. 827 (S.D. Texas 1972), *aff'd*, 493 F. 2d 408 (5th Cir. 1974); *Janney v. Housekeeper*, 70 Md. 162, 16 A. 382 (1889): (A husband's consent was not necessary for a surgical procedure on the wife).

[46]*Gravis v. Physicians' and Surgeons' Hospital of Alice*, 427 S.W. 2d 310 (Texas 1968).

elective sterilization, artificial insemination, or purely elective surgery adversely affecting the normal function of reproductive organs. For such treatment, elected by the patient, a spouse's consent is generally deemed advisable by conservative legal opinion because the spouse in his or her own right may otherwise have a valid cause of action for damages, based either upon the theory of unjustified interference with the marital relationship or upon the legal right of consortium.

When the patient's health and well-being is concerned, however, even if reproductive capacity is adversely affected, the consent of the spouse is not necessary. A recent Oklahoma case has held that the husband, who had not consented to a hysterectomy on his wife, had no cause of action for loss of consortium.[47] In short, the wife's right to health is paramount; and her decision alone, based upon the professional advice of her physician, is controlling. A reading of this case indicates that "health of the patient" will be very broadly construed, and that modern courts will be extremely reluctant to recognize a separate right in a husband to a fertile wife or vice versa. Moreover, as we will see in the chapter on abortion, a husband has no right of his own to prevent the surgical procedure on his wife. Whenever a surgical procedure of any nature affects the reproductive capacity of the patient, it is wise to obtain the spouse's consent, if possible, in deference to both conservative legal interpretation and sound physician-family relations. If a competent adult patient seeks and consents to such a procedure, however, and if the patient's physician can justify the surgery as necessary to the physical or mental health of his patient, or if the patient has a "constitutional right" to the procedure as in the case of an abortion, then consent of the spouse is not necessary.

It follows that if a competent adult has consented to treatment or surgery necessary to preserve his or her physical or mental health, including sterilization or other surgery likely to affect adversely the reproductive function, the refusal of a spouse's or relative's consent should not be honored to prevent treatment of the patient. Nor should such refusal prevent treatment considered necessary in any medical emergency involving a threat to life or health, where the patient is unable to give an effective consent. The reason is that a spouse or relative has no legal right to bar treatment necessary to preserve the life or the health of the patient when the latter has consented, or when an emergency exists and the law therefore presumes that the patient would choose the option of life, obviating

---

[47] *Murray v. Vandevander*, 522 P. 2d 302 (Okla. Ct. App. 1974).

the need for consent. To illustrate, in *Collins v. Davis* an adult patient who had sought medical attention became comatose and required surgery to save his life. The spouse refused to consent to the surgery, whereupon the hospital referred the matter to an appropriate court and obtained an order permitting the operation.[48]

If the spouse's consent or that of the nearest relative is sought and refused, the best advice would therefore be to proceed in the attempt to preserve life solely on the basis of the patient's own consent, if obtainable, or on the basis of a medical emergency if the patient's consent is not obtainable. If the patient is not competent to consent and if time permits, the hospital would be well advised to obtain a court order; but even in the absence of such an order the spouse would have no legal right to bar emergency care for the patient designed to preserve life and restore health. If the spouse or nearest relative has no right to refuse consent on behalf of the patient, a suit for damages by the spouse or relative is not likely to be successful.

The well-publicized 1975–76 litigation entitled *In re Quinlan* concerned difficult ethical and legal issues with an eventual result in the New Jersey Supreme Court that was unanticipated by many qualified observers.[49] The precedental impact and implications of the case with respect to future development of the law of an individual's right to live and to die are uncertain at this time of writing.

Miss Karen Quinlan, a 22-year-old patient who had sustained severe brain damage, perhaps as a result of consuming alcohol and drugs, became comatose and remained for several months in a chronic "vegetative" state. Attending physicians, presumably applying customary and prevailing medical standards, employed a mechanical respirator to aid her breathing. When the physicians and the hospital refused to terminate this life support system at the request of Miss Quinlan's parents, her father instituted suit requesting appointment as guardian of his daughter's person and court authorization to discontinue the use of the respirator. Prior to trial it was stipulated by all parties that the patient was incompetent and that she was not dead by either the classical medical definition of death in terms of cessation of the heart and respiratory functions or the criteria of "brain death" as articulated by the Ad Hoc Committee at Harvard University in 1968. It should also be noted that New Jersey does not have a statutory definition of death, nor had there been any

---

[48] 44 Misc. 2d 622, 254 N.Y.S. 2d 666 (Sup. Ct. 1964).
[49] 70 N.J. 10, 355 A. 2d 647 (1976).

prior litigation in the state involving the concept of "brain death."

The New Jersey trial court denied Mr. Quinlan's request to be appointed guardian of the patient's person and also his request to terminate the use of the respirator, holding in effect that the decision was solely that of the attending physicians acting in accordance with prevailing medical standards; and it rejected the argument that there is a viable legal distinction between "ordinary" and "extraordinary" measures to sustain life. The trial court further ruled that the constitutional right of privacy could not be the basis of a decision to "take" a life, although acknowledging that if the medical community later establishes customary practice as embracing withdrawal of treatment in cases like Miss Quinlan's then the physicians could not be prosecuted criminally for homicide.[50]

On appeal the decision was reversed; the New Jersey Supreme Court indicated that Mr. Quinlan was entitled to be appointed guardian of the person, could select a physician of his choice to care for his daughter, and could participate with this physician and the hospital's medical ethics committee in a decision to withdraw the mechanical respirator. The legal basis for the decision was the patient's constitutional right of privacy, specifically her right to decline treatment under the circumstances of her situation, as noted in the "right to die" cases discussed in the previous section of this chapter and as articulated by the United States Supreme Court in the abortion cases.

To put the matter another way, in the context of the right of privacy, a state may not intervene in a personal decision unless it has a "compelling interest" to protect life; and the interest of the state in preserving life was made weaker by the facts of the *Quinlan* case, which established the medical prognosis for the patient as "dim." The earlier New Jersey case of *John F. Kennedy Memorial Hospital v. Heston*,[51] which had held that the state could intervene and order a blood transfusion to preserve the life of a single adult woman, differed in that such an intervention was justified to preserve a meaningful, healthful life and thus did not apply to the facts presented in *Quinlan.* Most significantly, the New Jersey court went on to rule that where the patient is so grossly incompetent that she cannot express her right of privacy on her own behalf, her father as guardian may do so under the doctrine of substituted judgment. Hence the

[50]*In re Karen Quinlan*, 137 N.J. Super. 227, 348 A 2d 801 (Ch. Div. 1975).
[51]58 N.J. 576, 279 A. 2d 670 (1971).

father has standing to assert and implement the constitutional rights of the patient.

To guard against misuse of the substituted judgment doctrine, especially in situations less worthy on the facts or with respect to family motivations, the court spoke approvingly of relying on the hospital's ethics committee; and in fact it required the guardian and the attending physicians to consult with such a committee which would then review the medical evidence and opinion about the possibility that the patient might emerge from her chronic comatose state. In summary, the court ruled, upon concurrence of the guardian, the attending physician, and the ethics committee, the "life support system" could be withdrawn without the fear of civil or criminal liability.

The court did not define or give illustrations of "life support systems." This case involved the withdrawal of a mechanical respirator, leaving medical persons and the law to decide the further question: whether a guardian of the person of an incompetent patient, together with physicians, may withdraw the use of drugs and food that are sustaining life.

Consent for Minors

In treating minors several questions arise in connection with obtaining sufficient consent. Because of differences in the facts of each situation and in local state law, via case or statute, not all of these questions can be answered with legal certainty. On occasion, therefore, a physician and the hospital must rely upon their best judgment in the particular circumstances.

At the outset it will be recalled that no express or implied-in-fact consent at all is legally necessary when there is a medical emergency. As previously defined, an emergency usually involves an immediate threat to life or health where delay would cause permanent damage. For a minor it includes the impossibility or impracticality of obtaining consent from the parent or the person authorized to speak for the youth. Medical necessity for treatment, if delay to obtain consent would not permanently harm the patient, is not tantamount to an emergency.

Physicians and hospital staff should always as a general rule, even when they believe that the situation involving a minor constitutes an emergency, make a reasonable effort to reach the parents or the person standing in a parental relationship, if the patient's condition allows the effort. If there is opportunity to do so, the medical emergency should also be documented by professional consultation.

The case of *Luka v. Lowrie* illustrates an emergency where the patient was a minor.[52] A boy fifteen years of age was hit by a train. Five physicians determined that it was necessary to amputate his foot, and they acted without obtaining the consent of his parents. Their action was held to be justified, inasmuch as in the professional judgment of the physicians the patient's condition constituted a threat to his life or health unless immediate action was taken. The case shows the importance of consultation with other physicians before administering care.

AGE OF MAJORITY

Policies and practices in connection with obtaining proper consent for the treatment of minors when there is no emergency require that physicians and hospital personnel first determine the age of majority in their particular jurisdiction. The controlling law is probably that of the place of treatment. At common law the age of majority is twenty-one years. Majority is reached the day prior to the patient's birthday. This is still the law of many states. In some jurisdictions, however, by statute both males and females who are married are considered adults. A significant number of states (and England) have reduced the age of adulthood to eighteen for all persons. In short, the statutory and case law of each particular jurisdiction must be consulted to determine the age of majority. Once the age is attained, the patient is of course considered an adult.

In the absence of a local statute, the mere fact that an individual is authorized by law to marry without parental consent, to vote, or to purchase alcoholic beverages does not render him legally capable of entering into a binding contract as an adult or capable of giving an effective consent for medical treatment. Hence a married minor is not, legally speaking, an adult, and the fact of marriage does not in and of itself authorize a minor to give his consent to medical treatment unless a specific statute so prescribes. Similarly emancipation from parental control and support, which can occur with or without marriage, does not create adulthood. Physicians and hospitals in those states which have no statute speaking specifically on the matter must therefore not arbitrarily rely on the sole fact of marriage or emancipation as making it legally safe to proceed on the basis of the minor's own consent without obtaining parental consent.

In most states, obtaining the consent of married or emancipated

---

[52] 171 Mich. 122, 136 N.W. 1106 (1912).

minors for treatment should be approached in the same way as consent from unmarried, unemancipated minors living at home with their parents.

The fact of marriage or emancipation, even though it may not establish adulthood, may be most important, however, in determining the response to the next question, that is, whether the patient, even though a minor, is legally capable of giving effective consent without the consent of a parent or guardian. The answer may be provided by local statutory law or by judicial decision.

Consent by Minors

It has often been arbitrarily stated that in the absence of an emergency the consent of the parent, or the person standing in a parental relationship to the minor, is necessary before medical or surgical treatment can be administered to the minor. Analysis of the cases and a review of recent statutory laws indicate that this statement of the law is not always true.

Hospital policies and practices should be workable and practical, and at the same time they should provide maximum legal protection. The easiest rule perhaps would be to insist arbitrarily upon parental consent, or the consent of the person standing in a parental relationship, in all cases of medical treatment or surgery involving minors, except in medical emergencies or when a statute specifically eliminates the need for the consent of parents. Yet such a policy is not practical. There are too many situations in which medical or surgical care for a relatively mature and knowledgeable minor is advisable but where the parent is not readily accessible or is perhaps completely inaccessible. Moreover, a mature minor may seek care and object to obtaining parental consent, especially for treatment of medical conditions relating to pregnancy, for example, or family planning.

Analysis of the cases suggests that in most decisions the basis for the common law rule that a parent's consent is necessary for treatment is the belief that minors are incapable, by reason of their youth, of understanding the nature and the consequences of their own acts and must therefore be protected from the folly of their own decisions. If this is the true basis for the rule that the parent's consent must be obtained, then there is nothing magical about the arbitrary age of twenty-one, or any other age of majority. In other words, the test of the validity of a minor's own consent should be his maturity—as measured in part by age and his ability to comprehend the nature of his own decisions—and not the particular chronological age of majority. This judicial view is called the age-of-discretion doctrine.

Several cases of long standing as well as the *Restatement of Torts* recognize the legal validity of a minor's own consent and do not insist upon the parent's consent, providing the minor is capable of understanding and appreciating the nature of his consent.[53] Reliance on the minor's own consent, however, should be limited to situations where the medical treatment or surgery is for the minor's benefit, as distinguished from situations where the procedure is primarily for the benefit of another.[54] In the latter event the consent of the parent should always be obtained.

Moreover, as a matter of practicality the hospital should establish some age as an aid in determining whether the given patient is capable and sufficiently mature to understand the consequences of his act.[55] A workable rule might well establish the age of eighteen as a guideline in those states where twenty-one is still the age of adulthood, or sixteen in states where adulthood is reached at eighteen years.

If a minor is married or emancipated, this fact is evidence of his maturity and ability to understand. But, as previously noted, these facts are not in themselves enough to make it safe to ignore the advisability of obtaining a parent's consent as a matter of common law. Illustrating the importance of marriage and emancipation is the recent case of *Smith v. Seibly*, decided by the Supreme Court of Washington in 1967. It was here held that an eighteen-year-old married male could consent to a vasectomy.[56]

Another important factor in applications of the age-of-discretion doctrine is whether the minor has living parents who are readily available to grant consent. For example, in 1971 the Probate Court of the District of Columbia held that an eighteen-year-old girl who was without parents and without a legally appointed guardian could

---

[53] *Bishop v. Shurly*, 237 Mich. 76, 211 N.W. 75 (1926): (A 19-year-old could consent to administration of a local anesthetic). *Gulf & S.I.R. Co. v. Sullivan*, 155 Miss 1, 119 So. 501, 62 A.L.R. 191 (1928): (A 17-year-old could consent to vaccination). *Lacey v. Laird*, 166 Ohio St. 12, 139 N.E. 2d 25, (1956): (An 18-year-old girl could consent to a surgical operation). *Masden v. Harrison*, II 68651 Equity (Mass. 1957): (A 19-year-old twin could consent to a kidney transplant operation). *Restatement of Torts*, sec. 59 (1934).

[54] *Bonner v. Moran*, 126 F. 2d 121, 139 A.L.R. 1366 (D.C. Cir. 1941). (A 15-year-old's consent to skin grafting operation was held to be insufficient.)

[55] *Zoski v. Gaines*, 271 Mich. 1, 260 N.W. 99 (1935): (A 9-year-old's consent was insufficient). *Moss v. Rishworth*, 222 S.W. 225 (Texas Commission of Appeals 1920): (11-year-old).

[56] 72 Wash. 2d 16, 431 P. 2d 719 (1967).

consent to an abortion.[57] Another example occurs in *Younts v. St. Francis Hospital*, where a Kansas court held that a seventeen-year-old could consent to surgery on an injured finger. The patient's mother was herself hospitalized and in a semiconscious condition, and the father was unavailable.[58]

A strong judicial tendency is thus evident to permit minors to give an effective consent whenever they are mature enough to understand the nature of the contemplated treatment and the consequences of their action, whenever the patient is emancipated or married, and whenever the parents are not available. As a matter of fact, to the author's knowledge no judicial case has held a physician or a hospital liable for treatment that was beneficial to the minor in any of these circumstances. The ultraconservative policy of always insisting upon parental consent regardless of the minor's maturity or status in life is accordingly not justified.

Furthermore, when a minor seeks a legal abortion or contraceptive services, the trend clearly indicates that parental consent is not necessary. This trend is most evident in the enactment of state statutes authorizing such care on the basis of the minor's own consent, but it is also indicated by judicial decision. A recent decision of the Supreme Court of Washington is most significant. The court reversed a criminal conviction of a physician who had performed an abortion on an unmarried minor without first obtaining the consent of her parents. The basis of the reversal was that the patient had a constitutional right of privacy, and that accordingly the requirement of parental consent was an unjustified breach of the minor's rights. Arguments that the state could require parental consent because it had a legitimate interest in supporting parental authority, strengthening the family unit, and ensuring informed decision-making by minors were rejected by the court.[59] The courts are thus extending to minors an adult's right to privacy, which embraces the rights to contraceptive information and practices as articulated by the United States Supreme Court in *Griswold v. Connecticut*.[60]

---

[57] *In re Barbara Doe*, (*Unreported* case D.C. 1971).
[58] 205 Kan. 292, 469 P. 2d 330 (1970).
[59] *State of Washington v. Koome*, 84 Wash. 2d 901, 530 P. 2d 260 (1975). See generally: "Parental Consent Requirements and Privacy Rights of Minors: The Contraceptive Controversy," 88 *Harvard Law Review* 1001–20 (1975). See also: *Poe v. Gerstein*, 517 F. 2d 787 (5th Cir. 1975). (A Florida abortion statute which required written consent of the parents, custodian, or legal guardian of unmarried pregnant women under eighteen years of age was unconstitutional.)
[60] 381 U.S. 479, 14 L. Ed. 2d 510, 85 S. Ct. 1678 (1965). See also: *Eisenstadt v. Baird*, 405 U.S. 438, 31 L. Ed. 2d 349, 92 S. Ct. 1029 (1972), which held that unmarried adults have the same right of access to contraceptives as married adults.

In addition to the strong judicial trend under common law authorizing a mature minor to give his or her own consent for all beneficial medical or surgical treatment, there have emerged a number of specific statutes in the various jurisdictions which clarify the law with respect to treatment of minors in particular situations and for particular medical conditions. No effort is made here to list or categorize all of the relevant statutes. As noted previously, however, statutes in quite a number of states specifically provide that emancipated or married minors, regardless of age, may give their own consent for any medical treatment. Over half the states have recently enacted statutes providing that minors themselves may consent to treatment of conditions relating to pregnancy, family planning, venereal disease, and the use of drugs. It is important, however, for physicians and hospitals to analyze carefully each particular statute and to seek the advice of local counsel, because limitations based upon age, marriage, or other factors may affect the ability of the minor to give legal consent.

One of the better and more comprehensive statutes has been adopted in Mississippi. It specifically authorizes a minor to give consent in certain circumstances: marriage or emancipation enables a minor to consent to any medical care; a female, regardless of age or marital status, may consent to treatment of pregnancy; any minor can consent to treatment of venereal disease. The statute specifically enunciates the age-of-discretion doctrine by providing that any unemancipated minor of sufficient intelligence to understand and appreciate the consequences of the proposed surgical or medical treatment may consent for himself, again without any age limitations. Finally, a minor eighteen years of age or over may donate blood, and minor parents may consent to treatment of their children.[61]

Another example of clarifying statutes is a recently enacted Pennsylvania law specifically providing that any minor who is eighteen years of age or older, or who has graduated from high school, or who has married or been pregnant may give effective consent to all medical, dental, and health services. The statute also recites that in connection with pregnancy, or with venereal disease or any other legally reportable disease, the minor may give his or her own consent. Note that this latter provision sets no age limit. Furthermore, the statute clarifies the common law doctrine of treatment in an emergency by specifically permitting the physician to treat minors of any age without consent of the parent or legal guardian when in his profes-

---

[61]Mississippi Code 1972 Ann., sec. 41-41-1 et seq. and sec. 41-41-15 (Supp. 1974).

sional judgment a delay of treatment to secure parental consent would increase the risk to the minor's life or health.[62]

Both judicial and statutory law have thus contributed to a strong public policy to permit minors to receive health services without having to obtain parental consent, as long as the minor is mature enough to understand the nature of the contemplated treatment and the consequences of the action, and whenever the treatment is intended to benefit the patient.

Even in a jurisdiction which has not yet clarified the law by judicial decision or statute, necessary medical treatment should never be withheld from a mature and knowledgeable minor solely because parental consent has not been obtained. The withholding of services may well create more legal risk from charges of malpractice or negligence than would be incurred by furnishing the services in situations that might involve a technical assault or battery or the invasion of parental rights. More simply, damages for failure to treat might well be far greater than damages for treatment without consent. Accordingly each hospital and each provider of medical care should develop guidelines for the treatment of minors, based upon local law and upon recognized standards of clinical care.

It seems perfectly clear that a married minor can give consent for the treatment of his or her minor child. This common law has been clarified by statute in some jurisdictions, for example in Pennsylvania and Mississippi, where the statutes read that any minor who has been married or who has borne a child may give effective consent to all health services for his or her child. Note that these provisions authorize a married father or a married mother or an unmarried mother to give consent, but they do not authorize the unmarried father to give consent for the treatment of a minor child.

Several reported cases have considered the question of whether a parent or a court may authorize surgery performed on a minor for the benefit of another person. The typical example is the removal of a kidney for transplantation. Although, as noted previously, the Massachusetts courts have permitted kidney transplants to be performed on twins who were mature minors giving their own consent to the surgery, it is assumed here that parental consent should be obtained when the surgery has as its primary purpose the benefit of another. The issues still remain, however, whether or not a parent is authorized to consent to such an operation and whether a court

---

[62]Pa. Stat. Ann., Title 35, sec. 10101–5 (Supp. 1974).

may grant consent, especially if the patient is too young or otherwise unable to express his own wishes.

In Connecticut it was held that the parents of identical twins, eight years of age, could consent to a transplant of a kidney from one twin to the other.[63] In this case the risk to the donor was shown to be slight, and there were good prospects of sound health for both patients following surgery. In a situation such as that in the Connecticut case, it may be said that the donor does in fact benefit at least psychologically, in the sense that he is instrumental is saving the life or health of his twin.

In a few cases it has been held that a court has the power under local law to authorize a kidney transplant if the patient is a minor or incompetent or both of these. Georgia, for example, has held that a court may sanction the transfer of a kidney from a 15-year-old retarded child to her mother.[64] Similarly, a mother in Kentucky, acting as guardian of her son, a 27-year-old incompetent who was committed to the Frankfort State Hospital and School, sought a court order permitting a kidney transplant from him to a 28-year-old brother who was suffering from a fatal kidney disease, and the court authorized the surgery.[65] In this decision, however, a vigorous dissent was voiced on the basis that there was no evidence suggesting in any way that the surgery would benefit the patient. The dissenting judge was unwilling to allow either the mother or the court to make a martyr of one who was not competent to speak for himself. He clearly felt that the exercise of such parental and judicial power was unwise from the point of view of public policy. Following the same reasoning, in the more recent case of *In re Richardson* a Louisiana court held that neither a minor's parents nor the court could consent to the removal of a kidney from a 17-year-old retarded patient for transplantation to an adult sister.[66]

There are thus conflicting views of public policy, and different jurisdictions clearly have differing values. Is it wise for medicine and the law to maximize the rights of the helpless and the incompetent? Or alternatively, may they be subjected to treatment which will favor the patient who has a more immediate opportunity for regaining health?

[63] *Hart v. Brown*, 29 Conn. Super 368, 289 A. 2d 386 (1972).
[64] *Howard v. The Fulton-DeKalb Hospital Authority*, 42 U.S.L.W. 2322 (Georgia Super. Ct. 1973).
[65] *Strunk v. Strunk*, 445 S.W. 2d 145, 35 A.L.R. 3d 683 (Kentucky 1969).
[66] 284 So. 2d 185 (La. Ct. of App. 1974). See also: *In re Guardianship of Pescinski*, 67 Wis. 2d 4, 226 N.W. 2d 180 (1975). (Neither the guardian of an incompetent nor the court may authorize the removal of a kidney to save the life of the incompetent's sister.)

Concern for the patient has also been expressed in those cases which have held that the parent or guardian of a minor or an incompetent may not consent to a sterilization of the patient.[67] The basis for these cases has been generally that the interest of the patient must be protected until such time as he or she is in a position to be able to make an individual choice with respect to such an important matter as reproductive capacity.

When it is determined that parental consent is necessary, then an issue that frequently arises is whether both parents must consent. The answer is that the consent of either parent is sufficient if the parents are living together. If, on the other hand, the parents are divorced or voluntarily separated, then the consent of the parent having custody of the child should be obtained.

No individual having temporary custody of a minor child, whether a relative or not, is authorized at common law to give consent for treatment of the minor. Babysitters thus have no authority to consent to treatment of a minor. In the absence of the parents or a legally appointed guardian, the legal test of an individual's authorization to consent to treatment of a minor is whether or not the person having custody stands in place of the parent. This requires more than a showing of mere temporary custody.

REFUSAL OF CONSENT FOR TREATMENT OF MINORS

If the parent or guardian consents to treatment, but the minor patient possesses both maturity and understanding and refuses consent for treatment, the physician and the hospital should not proceed to render care. This policy is consistent with the thought that minors capable of understanding their own acts are capable of giving their own consent. Such cases should then be handled as if the youth were an adult who has refused or withdrawn consent.

Those who render care may encounter the reverse of such a situation: a mature and understanding minor may consent to treatment, and the parent or guardian may refuse consent. In this event one should rely on the mature minor's own consent and treatment should proceed. In both these situations the minor's rights are recognized to be probably paramount. The practical aspect of the dilemma is also recognized, that is, that invading the rights or interests of one who is not a patient entails less legal risk than a course of conduct which invades the interest of a patient.

---

[67]For example: *Frazier v. Levi,* 440 S.W. 2d 393 (Tex. Civ. App. 1969); *Holmes v. Powers,* 439 S.W. 2d 579 (Ky. Ct. App. 1968); *In the Interest of M.K.R.,* 515 S.W. 2d 467 (Mo. 1974); *In re Estate of Kemp,* 43 Cal. App. 3d 758, 118 Cal. Rptr. 64 (1974).

If the parent of a minor who lacks maturity and understanding, or who is otherwise legally incapable of expressing his own consent, should affirmatively refuse consent for treatment of the minor, the situation poses practical, ethical, and legal difficulties, especially when a medical emergency exists and the patient is likely to die if treatment is withheld. A number of legally and ethically sound guidelines can, however, be suggested.

The course of least resistance and least legal risk is to do nothing and permit the child to remain without care, even though he may die. It is doubtful whether the minor (or his estate) could later sue for damages in such a case on the grounds that the physician or hospital, or both of these, had a legal duty to override parental objections. It is possible, however, that the parents could be prosecuted criminally, and it is also possible by virtue of emerging tort law doctrine that the child would have a civil cause of action against his parents for damages.

Doing nothing to aid a child, at least in a medical emergency likely to result in death or permanent impairment of health, is of course contrary to ethical and moral doctrine. Sometimes the parents' refusal of consent is based upon their religious convictions, but parents may also refuse consent because of a fear of the risks involved, for example, or inability to pay for the care. Whatever the reason for parental refusal of consent, the following guidelines are suggested. The key issue is simply whether or not the condition of the minor will permit delay of treatment while the matter is referred to a court.

If the condition of the minor patient unable to express 'his own decision does not permit delaying treatment until a court order is obtained, the physician and the hospital should proceed with treatment despite parental objections. These will be situations where life is at stake, and humanitarian action to save life is preferable to inaction that may cause death, even if technically the parents are entitled to bring a lawsuit against the physician and the hospital. In most instances of this kind, the damages obtainable by the parents would be small. In any event, ethics and morals would seem to justify whatever legal risk there might be. The only possible exceptions would be situations where the medical treatment necessitates amputation or other permanent changes in the young person's bodily structure. Conceivably the damages awarded for such treatment undertaken without parental consent could be substantial.

If a professional medical opinion determines that the minor's condition will not be permanently harmed by a delay in treatment, then the physician or the hospital should seek a court determination of the matter. The delay may not be long; it would depend upon local procedure and upon the working relationship that the medical people can develop with the court. Courts have been known to act quite fast and at all hours.

Under the early common law—strangely, perhaps—parental denial of medical care was not parental neglect, and hence some doubted a court's power to order medical care for a minor over the objections of the parents. All the states now have statutes, however, which provide that the appropriate court has jurisdiction to protect the interests of dependent and neglected children. These statutes differ in their language and in the procedures specified to invoke the power of the court; but in general the state, a social agency, a hospital, a physician, and even other relatives of a neglected child may petition the court for an order removing the child from the parents' custody and placing custody in a court-appointed guardian.

The statutes are clearly a valid exercise of the state's police power to protect the general health and welfare of society. Hence they are constitutional, even when their application conflicts with or violates the parents' religious belief, at least when the life of a child may be at risk. In the leading case of *State v. Perricone,* the New Jersey Supreme Court affirmed the trial court's order that a blood transfusion should be administered to an infant child of parents who were Jehovah's Witnesses.[68]

With respect to the constitutional legal issue of religious freedom of the parents, the court said:

> Thus the amendment embraces two concepts—freedom to believe and freedom to act. The first is absolute, but, in the nature of things, the second cannot be.
>
> The right to practice religion freely does not include the liberty to expose . . . a child . . . to ill health or death. Parents may be free to become martyrs themselves. But it does not follow they are free, in identical circumstances, to make martyrs of their children before they have reached the age of full and legal discretion when they can make that choice for themselves. [Citations omitted.]

Accordingly, the primary legal issue raised by these statutes is one of court interpretation of applicability and effect. Influential on a case-by-case basis are the following factors: the precise statutory language, and specifically whether the statute expressly provides that

---

[68]37 N.J. 463, 181 A. 2d 751 (1962), *cert. denied,* 371 U.S. 890 (1962).

parental refusal to allow medical care is within the definition of
a "dependent and neglected" child; the medical condition of the
child and the probable result if treatment is withheld; the age of
the child and whether (even though a minor) his or her wishes
have been considered; and finally the basis for parental refusal of
consent.

Approximately half the statutes specifically provide that parental
denial of necessary medical care is within the legal definition of
a dependent and neglected child; the others do not, thereby leaving
the matter for judicial interpretation. In states with statutes of the
latter kind, most of the cases have construed the statutes liberally
to embrace situations where parents have refused medical care, at
least when a medical emergency existed and death or permanent
impairment of health was probable.

In such situations, where medical testimony has asserted that death
or irreparable injury was likely, most courts have readily made a
finding of neglect and have upheld orders of treatment, even if
the specific statute did not precisely define parental denial of medical
care as "neglect."[69] A New Jersey trial court has even ordered a
blood transfusion to be administered at birth for a child unborn
at the time of the court action, thereby extending protection of
the statute to the unborn.[70]

The legal result is less predictable where no emergency exists,
however needed and desirable the recommended treatment may be.
These are the cases where all of the other factors noted above are
weighed. In general, appellate courts will extend great discretion
to the trial court's determination and decision, since it is the court
which hears the testimony in a particular case and is closest to the
facts, although in some litigated cases higher courts have reversed
trial court decisions on the basis of either statutory interpretation
of legislative intent or constitutional issues. As noted by the New
Jersey court:

[69]Leading decisions are: *State v. Perricone*, 37 N.J. 463, 181 A. 2d 751 (1962), *cert.
denied*, 371 U.S. 890 (1962); *People ex rel. Wallace v. Labrenz*, 411 Ill. 618, 104 N.E.
2d 769, 30 A.L.R. 2d 1132 (1952), *cert. denied*, 344 U.S. 824 (1952); *Maine Medical
Center v. Houle* (Me. Super. Ct., Docket No. 74–145, Cumberland Co. 1974). (Parents
who withhold medically necessary and feasible treatment are guilty of legal neglect,
even if the physician's opinion is that the child has brain damage and that life is
not worth preserving.)
[70]*Hoener v. Bertinato*, 67 N.J. Super. 517, 171 A. 2d 140 (Juv. and Dom. Rel. Ct.
1961). See generally: Baker, "Court-Ordered Non-Emergency Medical Care for
Infants," 18 *Clev.-Mar. Law Review* (2) 296–307 (1969). See also: *Raleigh Fitkin–Paul
Morgan Memorial Hospital, et al. v. Anderson*, 42 N.J. 421, 201 A. 2d 537 (1964).
(The court ordered a transfusion when the life of an unborn child was threatened.)

True, not every refusal to consent to treatment for an infant constitutes evidence of unfitness or neglect to provide proper protection. For example, refusals to permit corrective surgery for a congenital arm deformity (*In re Hudson*, 13 Wash. 2d 673, 126 P. 2d 765 [Sup. Ct. 1942]) and to correct rachitis (*In re Tuttendario*, 21 Pa. Dist. 561 [Q.S. Phila. Co. 1911]) have been held insufficient grounds for taking custody from the parents.[71]

In *In re Hudson*, the case referred to in the above quotation, the Washington Supreme Court respected the mother's refusal of consent and reversed a trial court order, holding that it would not order nonemergency treatment of an eleven-year-old minor. Each of the following factors was probably of some significance: the statute granting the court "custody, care, guardianship and control" of "delinquent and dependent children" did not specifically provide that parental denial of medical care was encompassed within the meaning of "dependent" or "neglect"; the only medical treatment for the deformity of the arm was amputation of the arm, entailing considerable risk to the patient; finally, the court gave weight to the fact that the mother's refusal of consent was apparently sincerely based upon the genuine medical risk involved and upon a desire to postpone surgery until the patient might be mature enough to express her own wishes. Note that *In re Hudson* did not involve any such issues of constitutional law as freedom of religious belief. In a subsequent Washington case, in which the court refused to remove custody from a father who had failed to seek medical care for his child's speech impairment, the result was similar.[72]

In a like manner a New York court refused to order care for a minor needing correction of a harelip and cleft palate. The father possessed a fear of surgery and had apparently passed it on to his son. The influential factors in the trial court's opinion, which was upheld by the New York Court of Appeals, were that the child was old enough to have opinions of his own which should be respected, and that the surgery, although likely to be highly beneficial and free from risk, could wait.[73]

On the other hand, in a number of other cases the factual situation, the particular statute involved, and the philosophy of the judges have led courts to order nonemergency medical or surgical care for minors deemed to be "neglected." Illustrative are the Texas case

[71] *State v. Perricone*, 37 N.J. at 478, 181 A. 2d at 759.
[72] *In re Frank*, 41 Wash. 2d 294, 248 P. 2d 553 (1952).
[73] *In re Seiferth*, 309 N.Y. 80, 127 N.E. 2d 820 (1955).

of *Mitchell v. Davis,* involving a twelve-year-old suffering from arthritis and rheumatic fever, and the 1972 case of *In re Sampson,* in which a New York court ordered surgery to correct a serious deformity in a fifteen-year-old who had not attended school for several years.[74]

When issues of constitutional law are introduced into situations of nonemergency care, the matter becomes somewhat more complicated and perhaps even more emotional. In the 1972 Pennsylvania case entitled *In re Green* the minor patient, sixteen years of age, needed corrective surgery of the spine as a result of polio. The mother gave her consent to the surgery itself; but she refused permission to administer blood because she was a Jehovah's Witness. The superior court declared the minor to be "neglected" and appointed a guardian. This decision was reversed on the grounds that the state could not interfere with a parent's religious beliefs unless the patient's life was in immediate peril. Further, said the court, the lower court had not taken into account the minor's own wishes.[75] As in many such cases, there was a strong dissent this time by three judges who argued that the only concern should be the health of the minor and that parents should not be permitted to make martyrs of their children.

As we have seen, there are unresolved issues and conflicting philosophies regarding the intervention of a court when parents allegedly fail to provide adequate medical care for their minor children. When such fundamental constitutional rights as freedom of religion are at issue, the task of balancing the rights of all the respective parties becomes especially difficult and the differing philosophies of individual judges clearly apparent. The same conflict over the power of government to intervene is also evident in the cases dealing with the right of an adult individual to refuse medical care. With respect to governmental intervention designed to assure a minor child of proper care, the issues are likely to be resolved eventually in favor of the child's right to life and health.

Tests Requested by Law Enforcement Officials

Hospitals are frequently requested to draw blood or take samples of urine from a person in police custody or under arrest (or to perform a breath analysis test) in order to determine whether the prisoner is intoxicated or otherwise under the influence of drugs.

[74] 205 S.W. 2d 812, 12 A.L.R. 2d 1042 (Texas Civ. App. 1947); 29 N.Y. 2d 900, 328 N.Y.S. 2d 686, 278 N.E. 2d 918 (1972).
[75] 448 Pa. 338, 292 A. 2d 387, 52 A.L.R. 3d 1106 (1972).

Two major legal issues are presented by such requests.

The first is a question of civil law: does the taking of such a test constitute an assault and battery? Clearly, as a matter of common law, it would be a battery if the patient has not granted a proper consent as previously defined.[76] Even if he presumably consented, the consent might well be ineffective if the patient were intoxicated or so nearly unconscious that he did not understand the nature and effect of his act. Unless a statute specifically authorizes such tests without consent, a civil action in damages for assault and battery could consequently be brought against the physician, others who performed the test, or the hospital. Accordingly many attorneys advise their clients not to conduct such tests for law enforcement officials.

In most cases, however, no actual physical injury or harm would result to the patient subjected to a test contrary to his express or implied consent, as long as the test was conducted without negligence, and any damages recoverable in a civil action would probably be only nominal. Nevertheless the risk of legal liability requires that hospitals and their personnel refrain from administering these tests unless there is an adequate consent from the patient or unless the test is otherwise authorized by local law. This recommendation is particularly relevant to the withdrawal of blood, which of course necessitates physical contact with the patient's person.

Although law enforcement officials may request hospital personnel to conduct blood or similar tests in a variety of factual situations involving alleged criminal activity, the most typical situation concerns driving on public highways. To help the police promote highway safety, nearly all states have enacted "implied consent" laws. Many of these statutes do not, however, deal adequately with the civil liability of the hospital or of the personnel who administer the tests without consent of the patient.

Implied consent statutes differ considerably among jurisdictions, and the advice of local legal counsel about the effect of a particular law is absolutely mandatory. In general, however, the statutes provide that a person driving a motor vehicle on a public highway, by this act, "impliedly consents" to the administration of any or all blood, urine, and breath tests if he should be arrested and charged with

---

[76] *Bednarik v. Bednarik*, 18 N.J. Misc. 633, 16 A. 2d 80 (Ch. 1940). In general, under common law, medical and hospital personnel are under no legal duty to honor a request or command by law enforcement officials to conduct blood alcohol or other tests for possible intoxication. If a physician, for instance, is in the employ of a law enforcement agency, however, a duty is created by the employment contract. (The case cited was overruled on other grounds, *Cortese v. Cortese*, 10 N.J. Super. 152, 76 A. 2d 717 [App. Div. 1950].)

driving while intoxicated or under the influence of alcohol. Many of the statutes require that the driver be formally under arrest and officially charged pursuant to the relevant criminal statute before the implied consent law can be invoked by government.

However, the majority of the statutes provide that a driver may affirmatively refuse administration of the test or tests itemized in the statute to which he has presumably impliedly consented. The state in turn is thereupon authorized to revoke or suspend such a driver's license for a period of time without further criminal prosecution for alleged violation of the statutes pertaining to driving while intoxicated or under the influence of alcohol. The person under arrest may thus exercise his choice of submitting to the test in the hope of proving he was not legally intoxicated and so avoiding further criminal prosecution, or refusing the test and losing his driving privileges. Whether or not a given individual on given facts should submit to the test or refuse is a matter for him and his personal attorney to decide.

From the viewpoint of hospital personnel the main point is that, even though the test is authorized by the implied consent statutes and performed at the request of police, it should not be given in the face of an express refusal or resistance by the patient, if he has a statutory right of refusal, as is true in most states. On the other hand, if the person in police custody consents to the test, then the hospital should obtain the prisoner's approval in writing. Hospital personnel must also be certain that the patient is in fact formally arrested and charged, if that is a requirement of the local implied consent law. Further, some statutes require that the request from the police be in writing and that only certain persons—a physician, a registered nurse, or perhaps a licensed medical technologist—may perform the test. Statutory itemization of professional personnel authorized to conduct the requested test is especially likely for administering a blood test. Nurses' aides and orderlies are not usually authorized to withdraw blood.

Quite a number of the implied consent laws do contain certain provisions providing immunity from civil liability for medical personnel, nurses, and others, including the hospital itself in some states, if the blood is withdrawn or the test conducted at the request of police. However, the immunity provisions of each particular statute may not apply in many states if the driver has refused the test, or if the test was done "improperly." Immunity may thus be more apparent than real, thereby emphasizing once again the importance of having local counsel's opinion concerning hospital policy about tests that involve persons in police custody.[77]

When the test is administered to a driver who is dead, incapacitated by injuries, or unconscious, additional questions arise. He cannot exercise his right of refusal of an alcohol test. Some of the statutes provide that his implied consent to the test is effective, yet do not answer the precise question of possible civil liability of the hospital and its personnel. Unless local counsel advises otherwise on the basis of interpretation of a particular statute, a blood test for the sole purpose of determining alcoholic content should not be administered to an incapacitated or unconscious person. Medical care can and should be rendered to such a patient according to his needs and the general law of consent.

The second major legal issue in taking blood for alcohol and similar tests is whether the results of the examination are admissible as evidence in court in a criminal action against the alleged offender. The primary concern arises from state and federal constitutional provisions protecting individuals from unreasonable searches and seizures, from being a witness against themselves, or from providing self-incriminating evidence in criminal trials, and guaranteeing that all persons charged with a crime are entitled to due process of law. As a starting point, if an individual has granted a legally effective consent to the taking of the test, then the evidence is admissible in court since no constitutional right is violated so long as the test meets established standards of scientific reliability.[78] On the other hand, if the accused individual did not grant an effective express consent, or one implied in fact or in law, state courts have apparently differed in their interpretation of the rights involved under the state

---

[77]One of the more comprehensive immunity provisions would appear to be New York's statute. It provides that no physician, registered nurse, hospital, or other employer of a doctor or nurse shall be sued or held liable for any act done or omitted when withdrawing blood at the request of a police officer. N.Y. Vehicle and Traffic Law, sec. 1194(7)(b)(McKinney Supp. 1975-76). Accordingly, there appears to be immunity from liability even if the test is administered without consent of the patient. But, as the text cautions, not all immunity provisions are as protective of hospitals and their personnel.

[78]*Spitler v. State*, 221 Indiana 107, 46 N.E. 2d 591 (1943). See also: *State v. Werling*, 234 Iowa 1109, 13 N.W. 2d 318 (1944). (Results of blood test were admissible where there was no duress in taking the test and where the defendant voluntarily submitted, although he was mistaken with respect to his right to refuse the test.) Compare, however, constitutional rights with rights under local implied consent statutes: *People of State of Michigan v. Weaver*, 253 N.W. 2d 359 (Mich. Ct. App. 1977). (Results of a blood alcohol test administered pursuant to the implied consent statute with consent of patient in contrast to administration pursuant to common law were not admissible in evidence when the defendant was later arrested and charged with negligent homicide. The implied consent statute relates only to criminal prosecution for driving under the influence of intoxicating liquor or for driving while faculties were impaired by the consumption of liquor, citing *People v. Keen*, 396 Mich. 573, 242 N.W. 2d 405 (1976).

constitution, depending perhaps on the facts of each particular case. According to some courts the evidence was not admissible in state criminal proceedings, because it was obtained in violation of the right to be free from an unreasonable search or seizure, especially when the case concerned a test administered before the defendant's arrest.[79] On the other hand, other state courts permitted the evidence to be admitted in criminal trials, even if it had been obtained without consent, and even if the patient was not under formal arrest at the time the test was administered.[80]

The constitutional issues were resolved by two leading decisions of the U.S. Supreme Court, *Breithaupt v. Abram*[81] and *Schmerber v. State of California.*[82] In *Breithaupt*, a pick-up truck in New Mexico collided with an automobile and three persons were killed. A nearly empty whiskey bottle was found in the truck, and the smell of liquor was evident on the driver's breath. While Breithaupt, the driver, was unconscious in a hospital emergency room, a physician withdrew a sample of blood pursuant to the request of a police officer. Breithaupt was later charged with involuntary manslaughter, the evidence obtained from the blood test was admitted at trial, and he was convicted. The Supreme Court held that administering the test to an unconscious person and admitting the results of the test as evidence in the criminal proceeding did not violate the due process clause of the Fourteenth Amendment to the federal Constitution. Due process requires only conformance with the community's sense of decency and fairness; the concept is violated only by conduct that "shocks the conscience" or "offends a sense of justice." Since blood tests are routine, well accepted by society and state law in

---

[79] *State v. Weltha*, 228 Iowa 519, 292 N.W. 148 (1940): (A conviction for manslaughter was reversed when results of a blood sample taken from an unconscious patient were admitted in evidence). *State v. Wolf*, 53 Del. 88, 164 A. 2d 865 (1960): (Results of a blood test taken from an unconscious person not yet placed under arrest were not admissible in a criminal proceeding, because this would violate the provisions in the state constitution prohibiting unreasonable searches and seizures). *State v. Kroening*, 274 Wisc. 266, 79 N.W. 2d 810 (1956): (Taking a blood sample from a semiconscious person not under formal arrest does not violate a state constitutional provision against self-incrimination but does constitute an unlawful search).

[80] *State v. Pierce*, 120 Vt. 373, 141 A. 2d 419 (1958): (Taking of blood from defendant who claimed that he was unconscious at the time did not violate a state constitutional guarantee against unreasonable search; and admission of evidence did not violate the guarantee against self-incrimination). *People v. Duroncelay*, 48 Cal. 2d 766, 312 P. 2d 690 (1957): (Evidence of a blood sample taken from defendant without consent was properly obtained when no force was used, and when there was reasonable cause to believe that defendant had committed a felony and thus could have been lawfully arrested at the time. A search is not unlawful merely because it precedes rather than follows the arrest).

[81] 352 U.S. 432, 77 S. Ct. 408, 1 L. Ed. 2d 448 (1957).

[82] 384 U.S. 757, 86 S. Ct. 1826, 16 L. Ed. 2d 908 (1966).

a variety of factual contexts, and safe, and since they were administered in this case at a hospital by a physician, the "slight" intrusion on the individual's person must give way to society's interest in deterring the driving of motor vehicles while under the influence of alcohol.

The majority of the court distinguished between *Breithaupt* and a previous decision which had held that the forceable pumping of a prisoner's stomach, resulting in the discovery of narcotics, violated the rights of due process, since such conduct was "brutal," "offensive," and "shocked the conscience."[83] At the time of the *Breithaupt* decision, New Mexico did not have an implied consent statute, but it is clear from the reasoning of the decision that the court would have approved such a statute, at least the basic constitutionality of the law relative to the due process clause.

Additional constitutional issues were considered in *Schmerber v. State of California:*[84] a criminal defendant's right under the Fifth Amendment's guarantee against being compelled to be a witness against himself; and the Fourth Amendment's prohibition on unreasonable searches and seizures. First of all, these federal constitutional amendments were held applicable to state criminal prosecutions in decisions of the U.S. Supreme Court after the *Breithaupt* case and prior to *Schmerber,* since the two amendments are embraced within the Fourteenth Amendment.[85] In *Schmerber* the defendant had been arrested at a hospital while being treated for injuries received in an automobile accident; a blood sample was taken at the direction of a police officer despite the express objection of the patient. The results of the test were later admitted as evidence in a criminal prosecution for driving while under the influence of alcohol, and the defendant was convicted. The Supreme Court held that there had been no violation of Mr. Schmerber's constitutional rights.

The privilege against self-incrimination protects an accused only from being compelled to testify against himself, and this in turn relates only to obtaining evidence through a testimonial or communicative act. The defendant is entitled to remain silent unless he chooses to speak, and communications from him may not be compelled.

[83]*Rochin v. California,* 342 U.S. 165, 72 S. Ct. 205, 96 L. Ed. 183 (1952). See also: *People v. Bracamonte,* 15 Cal. 3d 394, 540 P. 2d 624, 124 Cal. Rptr. 528 (1975). (Administration of an emetic without the voluntary consent of a person suspected of violating narcotics laws, causing the regurgitation of balloons of heroin swallowed by the suspect, was not justified in the circumstances, and evidence thus obtained should have been suppressed.)
[84]384 U.S. 757 (1966).
[85]*Malloy v. Hogan,* 378 U.S. 1, 8, 84 S. Ct. 1489, 1493, 12 L. Ed. 2d 653 (1964) (Fifth Amendment); *Mapp v. Ohio,* 367 U.S. 643, 81 S. Ct. 1684, 6 L. Ed. 2d 1081 (1961) (Fourth Amendment).

But obtaining evidence through blood tests, fingerprints, photographs, or identification procedures does not violate the Fifth Amendment, since these activities of police officers do not compel "communications" or "testimony." Although the majority of the court concurred in this ruling, four justices vigorously dissented. The dissent of two was based primarily on the ground that administering the blood test over the objection of the defendant and subsequently using the evidence at his trial did indeed compel the accused to be a witness against himself. In short, this dissent rejected the majority's "shadowy" distinction between compelling him to give "physical evidence" like blood and "eliciting responses which are essentially testimonial."[86] A separate dissenting opinion agreed with the foregoing reasoning that the privilege of self-incrimination should apply and added the further argument that the due process clause prohibits the state from committing a tort upon the person of the defendant.[87]

With respect to the defendant's right under the Fourth and Fourteenth Amendments to be free from unlawful search and seizure, the *Schmerber* court ruled that the Constitution does not prohibit all intrusions but rather constrains intrusions "which are not justified in the circumstances or which are made in an improper manner."[88] There was probable cause in the case for the police to arrest the defendant without a warrant upon the charge of driving under the influence of alcohol. Following a lawful arrest the police can make a reasonable search without a warrant if they have reasonable ground for believing an emergency exists, in that evidence might be destroyed during the time necessary to obtain a search warrant. Since the percentage of alcohol in the blood diminishes soon after the person stops drinking, the search was an appropriate incident of the arrest. Further, the search was made or conducted in a reasonable manner; the administration of a blood test involves virtually no risk, trauma, or pain to the patient; the test was made by a physician in a hospital pursuant to accepted medical practices. Consequently defendant's right to be free from unreasonable searches and seizures was not violated.

---

[86] 384 U.S. at 775.
[87] *Id.* at 779.
[88] *Id.* at 768. *Cf.: People v. Williams*, 557 P. 2d 399 (Colorado 1976). (In the prosecution of Claudine Longet Williams for the fatal shooting of skier Spider Sabich the state acted improperly when it required her to give samples of blood and urine without consent or warrant, and in the absence of clear indications of intoxication or drug use.)

Physicians and hospital personnel should note carefully that the Supreme Court in *Breithaupt* and *Schmerber* did not deal with the issue of civil liability in tort for administering a blood test without the patient's consent. The issue of civil liability accordingly remains a matter for state law to determine through interpretation of the local implied consent statutes, as previously discussed.

The facts and legal issues in *Schmerber v. State of California* must be carefully distinguished from those in *Graves v. Beto.*[89] In *Graves* a suspect in a criminal proceeding consented to the taking of a blood sample at the request of police, who had apparently indicated that the sample was taken to determine the degree, if any, of the suspect's intoxication. In actual fact, the police wished to ascertain the suspect's blood type as possibly relevant to an alleged rape then under investigation. Since there had been misrepresentation concerning the need and purpose of the procedure, the consent was ineffective and taking the sample constituted a tort. Moreover the results of the test were inadmissible as evidence in a subsequent criminal proceeding against the patient. Proper conduct by the police to ascertain the blood type of the patient would be to obtain an appropriate court order for administering the test, since there was ample time for making the necessary application.

Courts, given the appropriate facts and circumstances, will order such tests and procedures as they deem necessary to promote the legitimate interests of society in gaining evidence which may help to establish the truth, providing society's interests outweigh individual rights. In the recent Georgia case of *Creamer v. State* the court upheld an order of the trial court permitting the removal of what was suspected to be a bullet from Creamer, a person under arrest for murder.[90] Creamer had allegedly been present when the double murder took place at the home of the victims, and had presumably been struck by a bullet fired by one of them. Although he voluntarily consented to a physical examination and apparently admitted that a bullet might be embedded in his body, he refused consent for its removal. Physical and x-ray examination indicated the presence of a steel object. Removal would require only a local anesthetic and entail minimal risk. The point of evidence, of course, was that retrieval of the actual object might well establish whether or not it was a bullet fired by one of the victims. Following the precedent of *Schmerber v. State of California*, the Georgia court held that a court order

---

[89] 424 F. 2d 524 (5th Cir. 1970), *cert. denied*, 400 U.S. (1970).
[90] 229 Ga. 511, 192 S.E. 2d 350 (1972), *cert. dismissed*, 410 U.S. 975 (1973).

authorizing removal of the object would not violate either the Fourth
Amendment, prohibiting unreasonable searches and seizures, or the
Fifth Amendment, guaranteeing that one shall not be compelled
to be a witness against himself.

Consistent with *Creamer* is *United States v. Crowder.*[91] This case
involved an attempted robbery of a dentist in which a struggle
occurred and the dentist was killed with his own .32-caliber revolver.
Crowder, who was charged with the crime, had been shot in the
forearm. An x-ray revealed that the bullet lodged in Mr. Crowder's
arm was .32 caliber. He refused medical treatment for the wound,
but a federal trial court granted the government's request for
authorization permitting surgical removal of what proved to be a
bullet fired from the dentist's gun. At the time the order was applied
for, expert medical testimony was submitted to the effect that the
contemplated surgery was "minor" and that it would not represent
any risk to the defendant's health. Subsequently Crowder was convicted of a second degree murder, robbery, and carrying a dangerous
weapon.

On appeal the court found that the defendant's right to be free
from an unreasonable search and seizure had not been violated,
and hence that the evidence of the bullet was admissible at trial.
The trial court's order permitting the surgical removal of the bullet
from Mr. Crowder's arm without his consent was reasonable since
the evidence was relevant and could not be obtained in any other
way. Moreover, the minor surgery was performed by a qualified
surgeon in a hospital, and a full hearing had been provided before
the operation was performed.

Even though courts will order reasonable medical or surgical
treatment over the objection of persons charged with criminal activity,
when it is deemed necessary to promote the legitimate interests of
society, both law enforcement officials and medical personnel must
be constantly alert to the general rule and philosophy that an informed
consent is necessary before rendering medical care or treatment,
including treatment intended to help enforce criminal laws, unless
on the particular facts and circumstances the interest of the public
outweighs the right of an individual to be secure in his person.
When the hospital provides care to persons in police custody, the
hospital attorney should advise the institution concerning practices
and policies which will be consistent with both local state law and
constitutional law.

---

[91] 543 F. 2d 312 (D.C. Cir. 1976).

Sometimes a competent person capable of giving consent will request or even demand a blood or urine test for alcohol or drugs, acting in the belief that the results are likely to provide evidence of his innocence. In such situations law enforcement officials should arrange for the test—and medical and hospital personnel would probably be advised by counsel to cooperate thoroughly—since failure of the police to comply with the request may well constitute a deprivation of the individual's right to due process of law.

IX

Abortion

That the common law of judicial decision, constitutional law, and statutory law proscribing certain behavior as criminal all reflect the consensus of society's moral beliefs as well as social and economic policy is indisputable. Since law is inseparably bound with moral, social, and economic values, laws will change as these values change. The law of abortion provides an excellent illustration of these fundamental observations of the Anglo-American legal system.

Historical Background

Prior to the nineteenth century the act of abortion during the early stages of pregnancy was not prohibited by the English or American law. Indeed, the common law courts had not considered abortion before "quickening," that is, when the first fetal movements are felt by the mother, to be a criminal act. Canon or church law, expressed by various philosophers and theologians, held that the soul entered the fetus at the time of quickening, and accordingly the early English common law apparently made abortion of a quick fetus a crime. Some opinions, consistent with the views of Bracton and Coke, maintained that an abortion after quickening was a serious criminal act, a felony in the category of murder, manslaughter, or other recognizable forms of homicide. Blackstone, however, the greatest of common law scholars, believed that an abortion of even a quick fetus was an offense no greater than a misdemeanor; and some scholars have maintained that it was never established in English law at all that abortion of a quickened fetus was a criminal act. In view of these apparently differing opinions in England, the American courts in deciding actual cases pursuant to common law

260

reached differing conclusions. Some held than an abortion of a quickened fetus was criminal, at least a misdemeanor; but others ruled that an abortion, regardless of the stage of pregnancy, was not a criminal act.[1] In any event, regardless of these differing common law views, the matter soon became a question solely of statutory law, since according to a generally well-accepted principle in Anglo-American jurisprudence criminal law must be established by statute and not by common law judicial decision.

The English Parliament enacted the first restrictive abortion statute in 1803. It provided that a willful abortion of a quickened fetus was a capital crime and further prohibited all abortions by establishing lesser penalties for abortions performed during earlier stages of pregnancy.[2] If the surgery was performed in good faith to preserve the life of the mother, however, then no criminal act had been committed.[3]

American jurisdictions soon adopted this viewpoint by passing restrictive abortion statutes. Connecticut was the first state to do so when it passed a statute in 1821 which accepted the English distinction between a quickened and unquickened fetus. Similarly, an 1828 New York statute provided that an abortion after quickening was a felony—that is, manslaughter—and a misdemeanor prior to that point of pregnancy. An exception was made to preserve the life of the mother.

By the Civil War or soon thereafter nearly all states had enacted restrictive abortion statutes of some type; and by and large most statutes in time abandoned the distinction between a quickened and unquickened fetus. In the 1950s and 1960s the various laws generally fell into these categories: A few states banned all abortions regardless of the stage of pregnancy and regardless of the reason for the procedure. Most, however, permitted termination of pregnancy to preserve the mother's life, although prohibiting termination under all other circumstances; and a few statutes were more liberal, in that they permitted the surgery to preserve the mother's health. Some of the laws specifically required that only a physician could

[1] See citations in footnotes 27 and 28 of *Roe v. Wade*, 410 U.S. 113, 115, 35 L. Ed. 2d 147, 167; 98 S. Ct. 705, 718 (1973). See also: Wasmuth and Chareau, "Abortion Laws: The Perplexing Problem," 18 *Cleveland St. L. Rev.* 503, no. 3, Sept. 1969.
[2] Lord Ellenborough's Act, 42 Geo. 3, ch. 58. Parliament reversed this position by enacting a very liberal abortion bill in 1967.
[3] The statutory language of "preserving the life of the mother" was very liberally interpreted. In *Rex v. Bourne* (1939) 1 K.B. 687 (1938), a physician who aborted a 14-year-old rape victim was acquitted of criminal charges after the judge instructed the jury that the doctor was acting within the law to prevent the patient from becoming a mental or physical "wreck."

perform the surgery; some required the attending physician to consult with other doctors; and from state to state there were similar statutory safeguards intended to assure that professional people were following the fundamental statutory prohibitions on abortion. Violation of these restrictive laws was, of course, deemed a criminal offense. Consent of the patient did not generally protect the one performing the illegal surgery from criminal prosecution. As to whether or not consent prohibited a civil cause of action for damages, the state court decisions on this issue differed. The weight of authority held that a civil action could not be brought unless the patient could establish professional negligence or malpractice in the conduct of the abortion.

During the 1960s a very noticeable trend developed to liberalize these restrictive state laws in accordance with a model law developed by the American Law Institute. By 1970 approximately one-third of the states had amended their respective statutes by permitting a licensed physician to terminate pregnancy when there was "substantial risk that continuance of pregnancy would gravely impair the physical or mental health of the mother, or that the child would be born with grave physical or mental defects or that the pregnancy resulted from rape, incest, or other felonious intercourse."[4] Termination of pregnancy under circumstances other than those described was a felony of the third degree if performed prior to the twenty-sixth week, and of the second degree if performed after that time. The model law futher required that all abortions take place in a licensed hospital, unless an emergency existed and such facilities were not available. Moreover, at least two physicians had to certify in writing the circumstances justifying the surgery. Some jurisdictions, while enacting essentially the model law, added additional requirements. Examples of such requirements were that the patient be a resident of the state for a specified time prior to the surgery, that the attending physician obtain the concurrence of a hospital medical staff committee, and that the hospital where the surgery was to be performed be accredited by the Joint Commission on Accreditation of Hospitals.

The reasons for the highly restrictive criminal statutes lie in moral and social values of the nineteenth century which are not entirely clear. Most modern legal historians and other investigators have concluded, however, that the primary legislative motive in the 1800s and the first half of the 1900s was to protect the interest and, indeed, the very life of the prospective mother rather than the life of the unborn. Medically the procedure of abortion was dangerous to the

---

[4]Model Penal Code, sec. 230.3(2) (1962).

pregnant woman in the nineteenth century. With the substantial lessening of risk to the mother through more recent advances in medical science, many have argued that at least this rationale for restrictive legislation no longer existed. It is of course common knowledge that social and economic environments and values have changed considerably in the current century, setting the stage for the abolition of restrictive abortion laws, so that by 1970 the only concern would be the welfare of the individual mother.

In actual fact, the restrictive abortion statutes permitting therapeutic abortions only to "preserve the life of the mother," or to preserve her "life or health," were very liberally construed by public prosecutors as well as by many physicians and hospitals, which followed a policy of providing therapeutic terminations of pregnancy. Actual criminal prosecutions against licensed physicians conducting in-hospital abortions were indeed rare. Such criminal prosecutions as were on record were against physicians or laymen who performed abortions outside a hospital and under circumstances where standards of professional care and competence were questionable.

By the end of 1970, liberalization of the law in New York, Washington, Hawaii, and Alaska had gone much further than the model law of the American Law Institute. These states had adopted in essence the principle of abortion on demand, at least up to a statutorily designated stage of pregnancy. New York, Hawaii, and Alaska accomplished this change by statute, whereas the state of Washington did so by popular referendum of the people. Again, however, these states imposed certain restrictions. For example, the procedure had to be done by a licensed physician in a licensed or an accredited hospital; and all these states but New York required that the woman must establish a period of residency in the state before she would be eligible for an abortion.

Then came the two landmark cases of *Roe v. Wade* and *Doe v. Bolton*, decided by the U.S. Supreme Court in January 1973, after considerable litigation in lower federal courts and some state courts concerning the constitutionality of the restrictive abortion statutes.[5] In the light of what the Supreme Court has held, or apparently held, no useful purpose would be served in reviewing the lower court litigation, except to note by way of generality that the various cases dealt with several different issues of constitutional law and had varying results; and they were, of course, concerned as in all

[5]*Roe v. Wade*, 410 U.S. 113, 35 L. Ed. 2d 147, 93 S. Ct. 705 (1973); *Doe v. Bolton*, 410 U.S. 179, 35 L. Ed. 2d 201, 93 S. Ct. 739 (1973).

appellate litigation with the constitutionality of particular provisions of particular statutes. Nevertheless, a significant issue in all criminal statutes is that the statute must not be too "vague" for meaningful understanding and objective enforcement. As a general doctrine criminal statutes must adequately define the crime so that the alleged offender is properly informed of standards to guide his conduct. On the matter of the "vagueness" of statutes permitting abortion only "to preserve the life" of the mother or her "health," the courts differed in result until this particular issue was finally resolved by the United States Supreme Court. In *United States v. Vuitch* in 1971 it held that the District of Columbia statute permitting abortions only to "preserve" the mother's life and health was not unconstitutional and violative of the Fourteenth Amendment's guarantee of due process of law.[6] The word "health," it was said, has a generally accepted meaning, at least among physicians, and accordingly the statute provided adequate standards that properly informed the populace of expected conduct and were capable of interpretation in defining criminal behavior.

Other cases prior to the Supreme Court decisions in *Wade* and *Bolton* raised a broader, more fundamental issue of constitutional law: Does a female person have a right to decide for herself whether or not to bear a child free from governmental regulation? It was this fundamental question that the court decided in *Wade* and *Bolton*, although as will be noted other specific questions or issues still await determination or clarification.

The *Wade* and *Bolton* Cases

The case of *Roe v. Wade* concerned the constitutionality of the very restrictive Texas statute, while the companion litigation of *Doe v. Bolton* raised issues relevant to the more liberal Georgia legislation.

The Texas law permitted an abortion at any stage of pregnancy only to save the life of the mother. The issue presented to the court was whether or not the state had a sufficient "compelling interest" in the subject matter of regulation to justify the nearly total prohibition on abortion. As will be recalled, a state may regulate matters of health and welfare under its police power only if the measures are necessary in the public interest, to protect the general welfare and

---

[6]91 S. Ct. 1294, 28 L. Ed. 2d 601, 402 U.S. 62, (1971). On this issue of vagueness the court reversed the federal district court for the District of Columbia, 305 F. Supp. 1032 (1969).

public health of the community. Otherwise, regulatory statutes violate the Fourteenth Amendment.

The test of a sufficient public interest to justify regulatory statutes and regulations may vary, depending upon the nature of the individual rights which are regulated. To justify exercise of the police power the state generally needs only to establish that the regulatory measures bear a rational relationship to legitimate governmental interest. When "fundamental" individual rights are involved, however, as articulated by judicial decision, then the state must convince the court that there is a "compelling interest" justifying the restraints. Since an individual's right of privacy is a fundamental right, the *Wade* and *Bolton* cases employed the compelling interest test when ruling on the constitutionality of the Texas and Georgia abortion statutes.

In *Roe v. Wade* the court held the entire Texas statute to be unconstitutional in violation of the due process clause of the Fourteenth Amendment. A "balancing of interests" between the state, acting on behalf of the general welfare, and the individual seeking an abortion results in the conclusion that the individual's rights of privacy are paramount to the provisions of the statute under consideration.

This does not mean that the state may not regulate abortion at all. The court viewed pregnancy as consisting of three trimesters, and the extent of permissible state regulation will vary depending upon the duration of the pregnancy. Even in the early stages of pregnancy, the Supreme Court ruled, the woman's right to obtain an abortion is qualified. During the first trimester the state may require that the abortion be performed by a duly licensed physician, and abortions conducted by laymen can be proscribed as criminal under a properly drafted statute.[7] But no other restrictions may be placed upon a patient's right to terminate her pregnancy. Essentially the decision to perform an abortion during the first trimester of pregnancy is solely that of the patient and her physician.[8]

Accordingly, a state or city may not enact local statutes or ordinances regulating clinics and other facilities for first-trimester abortions, even if such laws are intended to improve the care rendered. An

---

[7]Such a statutory provision is clearly constitutional. *May v. State of Arkansas,* 254 Ark. 194, 492 S.W. 2d 888 (1973), *cert. denied,* 414 U.S. 1024 (1973). This decision was rendered after the *Wade* and *Bolton* cases. See also: *State v. Norflett,* 67 N.J. 268, 337 A. 2d 609 (1975).

[8]*Drake v. Covington County Board of Education,* 371 F. Supp. 974 (N.D. Ala. 1974). (Cancellation of an unmarried teacher's contract on the basis that she was pregnant was held to be an unconstitutional invasion of her right of privacy, since she had the right to decide whether or not to have an abortion.)

authoritative decision to date on this matter is *Word v. Poelker,* decided by the U.S. Circuit Court of Appeals, Eighth Circuit in 1974.[9] The court invalidated a St. Louis ordinance requiring abortion clinics to obtain a city permit which called for disclosure of the names of the applicants, of all physicians using the facilities, and of nurses, as well as a resume of the qualifications of the personnel, and a description of the space and equipment available. The basis of the decision was that similar permits or licenses were not required for other clinics or facilities in which surgery of like risk was performed on ambulatory patients, and thus the regulatory ordinance substantially limited the doctor's right to practice medicine and the patient's freedom of choice in seeking a first-trimester abortion. States and cities thus seem virtually powerless to regulate facilities where abortions are performed in the very early stages of pregnancy when such regulations apply only to abortion procedures, even though the purpose of the regulations is to enforce standards of quality in the care rendered.

Following *Word* the Seventh Circuit Court of Appeals found that detailed regulations promulgated by the Chicago Board of Health and applied to a medical corporation offering first-trimester abortions were unconstitutional.[10] These regulations established the following requirements: abortions should be performed by a licensed physician; a complete medical history should be obtained from each patient; records should be kept of the admission and discharge of patients; certain laboratory tests should be conducted; twenty-four hours must elapse between the initial examination and the termination of pregnancy; all equipment and supplies must be maintained in proper working order; certain equipment must be available; an elevator large enough to accommodate a stretcher was required in any location above ground level; suitable furnishings and accommodations, including waiting and dressing rooms, must be provided; monthly

---

[9]495 F. 2d 1349 (8th Cir. 1974). Also see: *Coe v. Gerstein,* 376 F. Supp. 695 (S.D. Fla. 1974), *appeal dismissed and cert. denied,* 417 U.S. 279 (1974), *aff'd,* 517 F. 2d 787 (5th Cir. 1975). (Held unconstitutional a Florida statute requiring that abortions be performed in an "approved facility.")
[10]*Friendship Medical Center, Ltd. and T.R.M. Howard v. the Chicago Board of Health,* 505 F. 2d 1141 (7th Cir. 1974), *cert. denied,* 420 U.S. 997 (1975). See also: *Arnold v. Sendak,* 416 F. Supp. 22 (Ind. 1976). (Indiana statute requiring that all abortions be performed in a hospital or licensed health facility is unconstitutional), *aff'd mem.,* 50 L. Ed. 2d 579, 97 S. Ct. 476 (1976). *Cf.: Abortion Clinic of Michigan, Inc. v. Michigan Department of Public Health,* 426 F. Supp. 471 (E.D. Mich. 1977). (Licensing statute and regulations of "free standing surgical outpatient facilities" are not facially unconstitutional as applied to first-trimester abortion facilities simply because statute narrows the physician's choice in deciding where an abortion is to be performed.)

reports listing the number of patients requesting abortions, the number of abortions performed, and the names of patients suffering complications must be filed; and a written affiliation agreement with a licensed Chicago hospital for the use of laboratory facilities and the treatment of emergency cases had to be executed. Moreover the clinic had to be supervised by a physician who was either a qualified obstetrician or a surgeon, as determined by certification or eligibility by the American Board of Obstetrics and Gynecology or the American Board of Surgery, The American College of Obstetrics and Gynecology, the American College of Surgery, the American College of Osteopathic Obstetricians and Gynecologists, or the American College of Surgeons.

The foregoing regulations were said to be invalid since they were made applicable to abortion facilities without regard to the trimester of pregnancy. Enforcement would be inconsistent with the Supreme Court's decision in *Roe v. Wade* that the government has a "compelling interest" in the subject matter of regulations only after the first trimester of pregnancy. To put the legal test or criterion another way, a mere "rational relationship" between the regulations and governmental interest in public health is not enough to justify the regulations. Further, the Chicago Board of Health's regulations at issue applied only to facilities for abortions, and there was no comparable regulatory pattern for clinics performing other medical or ambulatory surgical services in which the risks to the patient were as great. By making the regulations applicable only to abortion facilities, the court held, the regulations violated the equal protection clause of the Fourteenth Amendment, since such a classification is unreasonable and arbitrary. In sum, a state or local government lacks the authority to regulate the first-trimester abortion services, even in the interest of maternal health and well-being, because such laws interfere unduly with the fundamental constitutional right of a woman to obtain the surgery. The most that government can require is adherence to general standards of sanitation and building codes.

During the second trimester of pregnancy, however, the state is held to have a sufficient "compelling interest" to issue regulations to protect the mother's health. Individual physicians may by proper statute be prohibited from performing abortions in their private offices. The clinic or other locale of the surgery can be required to have a license and observe rules and regulations related to the mother's health. Probably a licensed hospital could be designated as the sole permissible place of surgery, on the basis that only such an institution is properly equipped and staffed for an abortion at this stage of pregnancy in view of the risks. Such a ruling would be especially likely if medical opinion held that overnight admission of the patient should be required.

Finally, at the stage when the fetus is viable—the third trimester—the state may act to protect the "potentiality of human life," which now, in effect, outbalances the personal interests and desires of the mother and her physician. To terminate pregnancy at this stage can be made a criminal act unless it is necessary to preserve the "life or health" of the mother. Although further clarification of the standard of "health" will be needed, the courts are likely to interpret it liberally and consider mental as well as physical health, as long as the physician can offer documented medical support for his decision.[11]

It is to be especially noted that the court in *Roe v. Wade* did not decide when life begins or when the fetus becomes a "person" as far as the law of abortion is concerned. Physicians, theologians, and philosophers have long debated these questions. A Rhode Island statute (enacted after these landmark Supreme Court cases) which declared that life begins at conception, and that accordingly abortion at any stage of pregnancy is criminal, has been declared unconstitutional, even though the *Wade* case had sidestepped this particular question.[12] Hence the constitutional right to have an abortion, as articulated by *Wade,* may not be avoided by a state statute expressing another philosophy or other grounds that attempt to circumvent individual rights.

Doe v. Bolton involved the constitutionality of the Georgia abortion statute. This legislation, a "liberalized" restrictive enactment following recommendations of the American Law Institute, permitted termination of pregnancies by a licensed physician whenever continued pregnancy would endanger the woman's life or injure her health, when the baby was likely to be born with grave, permanent defects, or when pregnancy was the consequence of rape. In the interest of protecting the patient's health and well-being, however, the law required the physician to exercise his "best clinical judgment" when

[11] *United States v. Vuitch,* 91 S. Ct. 1294, 28 L. Ed. 2d 601, 402 U.S. 62 (1971). ("Health" includes psychological as well as physical well-being.)
[12] *Doe v. Israel,* 358 F. Supp. 1193 (D.R.I. 1973), *cert. denied,* 416 U.S. 993 (1974). Further, the *Wade* and *Bolton* decisions have been held to apply retroactively. A criminal conviction of a physician under an abortion statute now declared unconstitutional must be vacated even if it preceded the Supreme Court decision. *State v. Ingel,* 18 Md. App. 514, 308 A. 2d 223 (1973).

recommending an abortion. It also required that the procedure be carried out in a hospital accredited by the Joint Commission on Accreditation of Hospitals, that it be approved by an abortion committee comprising members of the hospital's medical staff, and that the judgment of the patient's physician be confirmed by two other independent physicians who had examined the patient. Further, the patient had to establish Georgia residency to be considered eligible for an abortion.

The Supreme Court upheld the statutory requirement that the patient's physician be required to exercise his "best clinical judgment" when evaluating the need for an abortion. However, it invalidated the three procedural requirements and the residency requirement, holding that they unduly restricted the rights of doctors and patients to decide on the surgery needed by the patient, and hence violated the Fourteenth Amendment. The court supported its conclusion regarding the procedural matters by noting that Georgia law did not require that other surgical procedures of similar risk take place only in hospitals accredited by the Joint Commission nor that they be preceded by consultation with other physicians. The decision to conduct the surgery is left to the professional judgment and advice of the patient's own physician. Although the court struck down the requirement that abortions could be performed only in hospitals accredited by the Joint Commission, it specifically recognized that that state might, if it wished, require that abortions after the first trimester be performed at licensed facilities and promulgate reasonable standards consistent with the state's legitimate interest in protecting maternal health. The residency requirement was said to be an invasion of the constitutionally protected right to travel, included in the privileges and immunities clause of Article IV, Paragraph 2 of the U.S. Constitution, and hence no state could limit local medical care to its own residents.

The Georgia statute expressly provided that no hospital, physician, or employee of a hospital should be compelled to perform or participate in an abortion. The intent of this provision is of course to protect the institution's and individual's rights to adhere to their moral or religious convictions, as well as to recognize in the law that not all hospitals are adequately equipped and staffed to perform abortions. Individuals had to state their refusal to participate on moral or religious grounds in writing, and such refusal could not form the basis of a claim for damages or other disciplinary action. In *Bolton* the court specifically approved this statutory language—at least by dictum, which means that the precise issue was really not directly involved in the litigation. Such provisions are sometimes referred to as "conscience clauses."

Insofar as such statutes pertain to individuals—physicians, nurses, paramedical personnel—they are certainly constitutionally permissible. The individual's moral convictions should be upheld and protected, although at least the physician should be bound—and would be bound under the general judicial law of malpractice—to refer the patient to another competent practitioner willing to perform an abortion whenever such referral was medically indicated. Whether making hospitals and other health care institutións subject to such statutes is constitutional is discussed in the succeeding section of this chapter. There is likely to be further litigation on the "conscience clause" legislation as it pertains to hospitals, in spite of the Supreme Court's apparent approval of the clause in the *Bolton* case.

A review of these 1973 Supreme Court decisions makes it apparent that some abortions, in certain circumstances, will continue to be criminal acts when the states rewrite their statutes,[13] especially with regard to termination of pregnancies during the second and third trimesters. Certain long-standing legal issues will hence continue to pose problems for hospitals and medical personnel.

The first to be noted here is that a hospital has a duty to prevent criminal acts from taking place on its premises. As the criminal statutes are rewritten, counsel must carefully advise the hospital and its medical

---

[13]At the time of writing nearly one-third of the states have rewritten and enacted new statutes pertaining to abortion. Several simply outline the basic guidelines of the Supreme Court decisions. Others attempt to define "viability" and add requirements, such as the necessity of obtaining the husband's consent or parental consent for an abortion for a minor patient. The unconstitutionality of the new Rhode Island statute was mentioned in an earlier footnote.

Representative decisions with respect to revised abortion statutes are: *Hodgson v. Anderson*, 378 F. Supp. 1008 (D. Minn. 1974), *appeal dismissed*, 420 U.S. 903 (1975): (A Minnesota statute defining a fetus as "viable" at twenty weeks after the beginning period of gestation and prohibiting abortion after this date unless necessary to preserve life or health of mother is held inconsistent with *Roe v. Wade* and hence unconstitutional). *Planned Parenthood Ass'n. v. Fitzpatrick*, 401 F. Supp. 554 (E.D. Pa. 1975): (A Pennsylvania statutory definition of "viability" and a prohibition of abortion subsequent thereto is held unconstitutional). *Wolfe v. Schroering*, 388 F. Supp. 631 (W.D. Ky. 1974): (The following provisions of a revised Kentucky statute are held invalid: A requirement that the physician inform a woman of the physical and mental consequences of having or not having an abortion after the first trimester; a provision requiring the patient's written consent, since abortion was singled out and not distinguished from surgical procedures of like risk; requirements of husband's or parent's consent; prohibition of the saline method of abortion after the first trimester; a provision requiring a 24-hour waiting period for first-trimester abortions. Held valid were provisions prohibiting all abortions after viability except to save the life of the mother and a requirement to report to the city and county in which the patient was a resident). *Cf: Planned Parenthood of Central Missouri v. Danforth*, 392 F. Supp. 1362 (E.D. Mo. 1975): (The following provisions of a Missouri statute are held constitutional: A definition of "viability" as the point of gestation when the fetus could survive outside

staff about changes in the legal status of pregnancy terminations. Administrative policies and procedures must then be developed, as before, to make sure that the institution and staff perform their duty with respect to prevention of criminal acts.

A second legal issue, which will concern hospitals and physicians even more in the light of the greatly liberalized law of abortion, is obtaining the patient's informed consent before a legal abortion is performed. All of the previous discussion of consent is clearly applicable to any procedure designed to terminate a pregnancy. Indeed there is probably more risk of a lawsuit claiming damages because informed consent was not obtained for abortions (and sterilizations) than exists in connection with many other surgical procedures. The hospital must insist that the attending physician explain the procedure and the attendant risks to the patient and obtain a written consent form from the patient as evidence that proper consent was obtained, although it should not carry out special procedures that pertain only to consent for abortions and are not applicable to surgery of like risk.

Thirdly, whether the abortion is or is not a criminal act, the physician, the attending personnel, and the hospital would be civilly liable in damages for negligence or malpractice in either the way the procedure was conducted or the postoperative care.[14] Hence all the general principles of the law of hospital liability and professional

---

the womb; a requirement that the patient's informed consent be obtained; a requirement that the husband's or parent's consent be obtained if the patient is a minor; prohibition of the saline method of abortion after the first trimester), *aff'd in part, reversed and remanded in part*, 96 S. Ct. 2831 (1976). Requirements concerning the husband's and parent's consent are further discussed in a succeeding section of this chapter. See also: *Shulman v. New York City Health and Hospitals Corporation*, 38 N.Y. 2d 234, 342 N.E. 2d 501, 379 N.Y.S. 2d 702 (1975). (A city health department rule requiring that a confidential pregnancy termination certificate include the name and address of the patient was ruled valid and did not constitute unconstitutional invasion of privacy.)

[14]Several cases have ruled on allegations that the failure to diagnose pregnancy in time for an abortion constitutes malpractice, and state a claim for damages for the costs of raising a healthy, but unwanted, child. Wisconsin has rejected such a claim on the basis of public policy. *Rieck v. Medical Protective Company of Fort Wayne, Indiana*, 64 Wisc. 2d 514, 219 N.W. 2d 242 (1974). *Cf.: Ziemba v. Sternberg*, 45 App. Div. 230, 357 N.Y.S. 2d 265 (1974). (When the physician knew that the patient did not want children and he negligently failed to diagnose pregnancy in time for an abortion, there is a cause of action. The patient and her husband may recover damages for pain and suffering incident to birth, loss of consortium, and educational and medical expenses of the child.) *Cf.:* Negligent failure to diagnose rubella during pregnancy and to inform the mother does not give the deformed child a cause of action for wrongful life. Parents, however, have cause for damages if they can prove as a fact that they would have obtained a lawful abortion. *Dumer v. St. Michael's Hospital*, 69 Wis. 2d 766, 233 N.W. 2d 372 (1975).

negligence are relevant. This fact should be of particular concern
to physicians performing abortions in their offices or in clinics not
possessing the supporting equipment and trained personnel of a
hospital.

Moreover, in an institutional setting, quality assurance programs
and medical audits of an individual doctor's competence to perform
surgery are clearly necessary and legally supportable in connection
with abortions, just as they are in connection with any surgery. In
other words, not all medical staff physicians need to be allowed
to perform this surgery. Privileges to perform abortions and sterilizations can be restricted pursuant to the substantive and procedural
law reviewed in the chapter on medical staff privileges. The judicial
and statutory requirements for institutional peer review of medical
staff performance have not been eliminated or diluted as a result
of these abortion cases, as long as the review system does not single
out abortion and impose restrictions not equally applicable to other
surgical procedures of similar complexity and risk.

In connection with a criminal abortion, the question can arise
of the civil liability in damages to the patient incurred by the physician
or layman performing the criminal act. Numerous cases have dealt
with this issue and judicial authority has differed. Quite a number
of jurisdictions, probably most, have denied recovery of damages
in the absence of proof of malpractice, simply on the basis that
the patient consented to the procedure and hence is equally at fault
in the performance of a criminal act.[15] Others have held otherwise
and allowed recovery of damages even when the patient freely and
voluntarily consented. This latter view is founded on the philosophy
that public policy should discourage criminal acts, and one way to
do this is to allow a civil lawsuit for damages by the victim, even
when she had consented.[16]

The Hospital's Role in Providing Abortions and Sterilizations

The question here is whether a particular hospital or other health
care institution is legally required to make abortion and sterilization
services available to its potential patients, assuming that it has the
facilities and staff for rendering such care.

As we have seen, specific state or federal statutes may contain

[15]For example: *Miller v. Bennett,* 190 Va. 162, 56 S.E. 2d 217, 21 A.L.R. 2d 364
(1949).
[16]For example: *Milliken v. Heddesheimer,* 110 Ohio St. 381, 144 N.E. 264 (1924).
(A patient who consented to a criminal act can nevertheless recover civil damages.)

a "conscience clause" like that in Georgia, which reads that "nothing in this section shall require a hospital to admit any patient . . . for the purpose of performing an abortion" and which was discussed by way of dictum in the case of *Doe v. Bolton.*[17] In the absence of such a clause, the legal issue to be judicially decided is whether the hospital that refuses to provide abortions or sterilizations is acting in the name of the state in denying to the patient the guarantees of due process and equal protection of law—and thus violating the Fourteenth Amendment—or whether it is acting under "color of law" in denying statutorily established civil rights. In short, a state or any agency thereof, or an institution acting in the name of government, must not prevent an individual from exercising constitutional or statutorily protected rights. An individual or an institution with a duty to implement a right may not refuse performance of the duty. As emphasized repeatedly in various contexts throughout this book, however, the Fourteenth Amendment applies only to state action and not to private action.

It now seems to be well settled that a hospital owned and operated by federal, state, or municipal government may not refuse to perform abortions and sterilizations that are lawful surgical procedures. Publicly owned hospitals clearly act in the capacity of government and are hence subject to the Fourteenth Amendment. The leading decision to date is *Hathaway v. Worcester City Hospital.*[18] In this litigation the patient's physician recommended that she undergo a therapeutic sterilization, since additional pregnancies might well threaten her life. The court entered an order declaring that hospital policy which prohibited all sterilization procedures was a denial of the patient's constitutional right to equal protection of the law. Local statutes creating Worcester City Hospital and pertaining to its operation were silent regarding the provision of sterilization services. That is, the statute neither permitted nor prohibited such surgery. The decision assumes that the hospital had the facilities and staff necessary for the sterilization operation; and it rules, in effect, that restrictions may not be placed on sterilization, a legal surgical procedure, that are not placed upon other surgery entailing similar risks.

Even prior to the abortion cases of *Wade* and *Bolton* a federal

---

[17]410 U.S. 179, 197 (1973).
[18]475 F. 2d 701 (1st Cir. 1973), *appeal for stay of mandate denied,* 411 U.S. 929 (1973), reversing the federal district court, which had held that the patient possessed no constitutional right to have a sterilization performed in a city hospital. 341 F. Supp. 1385 (D. Mass 1972). The decision of the circuit court of appeals was rendered subsequent to the *Wade* and *Bolton* cases on abortion.

274 of The Hospital-Patient Relation

court had held that a public hospital basing its policy regarding sterilizations upon a patient's age and the size of the existing family might well be open to a cause of action for damages. The arbitrary policy resulted in a denial of civil rights as expressed in federal statutes, the court held, although the statute relevant to this particular litigation did not, of course, specifically grant a right to sterilization.[19] In *McCabe* the patient had been denied a sterilization solely on the basis that her age and the size of her family did not meet the rules of the hospital regarding such surgery. Further, in *Doe v. General Hospital of the District of Columbia* a governmental institution was ordered to process applications for abortions to patients who met its rules and regulations, which presumably accorded with the then existing law of legal abortions in the District of Columbia.[20]

Consistent with the *Hathaway* case is *Nyberg v. City of Virginia*, where it was held that a city-owned hospital may not prohibit its staff physicians from performing legal abortions.[21] Although there is no affirmative duty on the part of the hospital to provide staff and facilities for abortion, it may not arbitrarily ban surgery that is not contrary to the legal criteria established by the Supreme Court of the United States. The plaintiffs in *Nyberg* were two staff physicians who were said to have a right to practice medicine, including the performance of abortions. It is assumed that there was no issue in this litigation relative to the doctors' professional competence to do the surgery.

The matter of whether the law should require a private, voluntary hospital to furnish family-planning services is more difficult. On the one hand, the moral and religious convictions held by the institution should certainly be respected. As a legal matter, however, private hospitals that have received Hill-Burton Act funds or other governmental funding in significant amounts have been made subject

---

[19] *McCabe v. Nassau County Medical Center*, 453 F. 2d 698 (2d Cir. 1971).
[20] 313 F. Supp. 1170 (D.D.C. 1970), and 434 F. 2d 423 (D.C. Cir. 1970).
[21] 495 F. 2d 1342 (8th Cir. 1974), *appeal dismissed*, 419 U.S. 891 (1974). See also: *Doe v. Hale Hospital*, 369 F. Supp. 970 (D. Mass. 1974), *aff'd*, 500 F. 2d 144 (1st Cir. 1974), *cert. denied*, 420 U.S. 907 (1975). (A municipal hospital which prohibited all elective abortions although permitting therapeutic abortions was subject to "state action," and hence the policy was in violation of the equal protection clause of the Fourteenth Amendment. It was noted in the district court's opinion that there were virtually no other hospitals providing elective abortions in the area. The cause of action in *Hale* was brought by prospective patients who were in the first trimester of pregnancy.) *Cf.: Poelker v. Jane Doe, etc.*, 97 S. Ct. 2390, 53 L. Ed. 2d 528 (1977). (City-owned hospitals do not violate the Constitution when they choose as a policy to provide publicly financed hospital services for childbirth without providing corresponding services for elective nontherapeutic abortions), *rev'g Doe v. Poelker*, 515 F. 2d 541 (8th Cir. 1975).

to the mandates of the Fourteenth Amendment in cases where "state action" has been found applicable. As emphasized in the chapter on medical staff privileges, this result has been reached in several leading cases which have held that the physician is entitled to the constitutional rights of due process and equal protection with respect to his staff appointment and clinical privileges. Accordingly some lower court and early decisions held that a voluntary hospital may not refuse the patient a sterilization (and by analogy presumably an abortion) that has been recommended by her doctor, if the hospital had received Hill-Burton Act funds and no other hospital with adequate staff and facilities was available in the immediate vicinity.[22]

However, the weight of authority to date has reached an opposite conclusion, namely, that a private hospital need not provide abortion or sterilization services, even if it has been funded to a significant extent by Hill-Burton Act monies and other governmental funds in addition to such benefits as tax-exempt status. The leading case asserting this position is *Doe v. Bellin Memorial Hospital*, decided by a federal circuit court of appeals in 1973.[23] As a private hospital it could prevent its staff physicians from performing legally permissible abortions, because no "state action" was involved. Similarly, relying on *Bellin*, *Allen v. Sisters of St. Joseph* held that a Catholic institution could ban a sterilization procedure requested solely to prevent future pregnancy.[24] It should be noted that hospital policy in the *Bellin* case prohibited abortion and continued to do so even after the *Wade* and *Bolton* cases, except to preserve the mother's life or health, to prevent the birth of an infant likely to be born deformed, or when

---

[22] *Taylor v. St. Vincent's Hospital* (D. Mont. 1972). The federal district court issued a temporary injunction enjoining a private hospital from enforcing a ban on sterilization on the basis that receipt of governmental funds resulted in "state action." Subsequently the injunction was dissolved and the initial decision was thereby reversed, *Taylor v. St. Vincent's Hospital*, 369 F. Supp. 948 (D. Mont. 1973), thus upholding the hospital's policy of not permitting sterilization surgery. The basis of the reversal was, as in the *Watkins* case discussed later, that no violation of constitutional or civil rights was involved in the light of congressional enactment of the Health Programs Extension Act of 1973, 42 U.S.C.A. sec. 300a-7 (1973), which specifically provides that receipt of governmental funds under certain federal acts does not authorize any court or public official to require the facility to provide abortions or sterilizations when a policy of prohibition is based upon religious belief or moral convictions. The district court's decision was upheld by the circuit court of appeal, 523 F. 2d 75 (9th Cir. 1975) and the United States Supreme Court denied certiorari, 96 S. Ct. 1420 (1976), thus upholding the Health Programs Extension Act of 1973. *Cf.: Doe v. Charleston Area Medical Center*, 529 F. 2d 638, (4th Cir. 1975), noted in n. 26, *infra*.
[23] 479 F. 2d 756 (7th Cir. 1973).
[24] 361 F. Supp. 1212 (N.D. Texas 1973). Moreover, the district court's decision is not now reviewable by the circuit court of appeals, since the patient in fact obtained a sterilization at another hospital. *Allen v. Sisters of St. Joseph*, 490 F. 2d 81 (5th Cir. 1974).

the patient was a victim of rape. Further, in *Bellin* the stage of pregnancy was such that an out-of-hospital abortion was contraindicated; and all three of the private general hospitals in Green Bay, Wisconsin, followed similar policies of refusing to admit patients for such surgery.

In another important case, *Watkins v. Mercy Medical Center,* a physician brought suit against a Catholic hospital which forbade both abortions and sterilizations.[25] The policy of the hospital was upheld by a federal district court, which said that state action was not involved by receipt of governmental monies, state licensure, or tax exemption. Significant in this decision was the fact that Public Law 93–45, the Health Programs Extension Act of 1973, specifically provides that receipt of Hill-Burton money does not require a hospital to provide abortions or sterilizations as long as refusal is founded upon institutional religious beliefs or moral conviction.[26] Although Mercy Medical Center was not required to permit the plaintiff physician to perform the surgical procedure he desired, it could not terminate his medical staff appointment solely on the basis of his personal beliefs. Unlike the situation in *Bellin*, it is interesting to note, in *Watkins* several other institutions within a reasonable distance pursued policies that permitted their medical staff to perform abortions.

In sum, most decisions pertaining to private hospitals have to date held that no "state action" is involved under the Fourteenth Amendment, nor do voluntary institutions act under "color of law" in denying civil rights established by federal civil rights statutes, when they prohibit abortion and sterilization procedures. This conclusion is based either on the grounds that receipt of governmental funds and other benefits does not require the hospital to recognize the constitutional rights of the patient, as in the *Bellin* case, or on the grounds that the Health Programs Extension Act of 1973 protects the religious and moral convictions that the hospital represents, as in *Watkins* and *Taylor*.[27]

---

[25] 364 F. Supp. 799 (D. Idaho 1973).
[26] Health Programs Extension Act, 42 U.S.C.A. sec. 300a–7 (1973). Where there is nothing in the record to establish that a private hospital's policy of prohibiting abortions is based upon institutional religious beliefs or moral convictions, the Health Programs Extension Act does not apply. Moreover, a private hospital is engaged in "state action" when it has received Hill-Burton and other governmental funds. *Doe v. Charleston Area Medical Center,* 529 F. 2d 638 (4th Cir. 1975).
[27] See also: *Chrisman v. Sisters of St. Joseph of Peace,* 506 F. 2d 308 (9th Cir. 1974) (Health Programs Extension Act, 42 U.S.C.A. sec. 300a–7 is constitutional.) *Greco v. Orange Memorial Hospital,* 374 F. Supp. 227 (E.D. Tex. 1974), *aff'd,* 513 F. 2d 873 (5th Cir. 1975), *cert. denied,* 423 U.S. 1000 (1975). (A private hospital is not engaged in "state action," even though it receives a significant amount of governmental funds, and thus may bar abortions. The denial of certiorari by the Supreme Court,

As mentioned previously, many states have enacted specific statutes which recite that designated institutions and individuals need not participate in abortion and sterilization procedures against their moral or religious convictions. Most of these state laws relate only to abortions but purportedly apply to all hospitals, governmental and private; but some are made applicable only to hospitals owned and operated by churches or religious orders. The provisions of the Georgia statute, quoted previously, were apparently approved as constitutional in the case of *Doe v. Bolton.*[28]

The Michigan statute enacted in 1973 is perhaps typical.[29] It reads, in essence, that a hospital, clinic, teaching institution, or any other medical facility need not admit a patient for the purpose of performing an abortion. Moreover, a physician or any other person connected with the institution may refuse to perform or participate in a termination of pregnancy, and a statement of refusal based upon professional, ethical, moral, or religious beliefs shall render the individual immune from any civil or criminal liability. A physician who refuses to give advice relative to an abortion shall not be liable to the hospital or other institution nor subject to discipline from any institution with which he or she is associated, nor shall there be liability in malpractice as long as the doctor adequately informs the patient of his refusal. Notice, however, that the Michigan statute relates only to the refusal of an abortion and does not apply to sterilization. In that respect it is similar to the Georgia statute.

In spite of the fact that the Supreme Court approved the "conscience clause" of the Georgia statute at least by dictum, further litigation is probable, especially with respect to statutes applicable to governmental institutions. The provisions pertaining to an individual's right of refusal to participate would seem clearly constitutional. Perhaps the same can be said of the statutes recognizing the moral and religious convictions of a private sectarian hospital, since these are valuable rights to be protected in a free society.[30] The previously discussed

---

in effect, permits conflicting decisions on "state action" to remain, without resolving the issue on constitutional merits.) *Cf.: Doe v. Bridgeton Hospital Association, Inc.,* 71 N.J. 478, 366 A. 2d 641 (N.J. 1976). (Nonsectarian, private nonprofit hospitals may not deny first-trimester elective abortions when they permit therapeutic abortions, when staff and facilities are available, and when they are the only general hospitals in their respective communities. As "quasi-public" institutions, they must exercise fiduciary powers reasonably and for the public good. A statute that no hospital shall be required to provide abortion services cannot constitutionally be applied to nonsectarian institutions.)
[28] 410 U.S. 179, 197, 35 L. Ed. 2d 201, 216, 93 S. Ct. 739, 750 (1973).
[29] Mich. Comp. Laws Ann., sec. 331.551–.556 (1975).
[30] *Chrisman v. Sisters of St. Joseph of Peace, supra* n. 27.

judicial opinions based solely on judicial law would be additional
grounds for approval of similar statutory pronouncements of public
policy.[31] On the other hand, insofar as the statutes pertain to
governmental hospitals serving the general community they are
probably unconstitutional, although the U.S. Supreme Court may
be called to rule precisely on the issue sometime in the future.[32]
In the final analysis, the Supreme Court is the ultimate decision-maker
with respect to constititional interpretation of statutory law, and the
decisions of the future may turn on the facts of individual cases.
It is all a matter of balancing the various public policy issues involved.

A somewhat related issue is whether a state may deny Medicaid
payments for abortions rendered to indigent patients when the
surgery is elective and not medically necessary. Such a policy, adopted
by the commissioner of social services of the state of New York,
was held to be a denial of equal protection of the laws by a federal
district court and hence invalid, although further proceedings will
be necessary to make the Medicaid statutory language relating to
patient eligibility for care consistent with the *Wade* and *Bolton* cases.[33]

In spite of the cases which hold that a private hospital need not
provide abortion services, if hospitalized patients are refused an
abortion or sterilization, they apparently have at least a right to

[31] *Doe v. Bellin Memorial Hospital, supra,* n. 23, apparently approved of a conscience
clause statute pertaining to a private hospital, although no such statute was involved
in that litigation and hence the approval would be considered dictum. *Cf.: Doe v.
Bridgeton Hospital Association, Inc.,* 366 A. 2d 641 (N.J. 1976). (New Jersey conscience
clause statute may not be constitutionally applied to private nonsectarian hospitals.)
[32] See: *Doe v. Mundy,* 514 F. 2d 1179 (7th Cir. 1975). In *Roe v. Arizona Board of
Regents,* 23 Ariz. App. 477, 534 P. 2d 285 (1975), a statute providing that no hospital
was required to admit any patient for an abortion was ruled overly broad and
unconstitutional when applied to public hospitals; further, a statute providing that
no abortions should be performed at any facility under the jurisdiction of the board
of regents unless necessary to save life of mother could not be upheld. Subsequently
the Arizona Supreme Court reversed the court of appeals, at least with respect to
the ruling on the statute relevant to the University Hospital. It was said to be
constitutional in the light of the institution's status as a teaching hospital and the
availability of other public facilities for abortions. *Roe v. Arizona Board of Regents,*
113 Ariz. 178, 549 P. 2d 150 (1976). *Cf.: Wolfe v. Schroering,* 541 F. 2d 523 (6th
Cir. 1976). (An institutional conscience clause in a Kentucky statute is unconstitutional
as applied to public hospitals and constitutional as applied to private hospitals,
physicians, nurses, and employees.)
[33] *Klein v. Nassau County Medical Center,* 347 F. Supp. 496 (E.D.N.Y. 1972), *aff'd
in part,* 412 U.S. 924, 37 L. Ed. 2d 151, 93 S. Ct. 2747 (1973), *vacated and remanded
in part,* 412 U.S. 925, 37 L. Ed. 2d 152, 93 S. Ct. 2748 (1973). Clarification of
the issue presented in the text was provided by the United States Supreme Court
on June 20, 1977. It was held that Title XIX of the Social Security Act does not
require a state participating in the Medicaid program to fund elective nontherapeutic
abortions as a condition of participation. *Beal, et al. v. Ann Doe, et al.,* 97 S. Ct.
2366, 53 L. Ed. 2d 464 (1977); moreover, the equal protection clause of the Fourteenth
Amendment does not require a state participating in the Medicaid program to pay
expenses of nontherapeutic abortion for indigent women even though it does pay
expenses of childbirth, *Maher, Commissioner of Social Services of Connecticut v. Susan
Roe, et al.,* 97 S. Ct. 2376, 53 L. Ed. 2d 484 (1977).

be fully informed of their condition and provided with sound medical advice indicating where proper and appropriate care can be obtained. If surgery is without question medically indicated for therapeutic reasons and transfer of the patient to another institution would foreseeably harm the patient's health, then liability in damages would probably follow if the surgery were denied or the patient transferred. These observations are based simply upon general principles of the law of hospital liability.

If abortion is denied in circumstances where there is no threat to the mother's life or health, the matter of civil liability in damages is unsettled. If the abortion is solely the personal choice of the mother, and the hospital has no duty to provide the service, then the hospital would not be liable in damages, as indicated in the preceding discussion. On the other hand, if an abortion is prompted by fear that the infant may be born deformed, for example, then failure to abort or failure to exercise reasonable care in advising the patient could lead to civil liability of the hospital, the attending physician, or both. Litigation to date on this question, however, is inconclusive.

In *Stewart v. Long Island College Hospital*, a patient was refused an abortion when some evidence showed that she was infected with rubella. The medical staff abortion committee was divided on the necessity or desirability of an abortion because two of the physicians on this committee doubted that the patient had rubella. Subsequently the patient gave birth to a malformed child. In a suit against the hospital and the physician, the trial court jury awarded damages in favor of both the infant and the parents. The verdict in favor of the parents against the hospital was permitted to stand by the trial judge, although he directed a verdict for the hospital notwithstanding the jury's decision in the infant's cause of action. The intermediate appellate division affirmed the judgment in favor of the hospital on the infant's cause of action and reversed the judgment awarding damages to the parents. Upon further appeal the highest court in New York affirmed the ruling of the appellate division. It held that neither the infant nor the parents had a cause of action on the facts presented. The law of New York does not recognize a cause of action by the malformed infant for failure to abort the mother. Moreover, the parents' claim for damages also failed because it would be virtually impossible to measure compensation for the mental anguish occasioned by the birth of the child.[34]

---

[34] 58 Misc. 2d 432. 296 N.Y.S. 2d 41 (Sup. Ct. 1968), *modified and aff'd as modified,* 35 App. Div. 2d 531, 313 N.Y.S. 2d 502 (1970), *aff'd,* 30 N.Y. 2d 695, 283 N.E. 2d 616, 332 N.Y.S. 2d 640 (1972).

Similarly, in a case against a physician, New Jersey has held that it was not malpractice for the doctor to fail to advise the patient of the risks of rubella, and further that the infant born malformed had no cause of action for "wrongful life."[35] In contrast, however, the Wisconsin Supreme Court has recently ruled that the parents of a defective child might have a cause of action for alleged failure to diagnose properly the mother's rubella during the first trimester of pregnancy and inform her of the availability of a legal abortion, if the trier of fact can be convinced that the mother would have sought and submitted to the surgery.[36] The child, on the other hand, does not possess a cause of action.[37] Even when a child is born healthy, an intermediate New York appellate court has held that if a physician negligently fails to diagnose pregnancy early enough to permit a first-trimester abortion, the resulting birth could give rise to a cause of action by the parents for damages for pain and suffering incident to the birth, loss of consortium, and costs of raising the infant.[38]

At the time of writing, negligence on the part of a physician or a hospital which causes a mother to give birth to an unwanted child does not give the infant, whether born healthy or deformed, a cause of action for "wrongful life." Assuming, however, the availability of a legal abortion, and further assuming that the failure of medical persons to diagnose properly the pregnancy and the state of the mother's health can be established as the proximate cause of an unwanted birth, some jurisdictions will recognize a cause of action by the parents for damages, especially if the child is born deformed.

Consent of a Minor's Parent or a Patient's Spouse

The common and statutory law relating to parental consent for medical or surgical care of a minor, as well as the general rule that consent of a spouse is not usually necessary for treating a competent adult, were discussed in the chapter on consent. To be considered here is the more specific question of whether a parent's or spouse's consent is legally necessary for an abortion. By analogy, the same principles to be outlined would apply to sterilization.

---

[35] *Gleitman v. Cosgrove*, 49 N.J. 22, 227 A. 2d 689 (1967).
[36] *Dumer v. St. Michael's Hospital*, 233 N.W. 2d 372 (Wisc. 1975). *Cf.*: *Rieck v. Medical Protective Co. of Fort Wayne, Indiana*, 64 Wisc. 2d 514, 219 N.W. 2d 242 (1974). (No cause of action arose when a clinic and an obstetrician allegedly failed to diagnose pregnancy in time for an abortion and a normal, healthy child was subsequently born.)
[37] *Dumer, ibid.*
[38] *Ziemba v. Sternberg*, 45 App. Div. 2d 230, 357 N.Y.S. 2d 265 (1974).

Neither the *Wade* nor *Bolton* cases spoke to these issues of parental or spousal consent directly, since such questions were not involved in those landmark decisions. The rights of spouses or parents, if any, were left for resolution by further litigation.

If the patient seeking an abortion is a competent adult as determined by state law and is unmarried, it is perfectly clear under common law that the consent of the probable father is not a prerequisite to the surgery. The decision is solely that of the patient and her physician, and the father cannot prevent the abortion even though state law would require him to support the child if born.[39] When the woman was married, on the other hand, conservative legal advice based upon general common law principles has usually held consent of the husband to be necessary or at least most desirable, unless the abortion was required to preserve the life or physical health of the mother. The reason for this conclusion was that the husband might well possess his own common law cause of action for damages for interference with the marital relationship, or for loss of a possible right to father children should his consent not be obtained. By the same token, it was advised that the spouse's consent be obtained before a sterilization procedure on a patient of either sex.

This philosophy was specifically adopted by a number of states which enacted new abortion statutes following the 1973 Supreme Court decisions. By way of example, the Florida statute required the written consent of the husband of a married patient for an abortion, unless the husband was voluntarily living apart from his wife, or unless continuation of the pregnancy threatened the life of the patient. Written parental consent (or consent of the custodian or legal guardian) was also required for any abortion of an unmarried minor under eighteen years of age.[40] A federal court held that both of these provisions were unconstitutional, at least as they applied to first- and second-trimester terminations of pregnancy, on the basis that if a state cannot regulate or interfere with an individual's right to seek an abortion, as articulated by the Supreme Court, then neither can the state delegate a right of interference to either the husband or the parent of the patient.[41] In the case of a minor patient this assumes of course that the individual was mature enough and mentally competent to understand the nature of her condition and the

[39]*Jones v. Smith*, 278 So. 2d 339 (Fla. Dist. Ct. App. 1973). (Patient was 19 years of age), *cert. denied*, 415 U.S. 958 (1974).
[40]Florida Stat. Ann., sec. 458.22(2)–(3) (Supp. 1975–76).
[41]*Coe v. Gerstein*, 376 F. Supp. 695, (S.D. Fla. 1974), *appeal dismissed* and *cert. denied*, 417 U.S. 279 (1974).

consequence of granting her consent for the surgery. Following the decision by the federal district court, in essentially the same litigation involving the same constitutional issues, the circuit court of appeals affirmed by holding the Florida statute unconstitutional.[42] On the matter of requiring the husband's consent, the court reasoned that the woman's right of privacy outweighs the state's interest in regulating the marriage relationship. Parental consent cannot be required prior to an abortion for a minor, since the patient's right of decision is more fundamental than the state's interest in controlling alleged illicit sexual conduct among minors, protecting minors from their own improvidence, and supporting the family as a social unit.

Other federal and state court decisions reached essentially the same conclusions.[43] The Supreme Judicial Court for the Commonwealth of Massachusetts held in *Doe v. Doe* that an estranged husband had no constitutional right or standing to prevent his wife from seeking and obtaining an abortion at approximately eighteen weeks of pregnancy—in other words, during the second trimester prior to viability of the child.[44] Medical testimony in this litigation established that the general health of the patient was good, and that accordingly there was no therapeutic reason for terminating the pregnancy. On the other hand, there was no medical risk to the patient if the surgery was performed. In such a case the decision to obtain an abortion is solely that of the wife. Two justices of the Massachusetts court wrote vigorous dissents: general common law principles and constitutional law, they said, extend to the father a right of family relationships and privacy worthy of legal protection.

Not all lower courts agreed with the judicial decision that statutory requirements for a spouse's or parent's consent were unconstitutional. In *Planned Parenthood of Central Missouri v. Danforth*, the court upheld such state-imposed restrictions on the basis that government had

---

[42] *Poe v. Gerstein*, 517 F. 2d 787 (5th Cir. 1975).

[43] *Baird v. Bellotti*, 393 F. Supp. 847 (D. Mass. 1975): (A Massachusetts statute requiring consent of both parents and the minor for an abortion was unconstitutional). *State v. Koome*, 84 Wash. 2d, 901, 530 P. 2d 260 (1975): (The criminal conviction of a physician who performed an abortion on an unmarried minor without first obtaining consent of the parents was reversed, said statutory requirement being unconstitutional). *Planned Parenthood Ass'n v. Fitzpatrick*, 401 F. Supp. 554 (E.D. Pa. 1975): (A Pennsylvania statute requiring spousal and parental consent was unconstitutional). *Wolfe v. Schroering*, 388 F. Supp. 631 (W.D. Ky. 1974): (Kentucky statutory provisions requiring spousal and parental consent were invalid). *Baird*, however was vacated and remanded by the United States Supreme Court because the district court should have abstained from deciding the constitutional issue and should have certified to the Massachusetts Supreme Judicial Court appropriate questions concerning the meaning of the statute and the procedure it imposed. *Bellotti v. Baird*, 96 S. Ct. 2857 (1976), *aff'd mem.*, 428 U.S. 901 (1976).

[44] 314 N.E. 2d 128, 62 A.L.R. 3d 1082 (Mass. 1974).

a sufficient "compelling interest" to protect the marriage and family relationships.[45] In view of this conflict among the federal courts, the Supreme Court accepted review of the constitutional issues involved in *Danforth* and issued an opinion in July 1976 which struck down the Missouri statute requiring the husband's consent for an abortion and parental consent for such surgery on an unmarried minor under eighteen.[46] With respect to requiring the spouse's consent, the majority of the court reasoned that if the state could not restrict the decision of a married woman to seek an abortion prior to viability of the fetus, it could not, in effect, grant to the husband a unilateral right to prohibit his wife from terminating her pregnancy. Three dissenting justices believed that the requirement of the spouse's consent was constitutional as a legitimate means of protecting the father's interest in having his wife bear children. Four of the members of the Supreme Court differed from the majority opinion, holding invalid the requirement of parental consent. They expressed a philosophy to the effect that a state may legitimately require parental consultation in situations where a minor seeks an abortion, arguing that an unmarried minor woman needs protection from making a decision which may not be in her own best interests and welfare.

Also relevant to the rights of fathers or parents of a minor is the obverse question of whether a husband can require his wife to undergo an abortion (or sterilization), or whether a parent can enforce a similar demand upon a minor child. This latter question was presented to a Maryland court in 1972 and answered in the negative. According to this decision, if one were to read Maryland statutes relating to "juvenile delinquency" in the light of law on minors' right to consent to medical care for themselves and the then applicable Maryland statute regulating legal abortions, the court had no power to order an abortion sought by parents contrary to the wishes of a 16-year-old unmarried minor.[47] The same principle

---

[45] 392 F. Supp. 1362 (E.D. Mo. 1975).
[46] *Planned Parenthood of Central Missouri v. Danforth*, 428 U.S. 52, 49 L. Ed. 2d 788, 96 S. Ct. 2831 (1976). (The court upheld the following requirements of the Missouri abortion statute: a definition of "viability" as "the stage of fetal development when the life of the unborn child may be continued indefinitely outside the womb by natural or artificial life-support systems"; a requirement that the patient give her written informed consent; reporting and record-keeping provisions. The court invalidated prohibitions on the saline method of terminating pregnancies and a statutory standard of care that a physician performing an abortion must exercise the same degree of diligence to preserve the life and health of the fetus as he would in the case of a live birth.)
[47] *In re Smith*, 16 Md. App. 209, 295 A. 2d 238 (1972).

would probably apply to a situation where a husband attempts to require his wife to have an abortion or sterilization.

It is now legally resolved that a mentally competent woman, regardless of her age and marital status, who understands the nature of and the consequences of her decision, possesses a constitutional right to determine whether she wishes to have an abortion, prior to viability of her unborn child. The necessary corollary is that neither her husband nor her parents have a common law or constitutional right of their own to be a father or a grandparent. As evidenced by the differing opinions by the individual justices of the Supreme Court, these conclusions are not readily acceptable to all of society. Yet in the Anglo-American system of judicial decision-making and constitutional interpretation, public policy is formulated by a majority. Clearly, the rights of a competent individual to determine private matters have emerged as paramount.

X

Sterilization

Sterilization is a surgical procedure intended to terminate the ability to procreate. For the male the most common procedure is termed a vasectomy; the operation for the female is called a salpingectomy.

In analysis from a legal point of view, it is desirable to distinguish between voluntary and involuntary sterilizations and to classify them according to their purpose. Voluntary sterilizations are in turn subdivided into those performed for the patient's convenience and those undertaken as therapeutic measures. Sterilization for convenience may be desired for family planning or simply for contraceptive purposes. On the other hand, there may be sound medical reasons why the procedure is advisable to protect or improve the general health of the patient.

Involuntary sterilizations are called eugenic, their purpose being to protect the patient and society in general from procreation where the likelihood of inheritable disability is thought to exist. The law of a few states, however, requires even a eugenic sterilization to be supported by the consent of the patient or his legally authorized representative.

Therapeutic Sterilization

There are no legal issues of unique significance in connection with a therapeutic sterilization. By definition this is a procedure to preserve the life or health of the patient or the spouse. Hence the decision is one for the patient and his or her physician. Surgery to remove diseased reproductive organs and incidentally resulting in sterility should not be termed sterilization. The term therapeutic sterilization is restricted to surgery whose express purpose is to

285

produce sterility in the interest of the patient's life or health.

The law of all the states will approve a therapeutic sterilization. A few states have statutes, cases, or opinions of the attorney general specifically approving this surgery. In most, the statutory and case law is silent, and hence it is a valid assumption that there is no public policy against therapeutic sterilization. The case law would permit a broad interpretation of the word health and grant wide discretion to the physician. Furthermore, the term therapeutic sterilization has been used to denote a sterilization of the male—for example, to preserve the life or health of his wife.[1]

Before recommending a therapeutic sterilization, however, a doctor may wish to consult with professional colleagues. The legal risks for the physician and for the hospital, however, are no greater than for any surgical or medical treatment, namely, the possibility of a lawsuit founded on alleged malpractice, lack of informed consent, or breach of contract. All the usual substantive and procedural laws of malpractice would of course apply to any lawful sterilization. Likewise, a suit could be based on breach of contract or on a promise to produce a particular result, and more will be said about this later.

The patient, as in any surgical or medical treatment, is entitled to be fully informed regarding the sterilization, and his or her consent should be evidenced by a well-drafted consent form. Since the ability to procreate is such a significant human function, it is particularly important for the physician to obtain a genuine, fully informed consent whenever any surgery will result in sterility, even if such an outcome is incidental to the primary medical purpose of the procedure.

The question of obtaining the consent of the patient's spouse frequently arises. Where there is truly a need for therapeutic sterilization to preserve the patient's life or health, the spouse's consent is clearly not a legal necessity. The spouse should have no legal right to prevent or bar surgery necessary to save the life or preserve the health of the other marriage partner. Nevertheless allegations that the sterilization unduly interfered with the spouse's own interests in the reproduction function are always possible, and it is recommended as a matter of preventive law that the consent of the spouse be sought and obtained. Such consent is also to be recommended simply in the interest of creating a sound relationship between the

---

[1] *Christensen v. Thornby*, 192 Minn. 123, 255 N.W. 620, 93 A.L.R. 570 (1934).

family of the patient, the physician, and the hospital. But medically necessary treatment should never be withheld from the patient because the marriage partner has refused consent. Moreover, as will be discussed, some recent cases have recognized a constitutional right of individuals to obtain contraceptive sterilizations, and therefore the consent of the patient's spouse is not required.

Contraceptive Sterilization or Sterilization for Convenience

With increasing frequency, perhaps because of changing social and moral values, patients are seeking and obtaining sterilization purely as a convenient form of contraception. As is true also of therapeutic sterilization, there are no significant legal problems or barriers to such surgery.

The state law—statutory and case—is and always has been silent on the matter in most jurisdictions. The procedure is hence lawful, and neither criminal nor civil penalties could be assessed against the physician, the hospital, or the patient for a properly performed sterilization requested by the patient for personal reasons, although the usual rules of civil liability for malpractice, breach of contract, or lack of an informed consent would apply.

A few states do have laws that affirmatively approve of contraceptive sterilization. The Virginia statute provides that a licensed physician may perform a sterilization procedure after receiving the written request of any person twenty-one years of age or older.[2] If the patient is married, the written request of the spouse is also required, unless the patient states under oath that the spouse has disappeared or that they have been separated continually for more than one year.

The statute further recites that a full and reasonable explanation of the medical consequences of the surgery must be given the patient. Moreover thirty days must elapse between the time of the request for a male vasectomy and the actual surgery; and a similar waiting period is required for the sterilization of a female who has not previously given birth to a child.

One should observe that Virginia's requirement of spousal consent may be unconstitutional in the light of the 1973 Supreme Court cases concerning abortion. A New Jersey trial court has ruled recently that a married woman, separated from her husband for five years, had a fundamental constitutional right to a tubal ligation and could

[2]Va. Code Ann., sec. 32-423 *et seq.* (Repl. Vol. 1973, Supp. 1975).

not be denied the surgery because her husband had refused to sign
the consent form which her physicians had required as a matter
of policy.[3] If such a right is fundamental, separation of the married
persons should be irrelevant.

Other states affirmatively approve of contraceptive sterilization
by statute,[4] judicial cases,[5] or opinions of the attorney general. The
Georgia statute provides that a licensed doctor may perform a
sterilization for any person twenty-one years of age or older, or
for married persons under twenty-one. The request for the procedure
must be in writing and must contain the consent of the patient's
spouse, if the patient is married and if the spouse can be located
after reasonable effort. The physician is also required to consult
with another licensed doctor. Like the Virginia statutory requirement
for the spouse's consent, the Georgia requirements relating to consultation and the spouse's consent may be unconstitutional, assuming
that a contraceptive sterilization is analogous to a first-trimester
abortion.

Some statutes which affirmatively approve of sterilization, including
Georgia's, add the provision that no hospital may be required to
admit a patient for a sterilization, and further that no physician
or hospital employee may be required to participate in the surgery.
The constitutionality of such "conscience clauses" is noted and
discussed in the chapter on abortion.

Formerly at least two states—Connecticut and Utah—expressly
prohibited sterilizations solely for purposes of contraception and made
the procedure a criminal act. In Utah the statutory language prohibited all sterilizations except those dictated by medical necessity. An
action for declaratory judgment challenged that statute in relation
to voluntary sterilizations for convenience, however, and it was ruled
that the statute was applicable only to institutionalized patients.[6]
Voluntary sterilization of other patients was said not to be criminal.
The court based this conclusion on the grounds that the statute
is a part of the Utah code dealing with eugenic sterilization and
is under the general statutory topic of "State Institutions."

Connecticut had a statute which prohibited the use of contraceptives

[3]*Ponter v. Ponter,* 135 N.J. Super. 50, 342 A. 2d 574 (1975).
[4]For example: Arkansas Stat. Ann., sec. 59–501 (M) (Repl. Vol. 1971), Colorado
Rev. Stat. Ann. sec. 25–6–102 (1973), Georgia Code Ann., sec. 84–932/935 (Supp.
1974), Oregon Rev. Stat., sec. 435.305 (Repl. Part 1971).
[5]*Jessin v. County of Shasta,* 274 Cal. App. 2d 737, 79 Cal. Rptr. 359, 35 A.L.R. 3d
1433 (1969), *Jackson v. Anderson,* 230 So. 2d 503 (Fla. Dist. Ct. App. 1970), *Christensen
v. Thornby,* 192 Minn. 123, 255 N.W. 620, 93 A.L.R. 570 (1934).
[6]*Parker v. Rampton,* 28 Utah 2d 36, 497 P. 2d 848 (1972).

and advice or assistance in their use. Voluntary contraceptive sterilization was thus, in effect at least, prohibited by implication. This statute
was declared unconstitutional in the landmark case of *Griswold v.
Connecticut*, in which the U.S. Supreme Court ruled that the statute
invaded a right of privacy protected by the due process clause of
the Fourteenth Amendment.[7] Another Connecticut statute, which
purported to authorize only sterilizations pursuant to *statutory* provisions for eugenic sterilization, was repealed in 1971. Voluntary
sterilization as a matter of personal choice is now firmly established
in law in all states on the basis of modern social mores and ideas
about family planning.

Although the law of most states was silent on the issue, fears
and arguments were expressed that sterilization could be considered
criminal mayhem; and many physicians—sometimes upon legal advice
from private counsel—refused to perform the surgery unless there
was medical necessity for therapeutic reasons. In general terms,
mayhem can be defined as an intentional or willful disfigurement
of the body. Criminal statutes frequently prohibit such acts regardless
of malicious intent of the agent or consent of the victim. At least
two cases, however, although not directly on the point, do indicate
by way of interpretation or dictum that a consensual voluntary
sterilization is not a criminal act,[8] the arguments being that criminal
statutes prohibiting mayhem implicitly or explicitly require malicious
intent, or, more broadly, that public policy does not prohibit population control and family planning.

When sterilization is requested for convenience or contraceptive
purposes, the consent of the patient's spouse should be obtained
if the spouse is reasonably accessible. One reason is to promote sound
relations between the physician and the family. Another is to eliminate
any risk of suit for damages by the spouse, alleging interference
with his or her individual interests in the matter of procreation.
As noted above, however, the spouse's consent is probably not a
legal necessity when the patient alone is competent to decide the
matter.

---

[7]381 U.S. 479, 85 S. Ct. 1678, 14 L. Ed. 2d 510 (1965). Also see: *Eisenstadt v. Baird*,
405 U.S. 438, 31 L. Ed. 2d 349, 92 S. Ct. 1029 (1972). (Unmarried persons have
the same constitutional right to privacy with respect to contraceptive measures as
married persons do.)

[8]*Shaheen v. Knight*, 11 Pa. D. & C. 2d 41 (Dist. Ct. of Lycoming Co. 1957). (A private
contract between a patient and a physician for sterilization is not void as being against
public policy, although an award of damages for alleged breach of contract if the
normal birth of a normal child followed such surgery would be contrary to public
policy.) See also: *Christensen v. Thornby*, 192 Minn. 123, 255 N.W. 620, 622 (1934).

Eugenic Sterilization

Eugenics is the science dealing with the influences that improve the inborn or hereditary qualities of a race or breed. Hence the term eugenic sterilization denotes surgery on persons alleged to be unsound or unfit to be a parent because of presumably inheritable disabilities.

A true, legal eugenic sterilization must be based on a state statute that is consistent with the protection of state and federal constitutional law. Approximately one-half of the states have never enacted statutes authorizing compulsory eugenic sterilization; and accordingly the practice has never existed in these jurisdictions, except for an occasional attempt to utilize judicial authority to justify the surgery, as will be noted. A few states—for example, Nebraska in 1969—have recently repealed eugenic sterilization statutes either altogether or in part.

In the other half of the states, provisions of the statutes on eugenic sterilization differ; but essentially the pattern is first to identify the persons subject to the law, and second to detail the procedures to be followed before the surgery. The typical operations that are statutorily permitted are male vasectomies and female salpingectomies.

Most of the authorized eugenic sterilizations can be called compulsory because the surgery, although the law requires proper recommendations and procedures, can be performed without the consent of the patient or guardian. On the other hand, a few of the statutes permit only voluntary eugenic sterilization, as for example in Minnesota and Vermont, which require consent of the patient or of the patient's legal representative.

Some statutes are applicable only to persons confined in state or governmental institutions, such as hospitals for the mentally ill, training schools, or prisons, but some apply to other individuals as well. In any event, the statutes usually identify the persons subject to the law, using such terms as the insane, the feeble-minded, the epileptic, the habitual criminal, the mentally defective, the sexual psychopath, the incurably incompetent, and similar designations presumably meaningful to medical science.

The basic constitutionality of the statutes as a matter of substantive law was established by the famous Supreme Court case of *Buck v. Bell*, decided in 1927.[9] Carrie Buck was a white woman duly committed

---

[9] 274 U.S. 200, 47 S. Ct. 584, 71 L. Ed. 1000 (1927). During the 1920s and 1930s there were also several state court decisions which upheld the constitutionality of

to the state colony for epileptics and the feeble-minded. She was the daughter of a feeble-minded mother who had been confined to the same institution, and she herself had given birth to an illegitimate feeble-minded child. Following statutory procedures, a circuit court in Virginia ordered the superintendent of the institution to have a salpingectomy performed upon Carrie Buck. As in previous cases upholding compulsory vaccination laws, the statute was held to be constitutional under the police power of the state to regulate the general health and welfare. The law, in effect, was said to have a direct relation to public health. In writing the opinion validating the Virginia law, Justice Holmes spoke his often-quoted "Three generations of imbeciles are enough."

In contrast, the Supreme Court held unconstitutional an Oklahoma statute which authorized sterilization of "habitual criminals" but exempted individuals described as "embezzlers." The constitutional point of law was that the exemption resulted in an arbitrary, unreasonable classification and accordingly violated the equal protection clause of the Fourteenth Amendment.[10] Substantive equal protection and due process require that statutory identification and classification of persons subject to eugenic sterilization be such that they can be applied without arbitrary or discriminatory bias.

To be constitutional the statutes must also protect the right of procedural due process of law. Statutes will differ in detail, but due process requires that certain elements of fundamental fairness be observed. In most instances the superintendent of the hospital or other institution which houses the patient, or the parent or guardian, will be empowered to initiate the proceedings for recommending the sterilization. The recommendation must ordinarily be supported by medical opinion, often that of a committee chosen from the hospital's medical staff. Formal notice must be given to the patient and his guardian or next of kin no matter who initiated the proceedings, and a hearing must be provided by the statutorily designated public authority. Depending on the state of residence or the circumstances, this hearing may be conducted by a court

---

eugenic sterilization statutes. A more recent case approving a statute as valid under the police power was *In re Cavitt*, 182 Neb. 712, 157 N.W. 2d 171 (1968), *appeal dismissed*, 396 U.S. 996, 24 L. Ed. 2d 490, 90 S. Ct. 543 (1970). In this situation compulsory sterilization was required as a precondition of the release of a retarded mother of eight children from a state hospital. See also: *In re Sterilization of Moore*, 289 N.C. 95, 221 S.E. 2d 307 (1976). (A statute permitting sterilization of persons who are victims of "mental illness," or who are diagnosed as "mental defective(s)" is constitutional when applied to sexually active persons.)
[10] *Skinner v. Oklahoma*, 316 U.S. 535, 62 S. Ct. 1110, 86 L. Ed. 1655 (1942).

or by an administrative board in the presence of the patient or
his proper representatives.

Depending also on the particular statute, an inquiry is made at
the hearing regarding the necessity of consents. Some statutes require
that the patient or his authorized guardian or representative consent
affirmatively to the proposed sterilization; but most do not, since
the sterilization is "compulsory" in nature. Some statutes, as in Iowa,
require a court hearing and order if consent is denied. Others grant
the hearing body authority to order the sterilization without consent
and without court intervention at this point. In connection with an
administrative order for sterilization, however, due process always
requires a right of appeal to an appropriate court. If the statutory
procedures for a eugenic sterilization are not minutely followed,
criminal and civil liability would follow.

As noted earlier, eugenic sterilization must rest upon a statutory
law expressly authorizing the procedure. Courts cannot order sterilization unless authority has been granted by statute. A court order
to have patients sterilized may be sought by relatives of the proposed
patient, for example, or by local governmental public health agencies,
but such attempts have been unsuccessful. In some states it was
thought at one time that the courts, through their general powers
of law and equity, would have the power to order sterilization, and
the probate court case *In re Simpson* in Ohio so held in 1962.[11]
The trial court, without benefit of a specific eugenic sterilization
statute, had granted an order to sterilize an eighteen-year-old female
alleged to be promiscuous and mentally defective. However, a later
federal court case, interpreting Ohio judicial law, effectively overruled *Simpson.* In this recent litigation a county children's service
board had petitioned the state court for an order of sterilization
for a hospitalized minor female who had been diagnosed as "feeble-
minded," and the sterilization was performed pursuant to an order
granted by the court. The order was challenged in a subsequent
case entitled *Wade v. Bethesda Hospital,* where the patient brought
suit against both the hospital and the probate court judge, alleging

---

[11] 180 N.E. 2d 206 (Ohio P. Ct. 1962). *Cf.: Holmes v. Powers,* 439 S.W. 2d 579 (Kentucky
1969) and *Frazier v. Levi,* 440 S.W. 2d 393 (Texas Civ. App. 1969). (Where no
statutory authority exists a court cannot order or sanction eugenic sterilization of
a legally incompetent person who was unable to consent for herself. In *Holmes* the
action was brought by a county health officer and medical society. In *Levi* the mother,
who was legal guardian of an adult incompetent daughter, sought court approval
of a proposed sterilization). See also: *In the Interest of M.K.R.,* 515 S.W. 2d 467
(Mo. 1974). (A court may not order involuntary sterilization of a minor when no
specific statutory authority exists.) Accord: *Kemp v. Kemp.,* 43 Cal. App. 3d 758,
118 Cal. Rptr. 64 (1974).

that she had not consented to the operation and that the judge's order was unauthorized. The federal court agreed, and hence the judge, the hospital, and the doctor could all be civilly liable in damages.[12]

The conclusion was justified on several grounds. First of all, as noted above, Ohio has no statute authorizing eugenic sterilization. Past proposals for such legislation in that state had failed of passage. General statutes conferring jurisdiction on probate courts to appoint guardians for the mentally incompetent and to grant orders relative to their "care" do not encompass or contemplate an order of sterilization, since such judicial discretion would be contrary to the public interest. The order here was hence totally without legal authority. Normally, judges are immune from civil liability when acting in their official capacity with appropriate jurisdiction over the person and the subject matter, and with the power to render a decision. But when there is total absence of jurisdiction and power the doctrine of judicial immunity does not apply. The action in this case presented more than just an excess of jurisdiction.

Moreover the hospital in which the sterilization was performed and the physician could be liable in damages. Consent forms signed only by county or state officials are not valid protection for the hospital when no statute exists authorizing involuntary sterilization for eugenic reasons. The invalid court order cannot be relied upon to shield the hospital from liability. This was especially true in *Wade*, where the court order did not refer specifically to Bethesda Hospital and direct it to make its facilities available for this surgery.[13]

The litigation involving Bethesda Hospital and other cases cited in reference to it demonstrate that hospitals should not permit eugenic sterilization of minor patients without a clearly valid court order, as determined by express local state statutory law, and without an order directed specifically to the hospital. To ignore such a specific order would, of course, risk contempt of court proceedings.

Hospitals which permit minor patients to undergo surgery to effect contraceptive sterilization not directly related to preservation of life or health when only parental consent has been obtained may incur serious risk of liability in a suit later brought by the minor. According to judicial law, parents do not have the right to authorize either

[12] 337 F. Supp. 671 (S.D. Ohio 1971).
[13] *Wade v. Bethesda Hospital*, 356 F. Supp. 380 (S.D. Ohio 1973). See also: *Relf v. Weinberger*, 372 F. Supp. 1196 (D.D.C. 1974). (Regulations issued by the Department of Health, Education, and Welfare authorizing sterilizations under certain circumstances for certain patients under governmental funding for family planning services are invalid as applied to minors and mentally incompetent persons, since there is no statutory authority for use of federal funds for "involuntary sterilization.")

a eugenic or contraceptive sterilization for their minor children.[14] Hence, as a matter of policy, hospitals should deny sterilization surgery to all minors legally incapable of giving their own consent, unless they have received a clearly valid court order. A hospital can of course permit the sterilization of an adult, or perhaps of a married minor or one judged to be mature, when the physician and the administration of the institution are convinced that local law relating to a patient's informed consent for treatment has been complied with.[15]

It is probable that the statutes authorizing eugenic sterilization will be subject to renewed legal attack during the next decade. The recent abortion cases, which recognize a woman's constitutional right not to bear children, may give rise to arguments that they have an analogous right to bear children, even if the mother is presumed to be mentally handicapped. At all events, any statute which might attempt to provide for compulsory sterilization on the basis of a patient's economic status or the number of children already born to the family would clearly be arbitrary and discriminatory—and hence in violation of the equal protection and due process clauses of the Fourteenth Amendment to the federal Constitution.

Liability and Damages for Unsuccessful Sterilization

Even if the surgical procedure of sterilization is itself perfectly legal, there can of course be liability in damages for failure to obtain the patient's fully informed consent or that of a legally authorized guardian, as has been discussed. Liability can also be imposed for malpractice or negligently performed surgery, just as in any medical or surgical treatment, and failure to follow the generally accepted standards of care exercised by other physicians in similar circumstances could be the basis for a suit for damages. But mere failure to accomplish the intended result—i.e., complete sterility—would not normally be malpractice; and pregnancy following a sterilization of either spouse would not normally be proof of negligence, since physicians and hospitals are not guarantors or insurers of a particular

---

[14]*A.L. v. G.R.H.*, 325 N.E. 2d 501 (Ind. Ct. App. 1975): (A mother has no common law right to consent to the sterilization of a 15-year-old son, even if she believes surgery to be beneficial to her son). *Cox v. Stanton*, 381 F. Supp. 349 (E.D.N.C. 1974), *aff'd in part, rev'd and remanded in part*, 529 F. 2d 47 (4th Cir. 1975): (On the basis that proper consent was obtained, a motion was made to dismiss an action for damages by an adult who, while a minor, was sterilized with his mother's consent. The motion was judged without merit).
[15]*Smith v. Seibly*, 72 Wash. 2d 16, 431 P. 2d 719 (1967). (An 18-year-old married male could consent to a vasectomy.)

result.[16] The consent form signed by the patient or a legal representative (and perhaps by the spouse) should recite that there are no promises or guarantees of result.

If it can be established, however, that recognized standards with respect to either the conduct of the surgery or the follow-up care of the patient were not met, then a cause of action in malpractice is presented. When a physician conducted only one post-vasectomy semen test, although expert testimony at the trial was to the effect that three tests are accepted practice in the community, the court left it for a jury to determine whether or not the required standard of care was met.[17]

A third legal theory or basis for suit involving an unsuccessful sterilization is breach of contract or warranty. If the physician should expressly by words or action guarantee or promise sterility, a breach of contract has occurred should pregnancy follow. Several litigated cases have alleged this theory as the basis of a cause of action and a few have succeeded. According to *Doerr v. Villate*, an Illinois decision, assurances that sterility would result from a vasectomy performed on the husband provided a cause of action in breach of contract when the wife later gave birth to a mentally retarded and physically deformed child, and it was further ruled that the contractual statute of limitations would apply to the action.[18] In *Doerr* the wife had previously given birth to two retarded children; for this reason the parents had sought the vasectomy. On the other hand, a recent Kentucky case held that a doctor's statements that a vasectomy is a "sure thing," a "fool-proof thing, 100 percent," were merely the expression of a professional opinion and thus could not be the basis of a cause of action in contract.[19] Even when the court rules that the evidence of promise or warranty is sufficient to present a jury question, however, the plaintiff must convince the jury that the promise of sterilization was in fact made expressly, in words or at least by the physician's action. As noted above, this legal theory of action can in most cases be successfully defended if a carefully

---

[16]For example: *Lane v. Cohen*, 201 So. 2d 804 (Fla. Dist. Ct. App. 1967); *Peters v. Gelb*, 303 A. 2d 685 (Del. Super. Ct. 1973).

[17]*Hackworth v. Hart*, 474 S.W. 2d 377 (Ky. 1971). *Cf.: Ball v. Mudge*, 64 wash. 2d 24, 391 P. 2d 201 (1964). (The plaintiff was not successful in a malpractice action alleging that the failure of a doctor to perform semen tests was the proximate cause of a later pregnancy of his wife, since the plaintiff was unable to show that the failure was a departure from accepted standards at the time in that locality).

[18]74 Ill. App. 2d 332, 220 N.E. 2d 767 (1966).

[19]*Hackworth v. Hart*, 474 S.W. 2d 377 (Ky. 1971). See also: *Herrara v. Roessing*, 533 P. 2d 60 (Colo. Ct. App. 1975). (Statements made by the doctor were opinions and not a guarantee of results.)

worded written consent form has been obtained from the patient and the spouse, with a full explanation of the proposed surgery, the risks, and the probable outcome.

Even after malpractice or breach of contract has been established, two legal issues remain when an unwanted or unexpected pregnancy follows surgery intended to accomplish sterilization: the measure of damages recoverable by the patient, and the point of time from which the statute of limitations to an action begins to run. In the 1957 Pennsylvania case of *Shaheen v. Knight* the court followed what could perhaps be termed the historical and traditional approach and denied recovery of damages for the normal birth of a normal child.[20] The theory was simply that such a normal human event cannot be considered "damage," even though there is a monetary cost involved in parenthood and the rearing of offspring, and that it would be contrary to public policy to allow recovery of damages. A recent decision in accord with this view is *Terrel v. Garcia*, which has held that the birth of a normal and healthy baby following an unsuccessful, negligently performed bilateral tubal ligation does not entitle the parents to recover damages for the future care and support of the child.[21] Again, as in the previous cases cited, the basis of this decision was public policy founded on a belief that the normal joy and satisfaction of having a healthy child offsets the economic cost of rearing the baby.

In contrast, however, if the surgery is unsuccessful and if physical pain and suffering can be established as resulting from an unwanted birth, damages can be recovered as long as the pain and suffering are considered in the realm of the extraordinary. To illustrate, *Bishop v. Byrne* allowed the mother to recover damages for physical pain and mental anguish when a "sterilization" of the mother was unsuccessful, and the baby had to be delivered by Caesarean section, although the father was denied recovery for his alleged mental distress.[22]

The view illustrated in *Shaheen, Christensen,* and *Terrel* has been rejected by other courts, and their decisions probably represent the trend of the law with respect to damages when a normal birth of

---

[20] 11 Pa. D. & C. 2d 41 (Dist. Ct. of Lycoming Co. 1957). See also: *Christensen v. Thornby*, 192 Minn. 123, 255 N.W. 620, 93 A.L.R. 570 (1934). (An unsuccessful vasectomy performed on the husband to protect the wife from risks of childbirth did not result in damages to the husband when his wife subsequently gave birth to a normal child without undue difficulty.)

[21] 496 S.W. 2d 124 (Texas Civ. App. 1973), *cert. denied*, 415 U.S. 927 (1974). See also: *LaPoint v. Shirley*, 409 F. Supp. 118 (W.D. Texas 1976). (In Texas there is no cause of action for wrongful birth of a normal or abnormal child after an unsuccessful bilateral tubal ligation even if the surgery was negligently performed. The birth of an abnormal child is not a foreseeable event.)

[22] *Bishop v. Byrne*, 265 F. Supp. 460 (S.D.W. Va. 1967).

a healthy child follows a negligently conducted sterilization or when other forms of negligence result in an unwanted pregnancy. Delaware, Florida, Michigan, California, and Connecticut courts have all allowed recovery of damages covering medical expenses, lost wages, the economic costs of raising the child, and the pain and suffering occasioned by the unwanted birth.[23] The amount of the damage awarded is normally a matter which the jury determines, and the judge may instruct them to balance the above costs against the monetary value to the parents of a healthy child, and so to arrive at a "net cost."[24] Thus, in a judicial view of damages that is probably growing more widely accepted, the changing values and attitudes of society in general are being given recognition.

Similarly, judicial decisions regarding the statute of limitations for the bringing of lawsuits are changing. Traditionally the statute began to run at the time of the alleged malpractice (or breach of contract, if the jurisdiction recognizes breach of contract as a cause of action), and hence the cause of action would be barred when the time, measured from the date of the alleged wrong, had expired. Since pregnancy and birth may occur years after the sterilization procedure, however, the tendency of recent decisions is to hold that the statute will run from the time the tort or breach of contract is discovered—or in the exercise of reasonable care ought to have been discovered—in other words, from the time that the pregnancy was or ought to have been known.[25] The plaintiff might otherwise be barred from action before the tort or breach of promise and the injury could be discovered. The application of the "discovery rule" to unsuccessful sterilization cases, of course, follows the development of the rule in other malpractice situations.

---

[23] *Coleman v. Garrison*, 281 A. 2d 616 (Del. Super. Ct. 1971), *appeal dismissed* 298 A. 2d 320 (Del. 1972): (Plaintiff established negligence in the conduct of a sterilization. A jury may give damages for the subsequent birth of a healthy child); *Jackson v. Anderson*, 230 So. 2d 503 (Florida Dist. Ct. App. 1970); *Troppi v. Scarf*, 31 Mich. App. 240, 187 N.W. 2d 511 (1971): (Suit was brought against a pharmacist for negligence in dispensing a tranquilizer instead of the prescribed contraceptive. The court allowed the jury to determine damages for the birth of the healthy, yet unwanted, child); *Custodio v. Bauer*, 251 Cal. App. 2d 303, 59 Cal. Rptr. 463, 27 A.L.R. 3d 884 (1967): (Damages may include compensation for "physical complications" and "mental anguish and suffering"). See also: *Bowman v. Davis*, 48 Ohio St. 2d 41, 356 N.E. 2d 496 (1976): (A consent form purporting to release physicians from liability for "unfavorable" results of sterilization surgery does not release defendants from liability for negligently performed tubal ligation. Further, public policy does not bar suit for damages when patient gave birth to twins, one of whom was born with congenital abnormalities).
[24] *Coleman v. Garrison*, n. 23 *supra;* Accord: *Anonymous v. Hospital*, 33 Conn. Sup. 125, 366 A. 2d 204 (Conn. Super. 1976).
[25] *Hackworth v. Hart*, 474 S.W. 2d 377 (Ky. 1971); *Hays v. Hall*, 488 S.W. 2d 412 (Texas 1972); *Vilord v. Jenkins*, 226 So. 2d 245 (Fla. Dist. Ct. App. 1969); *Teeters v. Currey*, 518 S.W. 2d 512 (Tenn. 1974).

XI

Medical Records

This chapter will review the legal aspects of three major questions relating to the patient's medical record. The discussion will first treat the source of law that requires a medical care institution or physician to compile and maintain a medical chart or record for each patient, with some observations about the importance of medical records in the modern legal environment. The second issue is the release or disclosure of recorded medical information to the patient and to third parties. Finally the use of the record in judicial or quasi-judicial proceedings will be discussed. These are the three most frequent concerns of physicians, medical record librarians, and hospital administrators.

The primary purpose of a medical record is to serve the interests of the individual patient and facilitate his medical care and treatment; a current and complete record is indispensable to the practice of medicine according to recognized professional standards of care. Secondarily, but also of utmost significance, the records of patients, compiled over an extended period, can be subjected to study and analysis that will reveal standards and patterns of care for an institution and for the individual physician, thus indicating the quality of care rendered to the community of patients by a hospital and by each physician on the staff. Accordingly, the medical records become an indispensable source of information for implementing effective peer review and quality assurance programs.

Form and Contents

The form, organization, and contents of the patient's record are best determined by physicians and other professional personnel and not by specific legal requirements. The statutory and regulatory law of the majority of states does not and should not specifically mandate in detail the organization and contents of a patient's chart. In most states the legal requirements for maintaining medical records will be found in the rules and regulations promulgated by the state administrative agency responsible for licensing hospitals and other medical care institutions. Many of these regulations simply state that the record must be "adequate" or "complete." Some states provide by regulation or by statute that the record contain certain minimum categories of information expressed in general language, leaving to the professional judgment of physicians, nurses, and paramedical personnel the details of organization and content of the record. For example, licensure regulations may require that the record contain data identifying the patient, a medical history, a provisional diagnosis, treatment notes, tissue reports, formal diagnosis, and autopsy findings. Still other jurisdictions—for example, Utah—specify in detail by statute or regulation the contents of the record: a clinical history, a description of the physician's examination, reports of laboratory tests, x-ray examinations, pathology reports, provisional diagnosis, progress notes, and a description of treatments, with their results.[1]

Although physicians and hospital administrative personnel must be familiar with local statutes and licensure rules and regulations governing the keeping of medical records, since violation of such provisions could lead to suspension or revocation of a hospital's licensure,[2] it is more important that the record-keeping policies of the institution and its staff should meet current standards of professional practice. These standards will in most instances exceed specific legal requirements.

The Joint Commission on Accreditation of Hospitals has promulgated standards for keeping medical records. Failure to comply with these standards could of course result in the loss of accreditation. Moreover, it could be evidence of a hospital's negligence, if a patient brought a civil lawsuit against a hospital alleging that he was injured

---

[1] Utah Code Ann., sec. 26–15–58 (1976). Some hospital licensure regulations go even further than Utah in specifying detailed contents of the medical record, requiring, for example, "physician's orders," "nurse's notes including temperature, pulse, respiration, conditions observed and medications given," "pre-operative medication," "the name of the surgeon and his assistants," "the method of anesthesia," and "the name of the anesthetist." Professional persons will recognize that an acceptable record will contain information of this kind even if the local law is not so specific. See generally: Springer, (ed.) *Automated Medical Records and the Law*, Aspen Systems Corp., 1971, pp. 119–67.

[2] See, for example: *Spears Free Clinic and Hospital for Poor Children v. State Board of Health*, 122 Colo. 147, 220 P. 2d 872 (1950).

or damaged, the proximate cause being the institution's failure to
adhere to recognized standards of care.[3] The standards of the Joint
Commission provide that an adequate medical record be maintained
for every person evaluated or treated as an in-patient, an out-patient,
an emergency patient, or a patient in a hospital home-care program.
The record must contain sufficient information to identify the patient
and to support the diagnosis and treatment, and it must furnish
accurate documentation of results. The records shall be confidential,
secure, current, authenticated, legible, and complete; the record
department shall be adequately directed, staffed, and equipped, and
it shall maintain a system of identification and filing to facilitate
prompt location of each record. Finally, the role of medical record
personnel in patient care evaluation programs shall be defined.[4]

Distinct from the general statutory or regulatory legal requirements
for compiling and keeping a clinical medical record for each patient
are the far more precise local laws that require certain information
to be reported to public authorities for purely statistical purposes.
State statutes will ordinarily require hospitals and physicians to
maintain records of births, deaths, autopsies, and similar events in
which the public has an interest. Local statutes will also require that
records be kept and reports made to appropriate public authority
when patients are diagnosed as suffering from certain contagious
diseases, when they may have been involved in crimes of violence,
when child abuse is suspected, or when public health and welfare
are otherwise involved. Any failure to be aware of such public health
laws, as specified on a state-by-state basis, and to comply with these
statutes can have grave consequences for medical personnel and
hospitals. More will be said later about these implications.

Both legal regulations and professional standards of medical
practice require that entries in the medical record be signed by the
physician. Hence a physician's spoken order must be later recorded
and signed. One physician may not sign for the responsible or
prescribing doctor unless both share the responsibility for the patient's
care, but house staff in teaching hospitals may write orders without
a countersignature. This general requirement is of course meant
to provide proper authentication of the record. It leads, together
with the common requirement that the record be written, to the
general conclusion that entries in the record are intended by current

[3]*Darling v. Charleston Community Hospital*, 33 Ill. 2d 326, 211 N.E. 2d 253 (1965),
cert. denied, 383 U.S. 946 (1966).
[4]*Accreditation Manual for Hospitals*, Joint Commission on Accreditation of Hospitals
(1976), 93–102.

law to be manually authenticated, either by the actual handwriting of the doctor or by another form of signature, such as a printed or stamped name or initials. Depending upon the specific language of a local statute or regulation, a "signature" does not necessarily have to be handwritten. In general, however, current law does require the manual production of a "signature," however that requirement is defined, and thus an automated authentication of entries in the chart is at present not legally acceptable in the majority of states.[5] Fully computerized medical record systems are therefore not yet legally sanctioned. To be certain that the signature requirements are met, the medical staff bylaws and rules and regulations should contain provisions relating to proper authentication of entries in the patient's chart.

Similarly, the staff bylaws should require that the physician attending the patient keep the record up to date, and especially that the record be completed promptly upon discharge of a patient from the hospital. Such a rule, like that of properly authenticating the record, is consistent with both local law and acceptable standards of practice. As will be noted in the chapter on medical staff appointments and privileges, a physician found to have violated such a rule of the medical staff of a hospital can be subject to appropriate disciplinary measures.

The failure to maintain complete, accurate, and current records can have severe adverse effects for a defendant in civil malpractice litigation. For example, a primary function of professional nursing is to observe and record the reactions and symptoms of a patient. Failure to be prompt and systematic in keeping a patient under observation in accordance with his condition, and to record the observations without delay can be evidence of negligence for a jury to consider. Since medical records are generally admissible in evidence in a malpractice suit, the absence of appropriate entries in the chart—or the inclusion of inaccurate information—can be the basis for an adverse jury verdict.[6] Similarly, inaccurate information or a changed diagnosis should be corrected in the medical record at once and in a proper fashion. That is, erasures or total obliteration of medical information in the patient's chart should never be permitted; instead, the person making the change should carefully draw a line through the original entry, leaving the writing legible, and

---

[5]Springer, *Automated Medical Records and the Law*, 49.
[6]See, for example: *Hansch v. Hackett*, 190 Wash. 97, 66 P. 2d 1129 (1937). (The hospital was liable for a nurse's negligence in failing to observe and record symptoms of eclampsia.)

authenticate the correction by signing the corrected entry. Alterations of information in the record should include the date and the reason for the change.

To put the importance of completeness and accuracy of the record in another way: one of the best possible defenses in malpractice litigation is to present in evidence a medical record that is obviously a complete and accurate record of the continuous care and treatment rendered the patient. Such a record is frequently convincing evidence that the patient received reasonable care under all the facts and circumstances.

The adverse implications of an incomplete medical record are seen in the recent case of *Carr v. St. Paul Fire and Marine Insurance Co.* The patient presented himself at a hospital's emergency room complaining of severe abdominal pains and vomiting. He was seen only by a licensed practical nurse and two orderlies, who made a record of the patient's vital signs. Although they tried unsuccessfully to reach the patient's personal doctor, hospital personnel failed to summon another physician and allowed the patient to return home, where he died the same evening. The medical records compiled during the patient's visit to the emergency room were thereupon destroyed. In a subsequent lawsuit against the hospital's insurance company the jury was allowed to know that the patient's records had been destroyed, contrary to acceptable hospital practice, and then to infer that the documents would probably have shown that a medical emergency was present, necessitating attendance by a physician. The jury award finding that hospital personnel had failed to exercise reasonable care under the circumstances was therefore justified.[7]

Information in the record must be readily available when the facts and circumstances of the individual patient's case require it. To illustrate, the victim of an automobile accident was given a physical examination by a hospital staff physician. The dictated information had not, however, been transcribed and affixed to the patient's chart when the defendant surgeon, Greenberg, performed nonemergency surgery on the patient's wrist, contrary to the rules of the hospital, which were known to the surgeon. Adverse results followed the surgery.

In such instances, if the patient can show that failure to have relevant medical information readily at hand was the proximate cause

---

[7] 384 F. Supp. 821 (W.D. Ark. 1974).

of his injury or damage, liability of both the hospital and the operating surgeon can be established. The surgeon could be negligent by undertaking surgery when he knew that the report of the patient's history and the physician's examination was not a part of the record, or when he assumed that no history was taken and no physical examination performed.[8] The hospital also could be liable for not having an effective system of compiling and making required medical information available at the time such information was needed.

Incident and accident reports compiled in the course of a patient's care should not be included as a part of his medical record. The primary reason is that the medical record is generally available as evidence in a malpractice suit, as will be discussed more thoroughly. Incident reports are likely to contain factual information which might indicate fault or negligence on the part of physicians or hospital personnel. If such reports are incorporated as a part of the medical chart they become available for consideration by a jury. Under some state laws, incident reports are subject to pretrial discovery proceedings and hence available to a plaintiff.[9] Even so, if they are separate from the medical record, they would not normally be admissible as evidence at trial, for the reason that they constitute hearsay evidence. Moreover, an incident-reporting system is maintained for educational purposes and to improve general standards of patient care and safety. To serve these ends there should be assurance that such reports will not be available to potential malpractice plaintiffs. On the other hand, information with respect to the diagnosis and the care and treatment of a particular patient following an accident or an incident should properly become a part of the medical chart.

Retention of Medical Records

Hospital policies regarding the length of time that medical records are retained in their original form and whether they should be preserved in other forms, by microfilm, for example, will depend on local law and standards of professional care of patients in the light of institutional purposes.

The latter point recognizes that the foremost purpose of maintaining and preserving the charts of patients is to provide a high quality

---

[8] *Howlett v. Greenberg*, 34 Colo. App. 356, 539 P. 2d 491 (1975).
[9] Pretrial discovery proceedings must be carefully distinguished from the use of records as evidence at trial. Whether incident reports are subject to pretrial discovery is a matter of local state law and there is a conflict of authority. An example of a decision that incident reports are *not* subject to discovery is *Sligar v. Tucker*, 267 So. 2d 54 (Fla. Dist. Ct. App. 1972).

of patient care from the point of view of both the individual patient
and the institution. Accordingly, governing bodies of hospitals and
other medical organizations must not only be familiar with local
legal requirements respecting the length of time that records must
be preserved; they must also analyze their own medical and administrative needs regarding future use of the records. Teaching hospitals,
for example, and other institutions engaged in significant and continuous medical research will wish to retain records longer than hospitals
not so engaged. All institutions will need to retain records long enough
to facilitate continuing programs of peer review and quality assurance.
Certain institutions may therefore preserve clinical records longer
than local laws require.

The law regarding the length of time that medical records must
be retained varies widely from state to state. Although a few states
may have statutory law on the subject, most commonly the matter
is found, if at all, in administrative rules and regulations bearing
on licensing hospitals or other institutions. Regulations range from
a total absence of rules about retaining medical records to requirements that patients' charts must be kept "permanently." The latter
would probably not effectively prohibit microfilming, and some
regulations affirmatively permit it. In general, if local law says nothing
about microfilming, the process is assumed to be permitted.

Some states provide for retention of records for a stipulated number
of years: for example, ten, fifteen, or twenty-five years, dating from
the discharge of the patient from the hospital, or perhaps from
the patient's known death. Regulations of this type may also permit
microfilming; or they may permit certain items in the record, such
as nurses' notes, to be destroyed earlier than others. Notes on a
patient's progress are important in malpractice litigation, and it is
hence suggested that the nurses' notes be retained as long as any
other part of the record, even if local law permits earlier disposal.
Regulations regarding the preservation of records may provide that
records of minors be retained in their original form or on microfilm
for a stipulated period after the patient has attained adulthood.

A minority among the states require approval of the licensure
authority before records may be destroyed. Some licensure regulations
say only that the period of retention shall be determined by the
state law of the statute of limitations pertaining to actions in contract
and in tort. Such a provision means that hospital and medical
personnel must know the relevant statutes of limitation and their
judicial interpretations. Because many states have recently been
revising their statutes of limitations in response to the malpractice

insurance "crisis," and also because of a continuing flow of judicial opinions concerning the interpretation of the statutes, hospitals are especially advised to consult legal counsel for current information on the length of time that the original records of patient care must be retained and on the legality of microfilm copies. In any event, when state statutes or regulations do not specify a longer period, the minimum period of retention should be determined by relevant statutes of limitations.

In summary, how long the clinical records of patients are retained and whether they are microfilmed will be determined by standards of professional practice, by the administrative and medical needs of the particular hospital, and by local law on a state-by-state basis. Institutional policies on these questions must be carefully developed and reviewed from time to time with the aid of legal counsel.

Many regulations provide that records be stored in fireproof or fire-resistant facilities. This requirement also emphasizes the need for medical and hospital personnel to be familiar with state administrative law. Since administrative regulations are subject to much amendment and modification, it is important to conduct frequent reviews of current requirements.

Private organizations such as the Joint Commission on Accreditation of Hospitals and the American Hospital Association have occasionally published statements of policy with respect to the retention and destruction of records. Hospital and medical personnel should watch for such statements of professional standards.

Ownership and Control of the Medical Record

The ownership of medical records rests with the hospital, or with the physician who keeps records of private patients in his office. Similarly x-rays, laboratory reports, reports of consultants, and other documents relating directly to the care of individual patients are owned by the hospital or by the private physician who ordered them in connection with his office practice. The owner of the record thus has the right of physical possession and control.[10] As a general rule, such owners should not permit removal of the chart from their control, except by court order. Neither a patient nor his authorized representative has a right to physical possession of the medical records.

[10] *McGarry v. J. A. Mercier Co.*, 272 Mich. 501, 262 N.W. 296 (1935); *Flaum v. Medical Arts Center Hospital*, 160(36) *N.Y. Law Journal* 2 (Sup. Ct., 1968). (The court would not order the actual hospital x-rays to be sent to a physician.)

These principles are included specifically in the hospital licensure regulations of some states.

Ownership and right of physical control does not mean, however, that the patient and various legitimately interested third parties have no legal right of access to the medical record and the information it contains. Indeed, an increasing number of jurisdictions are affirming that the patient has a right to view and copy his record and to appoint authorized representatives to examine the documents, as will be more fully discussed in the next section. Moreover, attending physicians of hospitalized patients may not prevent disclosure to them of information from the hospital record,[11] with the possible exception of cases where such disclosure might adversely affect the person's physical or mental health.

Physicians who retire from practice, those who have been replaced by other doctors selected by their patients, and the estates of deceased physicians are morally and ethically obligated to transfer the medical record or copies of it to the current physician, when the patient so requests. Hence, in a case involving unique facts, the court invalidated a provision in a deceased physician's will that all of his professional records be burned by his executor.[12] At the same time, the court recognized that the physical records belonged to the physician's estate and should not be delivered to the doctor's former patients.

Instead of delivering the entire original record to the new physician, the former doctor may wish to transfer a copy of the record or whatever excerpts or summaries are necessary for adequate treatment or diagnosis. This would be the normal procedure for hospitals when a patient is transferred to another institution or when a former patient seeks care elsewhere. When a hospital transfers a patient to another hospital—or when a private physician, for example, recommends a consultation with a specialist—the hospital or the physician has a legal obligation, as distinct from an ethical duty, to make available to the receiving institution or the consultant all medical information of record that is relevant to and necessary for the appropriate care of the patient.

The foregoing ethical and legal obligations to transfer information to succeeding practitioners or institutions may require some exceptions. If the patient requests transfer of the record or of information to a person known by the physician or hospital to be clearly unqualified

---

[11] *Matter of Weiss*, 208 Misc. 1010, 147 N.Y.S. 2d 455 (Sup. Ct. 1955).
[12] *In re Culbertson's Will*, 57 Misc. 2d 391, 292 N.Y. 2d 806 (Sup. Ct. 1968).

or unlicensed there is probably a duty to refuse the request. The physician or hospital, in the exercise of reasonable care consistent with recognized professional standards, should advise such a patient that the proposed recipient lacks the proper qualifications. [13]

The Patient's Right to Medical Information

An increasing number of states are recognizing that the patient has a legal right to the information in his medical record, even in the absence of currently pending litigation. This right has been established in some jurisdictions by statute; in others it has been articulated by judicial decision. Accordingly an assumption by medical and hospital personnel that medical records are not to be seen or inspected by the patient or his authorized representative may no longer be valid; and physicians and hospitals should review and modify their traditional policies of not allowing records to be viewed by the patient, his attorney, or representative without a court subpoena. As will be pointed out, however, the right of the patient to view the record is qualified to some extent; he must generally have a legitimate reason for inspection and must comply with reasonable safeguards established by the physician or hospital to assure the physical safety of the record while the inspection is taking place. Perhaps, also—at least in the opinion of some courts—the physician attending the patient may deny access to information in the record that would not be in the best interests of his health, according to the good faith and professional judgment of the doctor.

Statutory laws creating a right in the patient to receive medical information are illustrated in enactments in Connecticut, Massachusetts, and Wisconsin. The Connecticut statute, applicable to all hospitals that receive state aid, provides that a patient, his physician, or an authorized attorney may examine the medical record. [14] The right includes access to the patient's medical history, as well as bedside notes, charts, pictures, and plates. Copies may be made. In Massachusetts, all hospitals except those under the control of the Department of Mental Health must make the records available for inspection by the patient, or by his attorney with the written authorization

---

[13] *Batty v. Arizona State Dental Board*, 57 Ariz. 239, 112 P. 2d 870 (1941). (A dentist's license to practice may be revoked if he sends patients to persons known to be unlicensed for dental treatment. The court indicated that the licensed practitioner who knows that his patient is about to undergo care by one not licensed to undertake the needed care has a duty to advise the patient.)
[14] Conn. Gen. Stat. Ann., sec. 4–104, 4–105 (West. 1969).

of the patient.[15] As in Connecticut, the patient or his representative
is entitled to a copy of the record upon the payment of a reasonable
fee. Wisconsin's statute requires all physicians and hospitals which
have custody of the records and reports concerning care or treatment
to make them available for inspection and copying by the patient
or any authorized representative possessing written consent.[16] If the
patient is deceased, the right is given to the personal representative
or the beneficiary of an insurance policy on the patient's life. Denial
of the right shall render the physician or hospital liable for the
reasonable costs of enforcing the patient's right to discover. In
Louisiana all general hospitals administered by the state department
of hospitals are directed to furnish a "report," as distinguished from
a copy of the record, to the patient's doctor, the patient, his heirs,
or his attorney upon the written request of the doctor who referred
the patient to the hospital.[17] Such a report is to be available upon
the patient's discharge from the hospital (or his death) and shall
include diagnosis, laboratory and x-ray findings, and treatment.

A few states allow the medical record to be accessible to the patient's
attorney or his representative, whereas the foregoing statutes give
the patient direct access.[18] The attorney must have the patient's
written authorization, the consent of the parents or guardian of
a minor patient, or the consent of the personal representative or
heir of a deceased patient. In New Jersey, when compensation or
damages are claimed for a person who has been injured or has
died, the claimant may examine the pertinent hospital records.[19]

Thus to an increasing extent the states are recognizing by statute
that the patient or his authorized representative has a legally protected
right to information relative to his health and the care and treatment
provided by physicians and medical care institutions. Simultaneously,
the courts have been active in developing the right of access simply
as a matter of local common law. Several leading decisions are worthy
of emphasis.

---

[15]Mass. Gen. Laws Ann., ch. 111, sec. 70 (West. Supp. 1975).
[16]Wis. Stat. Ann., sec. 804.10 (West. Supp. 1976); see also: Miss. Code Ann., sec.
41-9-65 (1972). (Patients or representatives may have access to information in hospital
records upon showing of "good cause" and upon payment of reasonable charges.)
Young, et al. v. Madison General Hospital, 337 So. 2d 931 (Miss. 1976). (Dismissal
of bill of complaint was proper when request for access to information in medical
records was made by mail; statutory right of access requires patient's or representative's
personal appearance.)
[17]La. Rev. Stat. Ann., sec. 40:2014.1 (West 1965).
[18]Cal. Evid. Code, sec. 1158 (West. Supp. 1976); Ill. Ann. Stat., ch. 51, sec. 71
(Smith-Hurd 1969); Ill. Ann. Stat., ch. 51, sec. 73 (Smith-Hurd Supp. 1976); Utah
Code Ann., sec. 78-25-25 (Supp. 1975).
[19]N.J. Stat. Ann., sec. 2A: 82-42 (West 1976).

An Ohio decision held that a patient has a property right in certain information contained in the medical record. Accordingly the patient and her attorney were entitled to copy such parts of the record as were consistent with the beneficial interest of the patient as determined by the discretion of the hospital, taking into consideration the purposes for which such records are kept and maintained.[20] The hospital was granted the authority to supervise the inspection. Similarly, a federal court in Oklahoma held that an insurance company having current authorization from patients, and having an interest in determining the validity of claims, could inspect and copy hospital records during normal hospital business hours; and the court enforced the right by issuing a mandatory injunction.[21] As in Ohio, the court said that the information sought was the subject of a property right possessed by the patient, and that the insurance company had been placed in the patient's "shoes" by obtaining authorization. Supporting the decision, it was further argued that medical charts are "quasi-public": that is, since state law required the keeping of records, the custodian of the record had no power to prevent the patient from viewing his record. This right of the patient is not fulfilled by furnishing an abstract of the record or by requiring that inspection and copying take place under the supervision of a physician, although the record may be withheld if the doctor certifies under oath in good faith that release of information to the patient is not in the best interests of the patient's health.[22] A recent decision in New Jersey held that attorneys for hospitalized mental patients may copy the complete records relating to their commitment and care as long as the attorneys had written authorization from the patients.[23] The fact that the patients were mentally ill did not in itself invalidate such authorization, since New Jersey statutes provide that admission to a mental institution shall not constitute a presumption of incompetency. In New York a patient was entitled to see his records in order to identify medical personnel who had participated in his treatment.[24]

---

[20] *Wallace v. University Hospitals of Cleveland*, 164 N.E. 2d 917 (Common Pleas Court, Cuyahoga Co., Ohio, 1959), *aff'd and modified*, 170 N.E. 2d 261 (Ohio Ct. App. 1960), *motion to dismiss granted*, 171 Ohio St. 487, 172 N.E. 2d 459 (1961).
[21] *Pyramid Life Insurance Co. v. Masonic Hospital Ass'n of Payne County*, 191 F. Supp. 51 (W.D. Okla. 1961).
[22] *Bishop Clarkson Memorial Hospital v. Reserve Life Insurance Co.*, 350 F. 2d 1006 (8th Cir. 1965).
[23] *Bush v. Kallen*, 123 N.J. Super. 175, 302 A. 2d 142 (1973). See also: *Rabens v. Jackson Park Hospital Foundation*, 351 N.E. 2d 276 (Ill. App. 1976). (There is a common law and statutory duty to disclose medical data in hospital records to a patient or his agent.)
[24] *Matter of Weiss*, 208 Misc. 1010, 147 N.Y.S. 2d 455 (Sup. Ct. 1955).

The availability of medical information relating to the care and treatment of hospitalized mental patients is a matter of special concern. As noted previously, state statutes granting a right to a patient or his representative frequently do not cover governmental institutions for the mentally ill. In Michigan, however, as well as in the New Jersey case noted above, mentally ill patients succeeded in gaining access to their medical records. The Michigan Supreme Court held in *Gaertner v. State of Michigan* that the guardian of an incompetent patient who had been treated in state hospitals could view the hospital records, except in those instances where information in the record would severely disturb the patient.[25] Rejected was an argument by the state that the privileged communication statute prevented disclosure. Such a statute establishes a privilege in the patient of maintaining confidentiality of his medical record only under certain circumstances; further, the patient or the guardian may waive the privilege. As in the other cases discussed in this section, the hospital may require the guardian to present a written permission form from the patient.

All of the foregoing decisions are consistent with the fiduciary qualities of the physician-patient and hospital-patient relationships. As was pointed out earlier, a fiduciary is one who stands in a position of great trust and confidence in relation to another and hence is under an obligation to disclose all pertinent and relevant data to the patient when the information fulfills a legitimate need and purpose. The fiduciary relationship was the basis of the reasoning in two other cases, both of which recognized the right of the patient and his authorized representative to obtain information from medical records without first getting a court subpoena.[26]

Establishing that the information fulfills a legitimate need and purpose is extremely important, however. The courts will not authorize inspection of the record when the plaintiff's purpose is merely a "fishing expedition," or to satisfy curiosity. Hence, when an insurance company possessing the consent of the insured patients sought to review numerous medical charts relating to past hospitalizations for which the claims had long been paid, access was denied because the plaintiff's purpose did not relate to the processing of present and future claims.[27]

Moreover, constitutional law confers no general, unrestricted prop-

---

[25] 385 Mich. 49, 187 N.W. 2d 429 (1971).
[26] *Emmett v. Eastern Dispensary and Casualty Hospital,* 396 F. 2d 931 (D.C. Cir. 1967): (The son of a deceased patient and administrator of his estate was allowed to inspect records). *Cannell v. The Medical and Surgical Clinic,* 21 Ill. App. 3d 383, 315 N.E. 2d 278 (1974).
[27] *Pyramid Life Insurance Co. v. Gleason Hospital, Inc.,* 188 Kan. 95, 360 P. 2d 858 (1961).

erty right in the patient to inspect his medical charts. In *Gotkin v. Miller* a former voluntary mental patient sought access to her record with the intention of using the data in a book about her illness and her experiences during several periods of hospitalization. She asserted that denial of access constituted violation of her protected rights of freedom of speech and freedom from unreasonable searches and seizures, violation of her right of privacy, and deprivation of property without due process of law. The court rejected these arguments.[28]

"Legitimate need and purpose" may hence be taken to mean that plaintiff must show that the information will facilitate further health care or is needed for a proper evaluation of a contemplated legal measure. The *Gotkin* case should not be considered inconsistent with the several other decisions previously discussed or interpreted as a rejection of the patient's common law right to view and copy the medical record. Rather, the ruling should be confined to the facts of the case and the legal issues of constitutional law presented to the court for decision.

In the past, physicians and hospitals have traditionally refused the patient access to the medical record on the basis that records are technical and not understood by lay persons, that revelation of medical information might adversely affect the patient's health, and that the privacy of third parties who may be named in the chart should be protected. Clearly, the first and third of the foregoing reasons are no longer valid or supportable in the light of a growing social concern for the individual patient and his right to information that directly affects his health and welfare. The second reason has, as noted, been recognized by several courts as valid and honorable as long as the action is based on the professional judgment of the attending physician that in each case the patient's health might suffer, and as long as this judgment is properly documented.

Hospitals and their medical staffs must revaluate their former policies in the light of the new concern for the patient's rights. An arbitrary policy of routinely denying a request to inspect the chart unless a court order has been obtained is no longer acceptable. Such a policy can only cause conflict with patients and their bona-fide representatives, especially their attorneys.[29] Indeed, a policy of

---

[28] 514 F. 2d 125 (2d Cir. 1975).
[29] The Secretary's Commission on Medical Malpractice recommended in 1973 that medical records should be available to patients through a duly authorized representative. U.S. Department of Health, Education, and Welfare, *Report of the Secretary's Commission on Medical Malpractice*, Washington, D.C., U.S. Government Printing Office, 75–77.

denying access may even encourage malpractice suits, for then the medical record will always be available to the attorney and his client.

Hence, as a starting point in developing administrative policies, hospitals should generally make the medical chart available to a patient's attorney upon presentation of a current written authorization of the patient. In some communities the hospitals in the area and the local bar association have entered into agreements to this effect, thus improving the relations and the mutual understanding existing between the medical and legal professions. At the same time the hospital can and should exercise reasonable control and supervision over inspection of the record and is entitled to recover costs of the inspection.

Although under the law the attending physician cannot arbitrarily deny a patient access to the record, he should be consulted and his consent obtained prior to examination of the record by the patient or a representative. Not only is this a matter of professional courtesy; more significantly it protects the patient, since revelation of certain information may adversely affect his health or his willingness to continue treatment. Further, inspection of the record should be permitted only after the patient is discharged from the hospital and after the record has been completed.[30]

Especially important is the moral, if not legal, duty of a hospital or physician to make certain that the patient's consent is current and genuine when an attorney, insurance company, or other third party wishes to inspect the record. Although the prospect of legal liability for release of medical information without a patient's consent is not as great as is sometimes believed, a matter discussed in detail in the next section of this chapter, there is a growing social and legal concern about the confidentiality of information.

Sometimes patients have been required, in a sense, to grant blanket permission to a third party to receive medical information. For example, such a provision is typically included in applications for life or health insurance. The applicant may have no alternative but to sign if he desires insurance. The provision may have been executed many years before the insurance company actually seeks information from a physician or a hospital; it may be used to obtain information recorded years ago and hence not current; the patient may not have truly understood the significance of his authorization allowing

[30]With respect to recommended administrative policies regarding inspection of patients' charts see, generally: Horty, "The Patient's Right of Access to His Medical Record," ch. 5 in *Action Kit for Hospital Law*, Pittsburgh, Pa., 1974.

a third party to see his medical record. For all these reasons, especially in an era when medical information is frequently stored in centralized computers, misuse or misappropriation of information under the pretext that the patient has consented to its release is a significant possibility. Medical and hospital personnel must therefore be alert and sensitive to the validity and authenticity of documents which purport to be the patient's authorization to release information to third parties.

Release of Information Without Patient's Consent

To many persons the concept of confidentiality or privileged communication implies that private information entrusted to another shall not be divulged to a third party without the consent of the subject of the information. Since ethical considerations treat medical information as confidential, and since many states have privileged communication statutes pertaining to the physician-patient relationship, it is sometimes believed that the release of the information to a third party will generally constitute a civil wrong giving the patient a cause of action for damages unless the release is specifically ordered by a court or authorized by the patient. This commonly held belief is misleading from a legal point of view.

There are many situations where third parties have a legitimate interest in medical information respecting a particular patient and where they have a legal right to gain access to the information. In such situations the release of information by a physician or a hospital without the patient's express consent will not lead to liability in damages. Indeed, in some circumstances, a hospital or a doctor has a positive legal duty to disclose medical information whether or not the patient has consented.

First of all, a valid court order directing that medical records be made available to a given third party or revealed in a given circumstance must be honored, and the patient's consent is not required. Some typical situations where a court will order revelation are noted at the close of this chapter. Generally, the legal process for obtaining medical information of record is through a subpoena duces tecum ordering that a witness appear, together with records or documents specified by the subpoena, in a court or other duly constituted tribunal having jurisdiction of pending litigation.

Statutes also exist which require hospitals and medical personnel to report certain medical facts to public authority in particular circumstances. Statutory reporting requirements differ from state to state, and hospital personnel must be familiar with local law. Typically required, however, are reports on patients suffering from venereal and other contagious disease, and from knife wounds or wounds caused by firearms when circumstances suggest that they have been the victims or perpetrators of violent criminal acts. Treatment of infant patients who may have been subjected to child abuse must also be reported. Failure to comply with the statutes and report such cases to the appropriate public authority may lead to civil liability in damages or to a criminal penalty.

For example, California statutes require physicians, hospitals, public health nurses, school officials, and others to report suspected cases of battered children and grant civil and criminal immunity to the hospital or the individual who makes the report, protecting them from liability for defamation of character, invasion of privacy, or other civil wrong. On the other hand, failure to report is a criminal misdemeanor, subjecting the offender to a fine or imprisonment or both of these. Reports must be made whenever a child appears for treatment of injuries which seem other than accidental. Since the criminal statute requiring the report is intended to protect the allegedly battered minor, the child may have a civil cause of action for damages against a nonreporting physician and hospital if he can prove at trial that he appeared to have been battered and that the failure to report his case was the proximate cause of further injury. In short, physicians and hospitals have a positive duty by virtue of the statute to exercise reasonable care to observe symptoms and injuries and make the required report.[31]

A treating physician and the hospital could also be liable to a child in a malpractice action for negligent failure to diagnose the "battered child syndrome." As in other malpractice actions alleging liability for damages resulting from improper diagnosis, a plaintiff was permitted to call expert witnesses in an attempt to prove that standards of medical practice required a reasonably prudent physician to diagnose child abuse when an infant had a broken leg as well as bruises and abrasions and the mother could not satisfactorily account for the injuries. Release of the patient to the parent in this instance was followed by subsequent beatings; these assaults by the parent were not necessarily "intervening acts" sufficient to relieve the hospital or physician from liability if the subsequent acts were "reasonably foreseeable." The issue of foreseeability is a question

---

[31] *Landeros v. Flood,* 17 Cal. 3d 399, 551 P. 2d 389, 131 Cal. Rptr. 69 (1976). West's Calif. Ann. Penal Code, sec. 11160–62.

of fact for the jury to determine at trial on the basis of the testimony given by the plaintiff's expert witness.[32]

Quite apart from a statutory duty to report if a patient's medical or psychological condition represents a foreseeable serious risk to a third party or parties, the physician or hospital knowing of the risk has a duty to disclose and warn of the danger. In an unusual California case with a tragic outcome the facts were these: a patient was undergoing psychiatric treatment at a university hospital as a voluntary out-patient. Several psychotherapists employed by the hospital were aware that the patient had threatened to kill a particular individual. One of the psychologists determined that the patient should be committed to a mental institution. At his request the campus police detained the man but released him when he appeared to be rational. Subsequently the chief of the psychiatry department reversed the psychologist's order for detention.

Two months later the patient did in fact kill his intended victim. In a suit by the parents of the victim the California court held that the duty of disclosure was superior to the duty of holding the medical information confidential. According to the court, the psychotherapists and their employer had a duty to exercise reasonable care to give threatened persons a warning that foreseeable dangers could arise from the patient's condition or treatment.[33] Breach of the duty can result in liability for damages. The therapists and the police were not liable, however, for failing to detain the patient. California law of governmental immunity protected them from liability on this point, since the decision not to detain was a matter of governmental policy-making. In contrast statutory governmental immunity does not extend to nondiscretionary negligent omissions such as failure to warn third persons in danger. In a similar situation, a hospital operated by the federal government failed to disclose pertinent information about a mental patient at a trial court hearing to determine whether the patient should be discharged from the hospital. Following his discharge the patient killed his wife, and the hospital was liable in damages.[34]

A third party's legal right to receive medical information regarding a particular patient is further illustrated by hospital lien statutes, which exist in approximately one-third of the states. In simplest

---

[32] *Id.*
[33] *Tarasoff v. Regents of the University of California,* 17 Cal. 3d 425, 551 P. 2d 334, 131 Cal. Rptr. 14 (1976).
[34] *Hicks v. United States,* 367 F. Supp. 434 (D.D.C. 1973), *aff'd,* 511 F. 2d 407 (D.C. Cir. 1975).

terms, the lien laws grant to the hospital a legal claim under which the cost of hospitalization is paid from damages which the patient recovers from a third party whose negligence or civil wrong caused the patient's hospitalization. In turn, the third party is entitled to access to the patient's medical chart without the authorization of the patient.

When information from a patient's medical record is disclosed by a physician or hospital without the patient's express consent and in the absence of an affirmative statutory or common law duty to disclose, the patient may feel aggrieved and file suit seeking damages, claiming that his rights were violated. The general question then raised is this: what are the legal theories upon which the patient bases his cause of action?

Before undertaking a review of these legal theories we should note the ethical and moral obligations to respect the confidentiality of information obtained in the course of medical care and treatment. The Hippocratic Oath requires a physician to hold inviolate and confidential all information entrusted to and obtained by him. This ethical obligation may be incorporated in the rules and regulations of some states governing the licensure of physicians to practice medicine, and violation of it may be a cause for revoking or suspending a license to practice. Whether or not a physician's violation of licensure regulations creates a civil cause of action for damages in the patient is, however, very much an open question legally and will be discussed subsequently.

At common law there was no doctrine of confidential or privileged communication between patient and physician. The common law recognized a doctrine of privileged communication only in three relationships: attorney-client, husband-wife, and minister or priest and parishioner. Accordingly, the doctor had no obligation under common law to hold medical information about his patient secret or confidential.

To correct this situation and to establish a confidential relationship between physician and patient, the legislatures of approximately three-fourths of the states have enacted laws known as the privileged communication statutes. Although the statutes differ somewhat in detail, the essence of the legislation is to declare that medical practitioners shall not be allowed to disclose any information which was acquired in attending patients in their professional capacity and which was necessary to the care and treatment of their patients. As will be noted, a patient may waive this privilege; in that event the doctor would not be prohibited from making such disclosures and could even be compelled by a court order to do so.

The major point of emphasis here, however, is that the privileged communication statutes do not apply precisely to out-of-court disclosures of medical information. They are applicable only to disclosures made in the course of judicial or quasi-judicial proceedings. Hence an out-of-court disclosure of private medical information does not contravene the privileged communication statutes, and an aggrieved patient may not base a civil cause of action for damages on an alleged violation of the statutes.[35]

Accordingly, a patient bringing an action against a physician or a hospital, or both of these, for damages allegedly resulting from an unauthorized out-of-court disclosure of information must base the action upon a common law tort or upon a theory of contract law. There are two or possibly three theories of action: defamation of character; invasion of privacy; or, as noted in a few recent cases, breach of an implied contract to respect confidentiality.

DEFAMATION

The personal tort of defamation is a written or oral communication to a third party of information respecting a living person which injures his reputation by diminishing the esteem, respect, or confidence in which the person is held, or by exciting adverse or derogatory feelings against him.[36] A written communication injuring reputation is libel; an oral communication is slander. Libel is actionable without proof of actual pecuniary damage. To succeed in a suit for slander, the plaintiff must usually prove actual damage resulting from the communication, although oral imputations that he has committed a serious crime or suffers from certain loathsome diseases, and statements affecting the plaintiff in his business or profession, may be actionable without proof of actual damages.

In the context of the release of information from a medical record, however, the prospects of successful libel or slander suits against physicians and medical care institutions are slight indeed. In the first place, at common law the truth of the published statement is a complete defense to a civil cause of action for either libel or slander in nearly all jurisdictions, even if the publisher had no legitimate motive or reason for the publication. Since this rule creates immunity regardless of motive for publication and permits at least

[35]For example: *Noble v. United Benefit Life Insurance Co.*, 230 Iowa 471, 297 N.W. 881 (1941); *Simonsen v. Swenson*, 104 Neb. 224, 177 N.W. 831 (1920); *Boyle v. Northwestern Mutual Relief Ass'n.* 95 Wis. 312, 70 N.W. 351 (1897).
[36]Prosser, *Torts*, sec. 111, at 737–51 (4th ed. 1971).

a morally indefensible dissemination of information, some states have modified the defense either by statute or case decision to provide that truth will be a defense only when the publication is made with a good motive or for a justifiable end. The burden of proving the truth will normally be on the defendant.

Moreover, in general, publication of a retraction by the defendant, or the presentation of evidence that he published a defamatory statement with a proper motive and a reasonable belief that it was true, will provide a partial defense that can be considered in the reduction or mitigation of damages.

Further, even if a statement published about another without consent is quite untrue and affects adversely the subject's reputation, the law has long recognized two types of privilege: absolute and qualified. There is an absolute privilege to publish in judicial proceedings, legislative proceedings, and even in proceedings of executive or administrative officers of government. Hence, if the hospital honored a court subpoena and disclosed a medical record indicating that plaintiff was under the influence of alcohol, a statement alleged to be false, there could be no liability based upon defamation since the release was absolutely privileged.[37]

A qualified privilege exists where information is transmitted to a third party with proper motive or purpose and with the exercise of reasonable care that the information was true. Publications may be made in good faith to protect or advance the legitimate interests of the publisher, or to protect the interests of the recipient or the public where the publisher reasonably believes he is under a moral duty or social duty to speak and make "fair comment" on matters that concern the public interest. To illustrate specifically, a hospital or physician could normally release information to an insurance carrier, even without express consent of the patient, for the purpose of collecting hospitalization insurance benefits, without fear of being liable in damages for defamation. Similarly, governmental agencies having a legitimate interest in the care rendered a patient have a right to relevant information, and a qualified privilege to release it would exist. Even attorneys representing the patient's interest may be given medical information, although it is better administrative practice to require an express consent from the patient before allowing an attorney access to the medical chart.

Hospitals and physicians may use medical record information in

---

[37] *Gilson v. Knickerbocker Hospital*, 280 App. Div. 690, 116 N.Y.S. 2d 745 (1952).

their own defense when they are sued by a patient. The institution
and the medical staff may use the charts of patients for medical
research, for education, and for the proper implementation of peer
review and quality assurance programs. In several jurisdictions the
use of medical information for research is affirmatively approved
by statute, and some statutes provide further that data can be shared
with the state health commissioner or other public or private agencies
engaged in research.[38]

In a Nebraska case, *Simonsen v. Swenson*, a physician disclosed
to a hotel that his patient, a resident of the hotel, had a contagious
venereal disease. In a suit alleging unwarranted disclosure of confidential information the court held that, even if the diagnosis was
incorrect and hence untruthful, the defendant physician was protected
from liability by reason of qualified privilege as delineated by the
law of defamation. Since the transmittal of information was made
in good faith without malice to a legitimately interested party, with
a belief that there was a moral obligation to protect third parties,
there could be no liability.[39]

Likewise there was no liability when a life insurance company
shared medical information about a particular person with a central
agency serving the life insurance industry.[40] In a similar situation,
the plaintiff customer was injured in defendant's store and examined
by the store's physician, who gave a copy of his medical findings
to the attorney representing the store. Since the report was true
and since the communication was made in good faith to an interested
party, the plaintiff had no right of action in defamation.[41]

Whether a publication was made in good faith, with the exercise
of a reasonable belief and care respecting the truth, may be a question
for the jury to determine. It was so held in a Utah case entitled
Berry v. Moench.[42] A physician in Wyoming, acting on behalf of
the parents of a young woman, wrote to the defendant physician
asking for his impression of a young man, formerly one of his

---

[38]Mich. Comp. Laws Ann., sec. 325.131–134 (1975). See also: *Klinge, M.D. v. Lutheran
Medical Center of St. Louis*, 518 S.W. 2d 157 (Mo. 1974). (A hospital medical staff
committee may use medical records of patients of a staff physician without the patients'
consent to determine the qualifications and competency of the staff physician.)
[39]104 Neb. 224, 177 N.W. 831 (1920); See also: *Cochran v. Sears Roebuck*, 72 Ga.
458, 34 S.E. 2d 296 (1945). (No liability was held to exist when a company nurse
reported erroneously to her supervisor that an employee was suffering from a
communicable venereal disease and the employee was discharged. The nurse acted
in good faith and no malice was proved.)
[40]*Mayer v. Northern Life Insurance Co.*, 119 F. Supp. 536 (N.D. Cal. 1953).
[41]*Quarles v. Sutherland*, 215 Tenn. 651, 389 S.W. 2d 249 (1965).
[42]8 Utah 2d 191, 331 P. 2d 814 (1958).

psychiatric patients, since the ex-patient wished to marry the young woman. Without authorization from his former patient, the defendant physician wrote that the young man had a psychopathic personality and suffered from depression. His father had taken his own life. The patient himself had been married several times and had not supported his wives and children. He was in trouble with the authorities during World War II and was financially irresponsible. On receipt of this letter the Wyoming doctor passed it on to the parents of the young woman who thereupon refused to approve their daughter's marriage to the patient. When she married him anyway the parents disowned her.

In a suit founded upon libel the court observed that the publisher had no interest of his own to protect, although a privilege may still exist to protect or advance the interests of third persons. However, a judgment by the trial court as a matter of law for the defendant physician was error, since a factual issue was raised respecting his exercise of reasonable care to ascertain the truth of the communication. The physician had admitted that he was not entirely certain of the source of all the information he transmitted, apparently relying to some extent on statements by a former wife of the patient. Accordingly, the possible failure to exercise care could be malice-in-law, a libelous publication without legal justification, and this issue was to be resolved by a jury. With respect to qualified privilege the court said:

> Where life, safety, well-being or other important interest is in jeopardy, one having information which could protect against the hazard may have a conditional privilege to reveal information for such purpose. . . . But the privilege is not something which arises automatically and becomes absolute merely because there is an interest to protect. It has its origin in, and is governed by, the rule of good sense and customary conduct to people motivated by good will and proper consideration for others. This includes due consideration for the subject being informed about as well as the recipient being protected.[43]

When a publication is made with malice-in-fact motivated by spite or ill will, the publisher can be liable for punitive damages as well as compensatory damages. In a New Mexico case a physician, who was examining a patient to determine the reason for her absence

---

[43] Id., at 197, 331 P. 2d at 817, 818 (1958).

from school, falsely reported to the school authorities that the 13-year-old girl was pregnant, and he refused to retract or correct the report after learning it was false. His refusal to make the correction resulted in loss of privilege. Since a matter of alleged pregnancy is libelous per se when it is false, the plaintiff is entitled to compensatory damages without proof of actual monetary loss and is also entitled to punitive damages for malice-in-fact.[44]

In an action based upon defamation the question of malice may be one for the jury, and the proper standard for the jury to consider is whether a publication was made with knowledge of falsity or with a reckless disregard for its truth. In a recent Virginia case a pediatrician who had resigned from the medical staff of a hospital was quoted by a newspaper as saying that he had resigned because he "could not condone the quality of gynecological and obstetrical medicine" at the hospital. The pediatrician denied making such a statement, and the newspaper editor had not verified the story. The two physicians remaining on the obstetrical staff brought suit against the newspaper for libel. A jury verdict for punitive damages was reversed for the reason that the jury had been improperly instructed by the judge, and a new trial was ordered.[45] Since hospitals and physicians uphold ethical standards and do not normally publish information which they know to be false or show a reckless disregard for the truth, the prospect of their being held liable for punitive damages is minimal.

INVASION OF PRIVACY

Separate and distinct from the tort of defamation is the civil wrong of invasion of privacy. Invasion of privacy as a tort was recognized and developed by the courts following publication of a law review article in 1890—and thus illustrates the profound influence that legal scholars can have upon the process of judicial law-making.[46] Not all jurisdictions have had occasion to rule on invasion of privacy. Some states that have considered the matter have rejected the existence of the right; but the majority of courts have recognized the tort, imposing certain limitations to discourage unwarranted litigation and to balance properly an individual's right to privacy with freedom of the press and of speech. A few states have recognized the right of privacy by enacting statutes which carefully delineate limitations to the cause of action.

---

[44] Vigil v. Rice, 74 N.M. 693, 397 P. 2d 719 (1964).
[45] Newspaper Publishing Corp. v. Burke, 216 Va. 800, 224 S.E. 2d 132 (1976).
[46] Warren and Brandeis, "The Right of Privacy," 4 Harvard L. Rev. 193 (1890).

Broadly defined, the right of privacy is a person's right to be free from unreasonable and serious interferences in his personal affairs that exceed the limits of decent conduct and are offensive to persons of ordinary sensibilities. With respect to publication of private information to third parties or to the public, there is a legal wrong only when the recipient has no legitimate interest in the information. In contrast to actions based on the law of defamation, when a suit is founded on invasion of privacy, the truth of an unwarranted publication is not necessarily a defense. On the other hand, express consent to the publication is a defense.[47]

An Ohio court, affirming the principle that an individual has a legally protected right of privacy, defined the right in the case syllabus as follows:

> An actionable invasion of the right of privacy is the unwarranted appropriation or exploitation of one's personality, the publicizing of one's private affairs with which the public has no legitimate concern, or the wrongful intrusion into one's private activities in such a manner as to outrage or cause mental suffering, shame or humiliation to a person of ordinary sensibilities.[48]

To succeed in an action for invasion of privacy it is not necessary for the plaintiff to prove pecuniary or monetary loss. Damages can be awarded for mental suffering. The right, however, is a personal one; the privacy of a deceased person cannot be invaded, and hence surviving relatives have no cause of action. Nor does a person too young to be damaged by "mental distress" have any right of privacy to be invaded. Similarly, a corporation or a partnership cannot bring the action, although other legal theories will protect a business from unwarranted appropriation of its name or good will.

Cases of invasion of privacy can be classified into four groups or types of factual situations. The first are those involving the unauthorized commercial appropriation of plaintiff's name, personality, professional skills, or photograph. Most of the cases in this category concern the use of plaintiff's name or picture without consent

---

[47] *Smith v. Doss*, 251 Ala. 250, 37 So. 2d 118 (1948).
[48] *Housh v. Peth*, 165 Ohio St. 35, 133 N.E. 2d 340 (1956). Prosser, *Torts*, 4th ed., sec. 117 (1971) identifies four categories of cases: (a) appropriation, for defendant's advantage, of plaintiff's name or likeness; (b) intrusion upon plaintiff's seclusion or solitude, or into his private affairs; (c) public disclosure of embarrassing private facts; and (d) publicity which places plaintiff in a false light in the public eye. The author's classification of cases will vary somewhat from Prosser's.

in connection with the commercial sale of defendant's product or for the promotion of his business. Even in such a factual situation, however, the court in *Roberson*, an early New York case where the defendant used the photograph of a pretty young woman to advertise its flour, rejected the plaintiff's suit, fearing excessive litigation and limitations upon the freedoms of speech and the press, thus rejecting invasion of privacy as a tort.[49] Subsequently, however, Georgia and many other courts recognized the tort when commercial exploitation of a person's name or likeness had occurred.[50] Moreover, New York later reversed the *Roberson* case by enacting a statute affording a right of action in such circumstances.[51] Several other states followed, with the result that in these jurisdictions a cause of action for invasion of privacy is limited to commercial uses of name or likeness.[52]

Where the cause is not statutorily limited to commercial uses of name or likeness some courts have extended the right of privacy to a second group of cases: the using of plaintiff's name or likeness for the defendant's own purposes or benefit, even though the use was not commercial and even if the benefit to the defendant was not financial.[53] Perhaps in this category is the Pennsylvania case of *Clayman v. Bernstein*.[54] The plaintiff succeeded in preventing a physician who had photographed her facial disfigurement without her consent from using the photographs to show the effect of her disability for instructional purposes. Alternatively the *Bernstein* case can also be classified with—at least it is akin to—the physical intrusion cases noted below.

The use of a name or likeness for personal benefit is further illustrated by an Oregon case where there was liability when a corporation signed plaintiff's name to a telegram addressed to the governor urging his veto of particular legislation opposed by the corporation.[55] On the other hand, Ohio has held that no relief could be granted when a magazine publisher and credit card company sold subscription lists to direct mail advertisers without the consent

---

[49] *Roberson v. Rochester Folding Box Company*, 171 N.Y. 538, 64 N.E. 442 (1902).

[50] *Pavesich v. New England Life Ins. Co.*, 122 Ga. 190, 50 S.E. 68 (1904).

[51] N.Y. Civ. Pract., sec. 50–51 (McKinney 1976).

[52] For example: Va. Code Ann., sec. 8–650 (1950). See also: Utah Code Ann., sec. 76–9–405 (1973).

[53] *Restatement (Second) of Torts*, sec. 652C, and comments, 108 *et seq.*

[54] 38 Pa. D.C. 543 (1940). See also: *Estate of Berthiaume v. Pratt*, 365 A. 2d 792 (Me. 1976). (The taking of a photograph of a terminally ill patient for the purpose of medical science over the objections of the patient invades the right of privacy.)

[55] *Hinish v. Meier and Frank Co.*, 166 Or. 482, 113 P. 2d 438 (1941). See also: *Magouirk v. Western Union Telegraph Co.*, 79 Miss. 632, 31 So. 206 (1901); *Schwartz v. Edrington*, 133 La. 235, 62 So. 660 (1913).

of the subscribers. The sale of mere names did not amount to an "appropriation" of "personalities."[56]

Not all of the cases involving the use or appropriation of a person's name or likeness can be reconciled. However, it seems clear that no wrong is committed by the mere mention of an individual's name or by reference to newsworthy public activities. Hence a newspaper is not liable for simply publicizing the names or likenesses of individuals. Only when one seeks to take advantage of a person's reputation, prestige, or personal values does there appear to be an unwarranted appropriation of another's personality. Since hospital and medical personnel do not normally have any reason to exploit or take advantage of a patient's name or personal reputation, the first two groups of privacy cases do not represent a serious threat of liability to medical care institutions and physicians.

As noted above, however, they must exercise caution in their use of photographs obtained in the course of patient care. Normally the mere taking of a photograph of a person is not an invasion of privacy, just as the mere mention of a name is not a civil wrong. When photographs are taken in the course of routine patient care, for the benefit of the patient and in accordance with acceptable professional standards, and when the photographs are then made a part of the medical record, no appreciable legal issue is presented. Like other parts of the record such photographs can be used by the medical staff of the hospital in evaluating standards and patterns of care and for scientific or research purposes, at least when the patient's anonymity is preserved. To prevent any possible risk of liability, however, in the light of *Clayman v. Bernstein* and *Estate of Berthiaume v. Pratt*, noted above, it is sound administrative practice to have the patient consent to the taking of photographs, and to obtain the consent at the time of admission or prior to surgery. Such a consent to photograph can be incorporated into the regular hospital admission or the surgical consent forms, whichever is most appropriate.

The taking of a photograph that does not benefit the patient or that is contrary to professional standards of medical practice, if done without consent, could constitute an invasion of privacy and be within the third category of cases, a physical intrusion into one's private affairs. Moreover, the unauthorized use of and publication of the pictures might also fall within the fourth group of privacy cases: where private information is made public to those who have

---

[56] *Shibley v. Time, Inc.*, 45 Ohio App. 2d 69, 341 N.E. 2d 337 (1975).

no legitimate concern or interest in the information.

An unjustified and unwarranted physical intrusion into a person's private domain or affairs constitutes a well-recognized invasion of privacy. Tapping plaintiff's telephone wires and listening to conversations on a dictaphone were both held to be actionable wrongs.[57] Similarly, entry into a woman's bedroom, and a layman's intrusion to witness a childbirth without the patient's consent constituted wrongful acts.[58] More recently, the "bugging" of a bedroom by the landlord who had leased an apartment to a married couple was said to be an intrusion upon the plaintiff's right to physical and mental seclusion.[59] These litigated cases exemplify acts which cause mental suffering or humiliation to a person of ordinary sensibilities.

In the hospital setting such cases are relevant in situations where physicians or hospitals permit lay persons to be present at surgery or during diagnostic examinations of a patient. Such a practice is unwise and quite probably an invasion of the patient's privacy, unless the patient is made aware of the layman's presence and the reason for it, and has consented to it. Teaching hospitals should make clear to patients that medical students may from time to time accompany house staff and physicians who are administering care and treatment, and it should be explained that the opportunity to observe is an integral part of the students' education.

Perhaps the most difficult privacy cases are those in the fourth group: where private information is revealed to individuals or the public without serving a legitimate concern or interest. The courts must delicately balance several related issues. In a general sense, the tort of invasion of privacy is founded upon recognition of an individual's right to be let alone and to be free from unwarranted disclosure of private information, especially the mass dissemination of information. On the other hand, public policy frequently requires that information be made public in order to ascertain the truth and to promote justice. The ascertainment of truth is particularly important in litigation and in other adversary situations. Further, the legitimate interests of the publisher must be recognized on the proper facts, since his interests may outweigh those of the individual who asserts an invasion of privacy. Issues of freedom of speech and of the press are frequently present in cases claiming an invasion

[57] *Rhodes v. Graham*, 238 Ky. 225, 37 S.W. 2d 46 (1931); *McDaniel v. Atlanta Coca-Cola Bottling Co.*, 60 Ga. App. 92, 2 S.E. 2d 810 (1939).
[58] *Byfield v. Candler*, 33 Ga. App. 275, 125 S.E. 905 (1924); *DeMay v. Roberts*, 46 Mich. 160, 9 N.W. 146 (1881).
[59] *Hamberger v. Eastman*, 106 N.H. 107, 206 A. 2d 239 (1964).

of privacy, at least when medical information concerning an individual
is published in a magazine or newspaper.

It can be said that when publication of private information violates
concepts of ordinary decent conduct and serves no legitimate purpose
it is an invasion of privacy. In a leading case, a newspaper, a hospital,
and a photographer were enjoined from publishing pictures of a
deceased, malformed child.[60] When a national magazine published
a photograph and story of a young woman suffering from a metabo-
lism imbalance which caused her to consume a fantastic amount
of food there was an invasion of privacy.[61] In a Kentucky case a
store owner posted a large sign in the window announcing that
the plaintiff had not paid a debt; this act of publication went beyond
the limits of decent conduct and was held unreasonable and oppressive.[62]

On the other hand, a majority of courts have determined that
a creditor may notify an employer that an employee has not paid
a legitimate debt without invading the employee's privacy, since the
creditor has an interest in pursuing collection and the employer
also may have an interest in the credit standing of an employee.[63]
Moreover, Minnesota's Supreme Court recently ruled that there was
no invasion of privacy when a hospital's credit personnel in the
presence of several others demanded payment of an outstanding
hospital bill by the plaintiff, who was seeking to have her son admitted
to the hospital.[64] In the course of making the demand, the hospital
employee had noted that the debt had been included in a petition
for bankruptcy filed in court by the plaintiff. The Minnesota court
reasoned that the bankruptcy was a matter of public record. Furthermore only a few persons witnessed the demand, and under the
circumstances the behavior of hospital personnel did not amount
to undue or oppressive publicity.

[60] *Bazemore v. Savannah Hospital*, 171 Ga. 257, 155 S.E. 194 (1930). See also: *Douglas
v. Stokes*, 149 Ky. 506, 149 S.W. 849 (1912): (Publication of a photograph of the
nude bodies of twin children, who had been joined together, transgressed bounds
of decency); *Rinsley v. Frydman*, 559 P. 2d 334 (Kansas 1977): (Publicity which places
plaintiff in a false light and is highly offensive to a reasonable man is an invasion
of privacy).
[61] *Barber v. Time, Inc.*, 348 Mo. 1199, 159 S.W. 2d 291 (1942).
[62] *Brents v. Morgan*, 221 Ky. 765, 299 S.W. 967 (1927).
[63] *Hawley v. Professional Credit Bureau*, 345 Mich. 500, 76 N.W. 2d 835 (1956);
Gouldman-Taber Pontiac v. Zerbet, 213 Ga. 682, 100 S.E. 2d 881 (1957).
[64] *Hendry v. Conner*, 226 N.W. 2d 921 (Minn. 1975). *Cf.: Biederman's of Springfield,
Inc. v. Wright*, 322 S.W. 2d 892 (Mo. 1959). (It was an invasion of privacy when
a creditor's collection agent appeared on several occasions in the cafe where the
debtor was employed, announcing loudly in the presence of customers that the debtor
and her husband refused to pay their bills and that they were "deadbeats.")

Disclosure of private information may be privileged on the basis that revelation protects the interests of others. Release of medical information without the express consent of the patient to persons and organizations having a legitimate interest in the information would not ordinarily constitute an invasion of the patient's privacy, nor would a release of information to advance the legitimate interests of the hospital.

Individuals and organizations having such an interest include attorneys for the patient, insurance carriers, various governmental agencies, family members, and bona-fide research personnel. For example, during marriage a husband is entitled to full information relating to his wife's medical condition, and a court subpoena seeking that information in connection with a pending divorce proceeding is proper.[65] In another example, *Iverson v. Frandsen*, a child suffered from claustrophobia to such an extent that she could not attend school. She was taken by her mother to a state institution for evaluation and given an intelligence quotient test. In a suit against the institution for reporting the score to the patient's school, the court denied recovery.[66]

In addition to all of the foregoing circumstances where disclosure is permissible, the patient by his actions may waive any possible right he had to confidentiality of medical information. In a New York case a civilian employee of the United States Air Force who had been absent from work asked his physician to certify to his employer that he was ill. The physician did so on several occasions without revealing the diagnosis of the illness. In due course the Air Force requested additional information about the patient's condition. The doctor informed the employee that he would disclose the diagnosis and then reported to the Air Force that his patient was an alcoholic. An action against the physician was unsuccessful on the basis that the patient had requested partial disclosure and thus was estopped from asserting any civil wrong when full disclosure was later asked for by the employer.[67] On such facts the patient has waived any right to confidentiality of the information, although the court apparently recognized that had there been no waiver the physician would have a duty of secrecy. This duty derives from New York's privileged communication statute respecting courtroom

---

[65] *Pennison v. Provident Life and Accident Insurance Co.*, 154 So. 2d 617 (La. App. 1963). See also: *Curry v. Corn*, 52 Misc. 2d 1035, 277 N.Y.S. 2d 470 (1966). (A physician is privileged to reveal a patient's condition to the spouse.)
[66] 237 F. 2d 898 (10th Cir. 1956).
[67] *Clark v. Geraci*, 29 Misc. 2d 791, 208 N.Y.S. 2d 564 (Sup. Ct. 1960).

testimony, and from the medical practice act providing that "unprofessional conduct" is a basis for disciplining a physician. Privileged
communications statutes and their effect are discussed further below.

Utilizing the same theory of waiver, the New Jersey court denied
damages to the parents of a child when their pediatrician reported
to a life insurance company that the child had been born with a
defective heart. Not aware of the heart ailment, the father of the
newborn baby applied for and was issued an insurance policy on
the baby's life. Subsequently the child died and the parents claimed
death benefits. During the processing of the claim the physician
reported to the company that the child had suffered from ill health
since birth. On these grounds the company denied payment of the
claim. In holding that the doctor was not liable to the parents for
the disclosure, the court noted, first, that they had waived any right
of confidentiality by initiating the insurance claim; secondly, the public
interest in these facts would permit disclosure in order to achieve
justice in the handling of insurance claims, thus constituting a privilege
of disclosure.[68]

Persons who consent to publicity or who place themselves in the
public eye through their activities and exploits—for example, authors,
actors, or candidates for public office—curtail their rights of privacy
to the extent that the public has a legitimate interest in newsworthy
events.[69] This principle applies also to persons who are not public
figures but who voluntarily take actions or are victims of circumstances
which put them temporarily in the public eye. Unless news stories
and photographs exceed the bounds of ordinary decent conduct,
as discussed earlier, a person cannot complain when he is, for example,
involved in an accident that is reported to the press, or commits
a crime that is publicized, or figures in any other newsworthy event
so long as the publicity is not misleading or the facts misrepresented.

Ordinarily, therefore, a hospital's release to reporters acknowledging an individual's admission to the hospital, naming his physician,
and describing in general terms his medical condition presents no
legal risk of liability for invasion of privacy. If, however, the mere
fact of admission could reveal the presence of a shameful and
humiliating disease or mental illness—as might occur, for example,

---

[68] *Hague v. Williams*, 37 N.J. 328, 181 A. 2d 345 (1962). *Cf.: Felis v. Greenberg*, 51
Misc. 2d 881, 273 N.Y.S. 2d 288 (1966). (A physician who files an intentionally
false report with an insurance company could be liable in damages.)
[69] *Sinclair v. Postal Telegraph and Cable Co.*, 72 N.Y.S. 2d 841 (Sup. Ct. 1935). (An
actor may insist that presentations of himself and his work to the public preserve
the attribute of dignity; hence the defendant's use of an actor's picture without
permission, presenting him in an undignified light, was wrongful.)

when the hospital in question was known to treat only alcoholics or those suffering from mental illness—then an announcement of admission could lead to liability, at least if the patient was not a public figure.

Illustrative of the public's interest in a newsworthy event is the recent Ohio case of *Zacchini v. Scripps-Howard Broadcasting Company.* Plaintiff Zacchini was a "human cannonball" performing his act of being shot from a cannon into a net at a county fair. Without the consent of Mr. Zacchini, a television station filmed the performance and broadcast the film as a part of its newscast to the general public. Individuals like the plaintiff have a property right in their name, photograph, or performance, and this right may be sold. There is no invasion of privacy on these facts, however, if the defendant had no intent to appropriate the publicity for a nonprivileged private use and no intent to injure the plaintiff.[70] On the other hand, a news story on surfing in a national sports magazine is not privileged to disclose bizarre details concerning a surfer's private life, since freedom of the press and of speech do not extend to the publication of unnewsworthy and embarrassing private affairs.[71] As in many other invasion of privacy cases, the truth of the matters that were published was not a defense to the action.

An actionable invasion of privacy occurred when a newspaper story concerning a special education class in a public school included photographs in which pupils in the class were named and described as "retarded" and "trainable mentally retarded." The children had not become "public figures" by merely being enrolled in the class, and hence the publication offended concepts of ordinary decency.[72]

Publishers and others broadcasting newsworthy events to the general public—including hospitals who permit access to news reporters—must also be aware that they may be liable for the tort of defamation as well as the tort of invasion of privacy. It will be remembered that truth is a defense to a cause of action founded upon defamation, but what legal duty does the publisher have to ascertain the truth before publication? Normally, as noted earlier in this chapter, the burden of proving truth is on the defendant. However, in the publication of matters of general or public interest this rule has traditionally been relaxed somewhat in order to make meaningful the constitutional guarantees of freedom of the press.

---

[70] 47 Ohio St. 2d 224, 351 N.E. 2d 454 (1976).
[71] *Virgil v. Time, Inc.,* 527 F. 2d 1122 (9th Cir. 1975).
[72] *Deaton v. Delta Democrat Publishing Co.,* 326 So. 2d 471 (Miss. 1976).

Thus the New York Court of Appeals recently held that an action for defamation against a newspaper would be allowed only when the publisher acted in a "grossly irresponsible manner without due consideration for the standards of information gathering and dissemination ordinarily followed by responsible parties."[73] Such a rule gives a publisher of news great flexibility and minimizes his obligation to verify stories before publication.

A somewhat higher standard of conduct has been imposed by the Supreme Court of Washington. That court has held, in a case brought by a private individual who was not a public figure or a public official, that a recovery for actual damages would be allowed for publication of a defamatory falsehood where substantial danger to reputation was apparent, upon proof by the plaintiff that the defendant knew or should have known that the statement was false or would create a false impression in some material respect.[74]

These two decisions illustrate once more the conflict between opposing public policies in current society. On one hand, constitutional law encourages freedom of the press and the public's right to know. On the other hand is the duty to protect the individuals' rights to keep their private affairs from being known. A proper balance must be struck, but in an open, democratic society this is not an easy thing to do.

On the question of releasing medical record information without the consent of the patient, it can be concluded generally that the patient is given relatively little legal protection from the torts of defamation and invasion of privacy. To put the matter another way: hospitals or physicians have little risk of liability based upon either of these two torts if they release information to a third party without the consent of the patient, when the release benefits the publisher in some way, or when the recipient has a legitimate interest in the information.[75] The patient's primary protection is derived from the ethical standards accepted by the medical community, and not from the law of defamation or invasion of privacy.

----

[73] *Chapadeau v. Utica Observer-Dispatch, Inc.*, 38 N.Y. 2d 196, 341 N.E. 2d 569, 379 N.Y.S. 2d 61 (1975). See also: *James v. Gannett Co., Inc.*, 353 N.E. 2d 834, 386 N.Y.S. 2d 871 (1976). (A professional cabaret dancer was a "public figure," and publication of a feature article about her life and profession did not constitute libel in the absence of allegations and proof that statements made in the article were malicious.)
[74] *Toskett v. King Broadcasting Station*, 86 Wash. 2d 439, 546 P. 2d 81 (1976).
[75] *Horne v. Patton*, 291 Ala. 701, 287 So. 2d 824 (1973). (A physician's unauthorized disclosure to a patient's employer of embarrassing and humiliating details of the patient's illness may constitute an invasion of privacy if there is no legitimate reason for the disclosure.)

The relatively slight legal protection afforded the patient from the classical and traditional torts of invasion of privacy and defamation, the increasing array of third parties claiming access to medical record information, the development of automated systems of record keeping, and the growth of centralized computer data banks have occasioned much concern about the maintenance of confidentiality. Certainly the computer, together with the tremendously enlarged role of government and third parties in financing medical care, has increased the risk of misuse and unjustified disclosure of private information. Current economics of health care and modern technology have thus combined to heighten the possibility of damaging individuals' rights of privacy.

Hence the implementation of ethical standards of nondisclosure of confidential information—at least the implementation of hospital policies—needs to be strengthened to make certain that only legitimately interested third parties have access to medical information and that such parties use the information only for proper purposes. There is also a need to strengthen the patient's legal right to insist upon confidentiality. It now appears that some courts are willing to take that step by developing a third theory—as distinct from the torts of defamation and invasion of privacy—to protect the patient's interest. Legislative bodies too are exhibiting a greater interest in protecting confidentiality, and examples of these legal developments will be noted. The third theory being developed by judicial law can perhaps be labeled liability for breach of the physician-patient contract.

As long ago as 1851 a court in Scotland held that an implied term of the physician-patient contract required the physician to retain the confidentiality of medical information obtained by him in the course of treating the patient.[76] Until recently, however, no American cases provided such straightforward legal reasoning, in spite of the well-accepted ethical standards of the Hippocratic Oath and the American Medical Association.[77] Recently, however, an Alabama court has held that a physician could be liable for damages for breach of contract when he furnished medical information to a patient's

---

[76] *A.B. v. C.D.*, 14 Sess. Cas. 2d 177 (1851).

[77] Section 9 of the 1957 *Principles of Medical Ethics of the American Medical Association* reads as follows: "A physician may not reveal the confidence entrusted to him in the course of medical attendance, or the deficiencies he may observe in the character of patients, unless he is required to do so by law or unless it becomes necessary in order to protect the welfare of the individual or of the community."

employer without consent, as a result of which the patient lost his job.[78] Note carefully that the traditional law of invasion of privacy would undoubtedly insulate the doctor from liability by recognizing a privilege of disclosure, since the employer could be recognized as a legitimately interested party if there was a valid reason for the disclosure. But if breach of contract is acknowledged as a basis for liability no such privilege is granted. The same principle could be applied to the hospital-patient relationship as well.

In *Hammonds v. Aetna Casualty and Surety Company,* a federal district court applying the law of Ohio as it interpreted such law found a physician liable for disclosure of information on these facts. A hospitalized patient was injured when a bed collapsed. The same insurance carrier had insured both the hospital and the patient's attending physician; and when the patient filed a claim against the hospital, the carrier informed the physician that the patient intended to sue him also, although this was not true, and prevailed upon the doctor to make a medical report on the patient's condition. Both the carrier and the physician were held liable for actual damages, the doctor's liability apparently being based upon an implied contractual obligation to maintain confidentiality of the patient's medical record.[79] The court indicated that maintenance of confidentiality was more important as a matter of public policy than the granting of a privilege of disclosure based upon the interests of the insurance carrier. In reaching this conclusion the court made reference to the ethical standards of confidentiality of the medical profession, to the Ohio Medical Practice Act, which requires licensed physicians to refrain from betraying a professional secret, and to the Ohio privileged communication statute, which precludes a physician from testifying in court with respect to confidential information.

As noted previously in this chapter, most courts in the past have said that violation of licensing statutes and rules and regulations providing for confidentiality of medical information may justify suspending or revoking a license to practice medicine, but that violation does not form the basis of a private cause of action in the patient for damages.[80] The same has been said of the privileged

---

[78]*Horne v. Patton,* 291 Ala. 701, 287 So. 2d 824 (1973).
[79]237 F. Supp. 96 (N.D. Ohio 1965): (An insurance carrier who induces a breach of contract between a patient and his physician may be liable for consequences). 243 F. Supp. 793 (N.D. Ohio 1965): (An implied condition of a physician-patient contract is that confidential information acquired through the relationship will not be released without the patient's consent).
[80]For example: *Quarles v. Sutherland,* 215 Tenn. 651, 389 S.W. 2d 249 (1965). (The court also held that there was no contract between a customer who had been injured

communication statutes, since they apply only to court or quasi-judicial proceedings. Further, even if a patient can base a private damage action on a violation of licensure laws or privileged communication statutes, no liability for disclosure without consent results when the disclosure fulfills a more important moral or social duty to protect the interests of a third party or the public.[81] Both of these rules may be changed or significantly modified as time goes on and further litigation occurs.

To put the matter another way, there may be a future trend to impose a contractual duty of secrecy on the doctor and the hospital to maintain the confidence of medical records. This can be done simply by reference to professional ethical standards or to specific provisions of licensing statutes and regulations, or by implication from the privileged communication statutes. In that event privilege of disclosure, in the context of the defamation and invasion of privacy cases previously discussed, will be significantly curtailed.

Such a result is especially likely when information is released without the consent of the patient, and when the third party is adverse to the patient. In the course of a lawsuit a physician who had treated the plaintiff gave a report to an attorney representing the defendant, this fact being known by the doctor; the report stated that the patient-plaintiff's symptoms were aggravated by a preexisting anxiety neurosis. In holding the physician liable for the unauthorized disclosure, the court stressed that a physician stands in a fiduciary relation to his patient, that this relationship includes the duty of confidentiality, and that a physician has an obligation to refrain from aiding a patient's adverse party.[82]

STATUTORY PROVISIONS MANDATING CONFIDENTIALITY

Physicians and hospital personnel must be familiar with local and federal statutes (or regulations) which create a postive duty, in specific circumstances covered in the statute or regulations, not to release medical information except as specified. For example, New York's mental hygiene law declares that officials of state mental institutions shall not make case records available except as provided in the law.

---

on the premises of the store and the physician engaged by the store to examine the customer. Hence, when the doctor released a medical report to the store's attorney, the customer did not have a cause of action based upon breach of contract.)

[81] *Simonsen v. Swenson*, 104 Neb. 224, 177 N.W. 831 (1920). (There was no liability when a physician disclosed to a hotel proprietor that the patient, a resident of the hotel, was suffering from venereal disease.) See also: *Clark v. Geraci*, 29 Misc. 2d 791, 208 N.Y.S. 2d 564 (1960), cited in n. 67.

[82] *Alexander v. Knight*, 197 Pa. Super. 79, 177 A. 2d 142 (1962).

Violation of this state statute created civil liability to the patient when a hospital director released the record to an adverse attorney.[83] At the federal level the "Conditions of Participation for Medicare" provide specifically that only "authorized personnel" shall have access to the record and that written consent of the patient is necessary for release of medical information.[84]

Another example of a federal statute and the attendant regulations providing for confidentiality of medical information is the Comprehensive Drug Abuse Prevention and Control Act of 1970. This legislation imposes very stringent requirements for maintaining the confidentiality of records of patients participating in drug and alcohol abuse research programs.[85] Violation can result in a criminal penalty. The act applies to all general hospitals and other providers of care receiving federal funds, either directly for research on drug or alcohol abuse or indirectly for such programs through Medicare, Medicaid, or other government programs. In sum, medical information is not to be disclosed to anyone not connected with the program, including family members, law enforcement officials, and courts except as specifically provided for in the statutes and regulations, without the express written consent of the patient. The consent form must contain the name of the patient and the institution, the name of the recipient of the information, the purpose of the disclosure, the precise nature of the information to be released, the length of time the consent is valid, and, of course, a date. Specially drafted consent forms are thus necessary for each disclosure. These requirements apply to patients who are minors as well as to adults receiving treatment for drug and alcohol abuse. Not even the parents or a guardian of a minor can receive information without his consent unless his physical or mental condition or very young age makes him incapable of reaching a decision. Hospitals and other providers who violate the law may be subjected to fines.

In 1972, Congress enacted the Drug Abuse Office and Treatment Act which provides that upon court order showing good cause the records of patients under treatment for alcoholism and drug addiction who are participating in "drug abuse prevention functions" can be disclosed.[86] The 1970 act's regulations had made it unlawful to divulge information identifying a patient in a methadone maintenance treatment program in any civil, criminal, legislative, or administrative

---

[83]*Munzer v. Blaisdell*, 183 Misc. 773, 49 N.Y.S. 2d 915 (1944), *aff'd*, 269 App. Div. 970, 58 N.Y.S. 2d 359 (1945).
[84]*Medicare Regulations*, sec. 405.1026.
[85]42 U.S.C. sec. 242(a) (1974) and 21 U.S.C. sec. 872(e) (1974.)
[86]21 U.S.C. sec. 1175(b) (2) (c) (1972).

proceedings conducted by federal, state, or local authorities. The 1972 act allowing disclosure of medical information upon court order applies to "drug abuse prevention functions." In contrast, the 1970 act's provision for absolute confidentiality is applicable to "drug research programs," and patients participating in research are accordingly entitled to absolute confidentiality.[87]

A case in point involving the Comprehensive Drug Abuse Prevention and Control Act of 1970 and then relevant regulations is *People v. Newman,* decided by the Court of Appeals of New York in 1973. A witness to a murder told the police that she had seen the alleged killer in the waiting room of a methadone maintenance treatment clinic. The clinic's files included photographs of all patients, taken when each was accepted for treatment. These were used to identify patients and thus make sure that unregistered persons did not obtain methadone and that registered patients received the correct dose. A court granted a subpoena ordering the director of the clinic to produce the photographs of all black males between the ages of 21 and 35 who were patients during 1972; the director refused to honor this subpoena and accordingly was subjected to contempt proceedings. He was found not guilty, the subpoena being held invalid in the light of federal legislation which provides for absolute confidentiality of medical records for such patients, unless they consent to disclosure.[88]

Although the federal law granted confidentiality for patients participating in the methadone treatment program, the New York court in *Newman* also ruled that the state's privileged communication statute did not prohibit disclosure of the photographs because they served a medical and administrative purpose and were not "acquired in attending a patient in a professional capacity."

Medical Records as Evidence in Litigation

As mentioned previously, the common law did not recognize the physician-patient relationship as privileged; accordingly medical information entrusted to or acquired by the doctor was not confidential.[89] Approximately two-thirds of the states, however, have enacted

---

[87]Current disclosure provisions appear in 42 C.F.R. sec. 2 (1974).

[88]32 N.Y. 2d 379, 298 N.E. 2d 651, 345 N.Y.S. 2d 502 (1973), *cert. denied,* 414 U.S. 1163 (1973).

[89]Apparently the first exception to the assertion in the text is the recent appellate court case of *Allred v. State,* 554 P. 2d 411 (Alaska 1976). The Supreme Court of Alaska has recognized a common law privilege with respect to communications made in the course of psychotherapeutic treatment rendered by psychiatrists and licensed psychologists.

privileged communication statutes which prohibit the physician (and
perhaps other professional medical personnel, depending upon the
coverage of the particular statute in question) from disclosing information in judicial or quasi-judicial proceedings unless the patient
has waived the privilege or has consented to the disclosure. A typical
statute reads as follows:

> The following persons shall not testify in certain respects
> . . . a physician, concerning a communication made to him
> by his patient in that relation, or his advice to his patient,
> but . . . a physician may testify by express consent of the
> . . . patient or if . . . patient be deceased by the express
> consent of the surviving spouse or the executor or admin-
> istrator of the estate of such deceased . . . patient; and if
> the . . . patient voluntarily testifies, the . . . physician may
> be compelled to testify on the same subject. . . . or if the
> patient, his executor, or administrator, files a medical claim
> such filing shall constitute a waiver of the privilege with
> regard to the care and treatment of which complaint is made.[90]

In general, privileged communication statutes are applicable to
pretrial proceedings such as motions for inspection and discovery
of records; and they are also applicable to investigations conducted
by state legislative bodies. Thus the privilege is not confined to actual
courtroom trials. Further, as a general rule the privilege of confidentiality continues after the death of the patient and may be asserted
by his estate.[91]

To create a privilege of confidentiality a patient-physician relationship must exist, and the information acquired by the physician must
relate to the care and treatment of the patient. No privilege will
be recognized if either element is absent. In *State of Washington v.
Kuljis* a hospital staff doctor who drew a sample of a patient's blood
to test for intoxication, at the request of the police and with the
apparent consent of the patient, had not established a patient-physician relationship, nor had he obtained information for the purpose
of treating the patient. Consequently the results of the test were
admissible in evidence in a criminal prosecution.[92] The effect of
a privileged communication statute is to prevent a physician or other
professional person possessing confidential information from disclosing it in court or in quasi-judicial proceedings if, as will further
be explained, the patient asserts the privilege.

---

[90]Ohio Rev. Code Ann., sec. 2317.02(B) (Page's Supp. 1975).
[91]*Boggess v. Aetna Life Insurance Co.*, 128 Ga. App. 190, 196 S.E. 2d 172 (1973).
[92]70 Wash. 2d 168, 422 P. 2d 480 (1967).

In states without a privileged communication statute or when the privilege does not apply or cannot be asserted by the patient, medical records are generally admissible as evidence in litigation under one or more of the exceptions to the rule of evidence prohibiting hearsay testimony. Medical records are considered hearsay evidence for several reasons. First, the information contained in a medical chart is compiled by persons not under oath. Further, these persons are frequently not available to testify in person in a trial, and thus their recorded statements are not subject to cross-examination by the adverse party.

However, the law of evidence has long recognized statutory and judicial exceptions to the hearsay rule. The foremost exception is the business record rule, which is recognized in the statutes of more than forty states as well as in federal law. These statutes provide that records compiled in the regular course of business, at or near the time of the act or event, and for the purpose which such records are intended to serve, are admissible as long as their authenticity is properly established. Medical records maintained by a physician or a hospital have frequently been held to fall within the business record statutes.[93] Medical records may also be admissible under a rule very similar to the business records rule, namely, the shopbook rule, a shopbook being an original record kept by tradesmen or shopkeepers to indicate accounts due for work or service performed. A third basis for admitting medical records in evidence is the view that they consitute public or official documents.[94] This is especially relevant in states which require by statute that particular forms of medical records be kept and which itemize the types of information to be recorded. Finally, a few states have statutes providing directly and specifically that medical records of certain hospitals are admissible. If the original records have been destroyed following microfilming, then the microfilms would normally be admissible as evidence in accordance with the foregoing criteria. Computer printouts have also been accepted as evidence.[95]

Even if records or parts of records are admissible in court under

---

[93] *Weis v. Weis*, 147 Ohio St. 416, 72 N.E. 2d 245 (1947); *Sims v. Charlotte Liberty Mutual Ins. Co.*, 257 N.C. 32, 125 S.E. 2d 326 (1962); *Estate of Searchill*, 9 Mich. App. 614, 157 N.W. 2d 788 (1968): (In a will contest where the mental competence of deceased at the time of execution of the will is at issue, a hospital's medical records are admissible under the Michigan Business Records Act); *Rivers v. Union Carbide Corp.*, 426 F. 2d 633 (3d Cir. 1970): (Hospital records disclosing a history of alcoholism and intoxication at the time of an accident are admissible by virtue of Federal Business Records Act, 28 U.S. C. sec. 1732).

[94] *City of Bay St. Louis v. Johnston*, 222 So. 2d 841 (Miss. 1969).

[95] *United States v. Russo*, 480 F. 2d 1228 (6th Cir. 1973), *cert. denied*, 414 U.S. 1157 (1973).

one of the exceptions to the hearsay rule, their authenticity and
reliability must be established. In other words a proper foundation
must be laid for admissibility, and normally this is done by having
the medical record librarian or other custodian of the documents
testify in court as to the procedures used in compiling and maintaining
current medical information. To be admitted, evidence must meet
the additional rules that all courtroom testimony be relevant to the
issue at hand, and that only a medical expert may state a diagnosis
or an opinion regarding the patient's medical or mental condition.
For example, a hospital record containing a patient's history, including
the statement "hit by a truck that was passing properly on the right,"
is not admissible as evidence in personal injury litigation as a business
record, because the statement pertains to a cause of the accident
and not to the medical or surgical treatment of the patient. Moreover,
the statement is opinion evidence based on hearsay from a lay person.[96]

There is legal authority in some jurisdictions to the effect that
records or excerpts from them will be received as evidence only
when the person who made the entry in the chart is not available
to testify in person. It should also be noted that the parties to litigation
may affirmatively agree or stipulate that medical records will be
received in evidence. In that event the hearsay rule and exceptions
to it become irrelevant.

The relative liberality of statutory and judicial law admitting records
in evidence during litigation, subject to the safeguards of materiality
and relevance, when no privileged communication statute exists or
when the patient has waived his right of confidentiality, constitutes
sound public policy. The fundamental purpose of litigation should
be to ascertain the truth and accomplish justice between the parties
in an adversary situation. Records maintained in the regular course
of patient care will presumably help establish that truth. Since
physicians, nurses, and hospitals do not normally falsify information
describing the diagnosis and care rendered a particular patient, courts
and quasi-judicial bodies receiving medical records may be confident
that the information accurately reports the facts and medical opinions
regarding the case. In addition, the records are frequently more
reliable than personal recollections: witnesses may be forgetful; they

[96]*Dorsten v. Lawrence*, 20 Ohio App. 2d 297, 253 N.E. 2d 804 (1969); *Ce Buss, Inc.
v. Sniderman*, 171 Colo. 246, 466 P. 2d 457 (1970): (Hospital records which antedate
the injury in litigation by as much as five years are not relevant); *Kelly v. Sheehan*,
158 Conn. 281, 259 A. 2d 605 (1969): (A statement in the hospital records that
a "16-year-old boy was driving the car" was not admissible, since the statement was
not that of the patient, nor did it relate to his medical care and treatment).

may not be available to testify in person; and even if they are available, the entries may have been made by so many different persons that it would be extremely time consuming and expensive if they all had to appear as witnesses. To exclude medical records from evidence on the basis that they are hearsay would defeat the legitimate goals of the judicial process.

Privileged communication statutes are thus contrary to the policy that the purpose of litigation is to determine the truth. By providing that medical information is to be held confidential and that a physician shall not be permitted to testify, they deprive a court or quasi-judicial body of the opportunity to receive evidence that could be relevant and material to the issues being litigated. As will be noted shortly, however, the privileged communication statutes have many exceptions which in effect recognize that disclosure is frequently preferable to secrecy.

The privileged communication statutes differ in detail and sometimes in major respects from state to state. All, however, extend the confidential privilege only to the patient, and not to the physician.[97] In other words, the physician may not assert a refusal to testify for reasons of his own. Further, as noted earlier, the statutes pertain only to judicial or quasi-judicial proceedings and do not generally prohibit a doctor from disclosing medical record information out of court; nor does such disclosure give the patient a cause of action for civil damages for alleged violation of the privilege statute. Some modern decisions involving civil liability, however, have cited the privilege statute as one more reason why a contractual duty of confidentiality should be imposed upon a physician (and by analogy a hospital) by implication.

The use in court of confidential information, contrary to the privilege statute, does give the patient a civil cause of action against

---

[97]*In re Lifschutz*, 2 Cal. 3d 415, 467 P. 2d 557, 85 Cal. Rptr. 829 (1970). (Although there is a psychiatrist-patient privilege under California statute, the psychiatrist may not assert privilege and refuse to disclose a relationship with a particular patient when sued by the patient for assault. The psychiatrist may be placed in jail as punishment for contempt of court if he refuses to honor a subpoena.) See also: *People v. Williams*, 39 Mich. App. 91, 197 N.W. 2d 336 (1972): (The state may not claim privilege. In a criminal prosecution for statutory rape, where the victim testified for the prosecution that she became pregnant and gave birth subsequent to an alleged assault by the defendant, the state could not prevent the defendant from calling the victim's physician as witness. He offered testimony that he treated her for possible miscarriage at the time of the alleged rape, thus casting doubt on the truthfulness of her testimony); *Klinge v. Lutheran Medical Center of St. Louis*, 518 S.W. 2d 157 (Mo. 1974): (Although hospital records are within the physician-patient privilege, the hospital medical staff committee may examine medical records of patients of staff physician without patients' consent to determine qualifications and competence of staff physicians, since the privilege is that of the patient and not the physician).

the medical practitioner who discloses it, in the view of the South
Dakota Supreme Court. In *Schaffer v. Spicer,* a divorced woman was
successful in an action against her psychiatrist, at least to the extent
of obtaining a decision that issues of civil liability were presented.
The case arose while the woman and her former husband were
preparing to engage in custody proceedings and because the wife's
psychiatrist prepared an affidavit for the husband's attorney, disclosing confidential information which reflected unfavorably upon her
fitness as a mother. The affidavit was intended for use in the pending
custody proceedings and had not been ordered by the court.

By a majority ruling, South Dakota's Supreme Court held that
the privilege statute had been violated, since the information had
been acquired by the doctor in the course of treating the patient
and the patient had not consented to the disclosure or waived her
right of privilege, even though she had stated in the divorce action
that she had been treated by the psychiatrist.[98]

The court also ruled that the concept of privilege and confidentiality
was paramount to the interests and welfare of the children who
were the subjects of the pending custody hearing. Despite this ruling,
however, the doctor could perhaps be called as a witness in the
actual hearing of the custody dispute, and be compelled to testify
then on matters affecting the children's welfare and best interests.
This would be possible if it were held that by seeking custody of
her children the patient had waived her privilege of confidentiality.

Applicability of the privileged communication statutes differs considerably according to the type of practitioner, the nature of the
information considered to be privileged, and the court (or tribunal)
in which the privilege is asserted. At least one state limits the privilege
to the psychiatrist and applied psychologist-patient relationship; no
privilege applies generally to medical practitioners.[99] New Mexico
requires a patient to submit a malpractice claim to a medical review
commission prior to the filing of an action in court, grants the review
panel access to all medical and hospital records pertaining to the
matter, and provides for waiver of any claim of privilege during
this review.[100] Some states exclude from privilege all proceedings
before workmen's compensation boards or other specifically designated administrative tribunals.[101] In West Virginia the privilege applied

---

[98]215 N.W. 2d 134 (S.D. 1974).
[99]Ga. Code Ann., sec. 38–418 (1974)(psychiatrist privilege); Ga. Code Ann., sec. 84–3118
(1975)(applied psychologist).
[100]N. Mex. Code, sec. 58–33–15/16 (1976).
[101]*Skelly v. Sunshine Mining Co.,* 62 Idaho 192, 109 P. 2d 622 (1941); *Hamilton v.
P. E. Johnson and Sons,* 224 Iowa 1097, 276 N.W. 841 (1937).

formerly only to cases in the Justice Court but this limitation was recently dropped.[102] Pennsylvania permits a patient to claim privilege only with respect to medical information which may blacken his character.[103]

A few states broaden the privilege by extending the patient's right of confidentiality to relationships other than those established with a medical practitioner. The privilege may apply to nurses, psychiatrists, psychotherapists, or even marriage counselors, although applicability to these professional persons is certainly not the general or majority view.[104] In some states the privilege may apply only to criminal cases, excluding civil actions.

Where it is otherwise applicable, the privilege generally applies to a hospital's medical records, on the grounds that they contain information acquired by the physician in the course of treating the patient.[105] However, since the privilege can be asserted only by the patient, the privileged status of hospital records is not directly relevant to the hospital in litigation between the patient and third parties. In other words, a hospital may not assert confidentiality of records on its own behalf when the court proceedings involve third parties, although it may claim confidentiality on behalf of a patient who is not able to assert his own claim of privilege. In most cases between patients and third parties the matter of privilege must be determined by the litigating parties and the court.[106] On the other hand, if the hospital is one of the litigating parties, the statute directly concerns the hospital's position, for then the hospital cannot use the records as evidence if the patient asserts a proper claim to the privileged status of the information. As will be emphasized shortly, however, the patient will be deemed to waive his right of privilege if he brings suit against the hospital.

---

[102]W. Va. Code, sec. 50–6–10 (1976).

[103]Pa. Stat. Ann., Title 28, sec. 328 (Purdon 1958).

[104]The privilege of confidentiality in Ohio does not extend to dentists. *Belichick v. Belichick*, 37 Ohio App. 2d 95, 307 N.E. 2d 270 (1973). The Ohio statute was quoted earlier in this section.

[105]*State of Iowa v. Bedel*, 193 N.W. 2d 121 (Iowa 1971); *Unick v. Kessler Memorial Hospital*, 107 N.J. 121, 257 A. 2d 134 (1969). See also: *Klinge v. Lutheran Medical Center of St. Louis*, 518 S.W. 2d 157 (Mo. 1974), n. 97, *supra.*

[106]The hospital is frequently an innocent bystander when adversary parties are contesting the confidentiality of records. In *Nelson v. Grossom*, 152 Colo. 362, 382 P. 2d 991 (1963), an ex-husband brought an action to prevent his former wife from removing their children from the state. The woman had remarried, and plaintiff challenged the fitness of the stepfather to care properly for the children. Accordingly, he sought to examine medical records bearing on the stepfather's physical and mental condition. In such a situation the hospital should await a court order before releasing medical information; in determining whether to grant an order or not the court will decide the issue of privilege in accordance with relevant local law.

There is no privilege of confidentiality under federal law. Hence the Internal Revenue Service was granted access to the medical records of a deceased person to ascertain whether the patient had made gifts of property during his lifetime in contemplation of death, thus subjecting the property to the federal estate tax. Since privilege is solely a matter of statute, and since the Congress has never enacted such a statute, the estate of the deceased could not claim a privilege.[107]

The privileged status of medical records is exemplified in a California case where the plaintiff sought damages following an automobile accident allegedly caused by the defendant's negligence. Through the pretrial process of an interrogatory obtained by the defendant, the plaintiff stated that she had been involved in an earlier automobile accident in 1969, that in the same year she had attempted suicide and had later been under the care of a psychotherapist. The defendant then obtained a court subpoena for all of her medical records, but she asserted privilege under California's statute. The supreme court held that the records were privileged and not subject to discovery.[108] Plaintiff had not waived her right to confidentiality, since her current suit against the defendant raised no issue regarding her mental health.

Many plaintiffs in lawsuits will seek by means of pretrial discovery to obtain information from the medical charts of other patients not parties to the litigation, or from hospital documents which they believe will aid the preparation and trial of their case. Depending upon interpretation of local law, the type of information sought, and the issues raised by such plaintiffs' suits, they may or may not be successful. An unsuccessful attempt to gain access to the charts of other patients was made in a recent Arizona case. The plaintiff had filed a malpractice action against a hospital following complications during childbirth when her private obstetrician was absent from the delivery room, although he was allegedly on the hospital premises. Arguing that under the circumstances the hospital had a duty to reach the physician, who was not a defendant in the action, plaintiff sought access to the hospital records of another patient of the doctor in an effort to find out what he was doing at the time in question. The trial court granted discovery of the records, but this decision was reversed by the intermediate court of appeals, which held that when neither the doctor nor the other patient was a party to the litigation the

---

[107] *U.S. v. Kansas City Lutheran Home and Hospital Association*, 297 F. Supp. 239 (W.D. Mo. 1969).
[108] *Roberts v. Superior Court of Butte County*, 9 Cal. 3d 330, 508 P. 2d 309, 107 Cal. Rptr. 309 (1973).

information was privileged.[109] Moreover, the court ruled that the hospital had a duty to assert the privilege on behalf of the absent patient.

Similarly, in New York, the medical records of all parties undergoing hysterectomies during a two-year period prior to an alleged act of malpractice by a defendant physician were privileged, and the defendant hospital could not be required to disclose the records without the express consent or waiver of the other patients.[110] In New Jersey, a defendant physician in a malpractice action did not need to disclose the names, addresses, and illnesses of his other patients treated with a particular drug, since the records of these third parties, who were not involved in the litigation, were privileged communications.[111] Further, a hospital need not reveal to the plaintiff its operating room schedule and record book for the day that alleged negligence took place, since the documents would contain medical information regarding patients who have not waived their privilege.[112]

In other cases illustrating the applicability of privilege, however, the courts have held that certain records revealing information about third parties are not confidential and that plaintiff is entitled to the information he seeks. When a patient sues a hospital in a malpractice action he has a right to discover the names of other patients who may be in possession of information regarding the alleged negligence or malpractice, and their consent to such disclosure is not necessary.[113] Without this ruling, the hospital could seek witnesses favorable to its side while denying plaintiff a like opportunity. The release of the names of patients in itself does nothing to reveal the nature of their illnesses or the treatment rendered. In a suit against a hospital that allegedly fails to supervise dangerous patients, the victim of an assault by a hospitalized mental patient

---

[109] *Tucson Medical Center, Inc. v. Rowles*, 21 Ariz. App. 424, 520 P. 2d 518 (1974).

[110] *Boddy v. Parker*, 45 App. Div. 2d 1000, 358 N.Y.S. 2d 218 (1974).

[111] *Osterman v. Ehrenworth*, 106 N.J. Super, 515, 256 A. 2d 123 (1969).

[112] *Unick v. Kessler Memorial Hospital*, 107 N.J. 121, 257 A. 2d 134 (1969). (However, a physician can be required to answer a plaintiff's interrogatories asking whether he has ever been a party to previous lawsuits and, if so, to name the parties to such suits and the courts in which they were filed, since this information does not relate to the illness or treatment of other patients.) See also: *Marcus v. Superior Court of Los Angeles County*, 18 Cal. App. 3d 22, 95 Cal. Rptr. 545 (1971). (A physician need not disclose names and addresses of other patients given tests and treatment similar to the plaintiff's, since this information is privileged.) *Cf.: Hodgson v. Nacogdoches County Hospital District* (E.D. Tex., *unreported* 1972). (In states with no privileged communication statute the courts may grant plaintiff a broad order of discovery to review and copy medical records of patients not parties to a suit, as an aid in developing evidence in pending malpractice litigation. There is no general common law privilege.)

[113] *Connell v. Washington Hospital Center*, 50 F.R.D. 360 (D.D.C. 1970).

is entitled to records relating to prior assaults by the same patient.[114] Clearly, nonmedical data regarding other assaults by such a patient are discoverable by a plaintiff, the disclosure not being a violation of either the privileged communication statute or the New York mental hygiene law, which provides that the medical records of patients of state mental institutions are confidential.[115]

Another issue, raised in the New York case of *Bremiller v. Miller,* was whether a registered nurse charged by the New York Department of Education with unprofessional conduct could have access to a mental patient's medical record for the purpose of aiding her defense. The nurse was alleged to have assaulted the patient who was the complaining witness. In seeking this patient's records, the nurse contended that they would show a pattern of aggressive conduct on the patient's part and thus perhaps establish a defense for her. On behalf of the Department of Education, the New York Attorney General maintained that the mental hygiene law, providing for confidentiality of the medical records of patients confined to state mental institutions, prevented access to the records unless the patient waived the privilege. On the issue of waiver the New York court observed that since the patient's mental competency was questionable it could not rule for the nurse on this basis.

Nevertheless, in the interest of fairness, the nurse was permitted to use the records in her defense.[116] The ruling recognized, in effect, that under any sound public policy a privilege of confidentiality should not be absolute, to the detriment of persons having a legitimate interest in obtaining medical information pertaining to another. The pending disciplinary action against the nurse placed her license to practice in jeopardy and hence involved her right to earn a living. In the view of the court, she had a right to question the credibility and capacity of the complaining witness. Further, the hearing procedure before the Department of Education was not a public hearing, and hence the patient's identity could be protected and disclosures from the record could be limited to those matters that were material and relevant to the pending allegations of unprofessional conduct.

A patient who files suit for damages and thereby places in issue his physical or mental health has clearly waived his privilege of confidentiality, and the medical records will be available to the adverse

---

[114]*Mayer v. Albany Medical Center Hospital,* 37 App. Div. 2d 1011, 325 N.Y.S. 2d 517 (1971).
[115]*Katz v. State of New York,* 41 App. Div. 2d 879, 342 N.Y.S. 2d 906 (1973).
[116]79 Misc. 2d 244, 360 N.Y.S. 2d 178 (1974).

party and admissible in evidence at trial, subject to the usual law of evidence as previously reviewed. When a person who claimed to have been injured in an automobile accident brought an action against both the state of Vermont and an individual, alleging that the defendants were negligent in causing the accident, the Supreme Court of Vermont affirmed the trial court's order of discovery of the medical records compiled by a physician in treating the alleged injuries.[117] Similarly, in a divorce action the wife's medical records are subject to subpoena if the information is relevant to the issues to be litigated.[118] Although a waiver of privilege in a given situation may depend on the particular wording of the state statute, a waiver by a patient can usually become effective in two ways: it may be made expressly by words or conduct, or it may be implied by acts of the patient or his legal representative.[119]

In determining whether information contained in a medical record or possessed by a medical practitioner is subject to pretrial discovery proceedings or is admissible in evidence in judicial or quasi-judicial proceedings, a court must therefore first interpret the local statute relating to privileged communications, if such a statute exists, and then apply it to the particular circumstances and facts of the litigation. If no statute exists or if the statute does not prevent access to medical information, the court must determine the admissibility of the information by application of the general rules of evidence respecting hearsay testimony and their exceptions, and then evaluate the authenticity, reliability, credibility, materiality, and relevance of the record. In jurisdictions with privileged communication statutes, the public policy issue of balancing the rights of patients to confidentiality against the rights of other parties to ascertain the truth in order to protect their legitimate interests is a sensitive matter. As is evident throughout this discussion, the courts attempt to deal fairly with these conflicting interests on a case-by-case basis, presumably accomplishing a high degree of justice in the light of the facts.

---

[117]*Mattison v. Poulen*, 353 A. 2d 327 (Vt. 1976).
[118]*Pennison v. Provident Life and Accident Insurance Co.*, 154 So. 2d 617 (La. Ct. of App. 1963).
[119]81 Am. Jur. 2d *Witnesses*, Sec. 268 (1976). See also: *Greuling v. Breakey*, 391 N.Y.S. 2d 585 (Sup. Ct. App. Div. 1977). (In a malpractice action against a physician, plaintiff must furnish defendant with medical records of her treatment by other physicians; patient could not refuse access to her medical records when placing her physical condition in issue.)

XII

Hospital Liability

Following the rapid decline of charitable immunity from liability for tort during the 1950s and 1960s, hospital liability has been one of the most dramatically changing areas of personal injury law. This chapter will explore the extent of the legal responsibility which has recently been imposed upon the private nonprofit community hospital. No attempt will be made here to trace the fall of charitable immunity or to cite the remnants of that doctrine that remain in a few jurisdictions. Nor will governmental immunity from tort liability be analyzed; the position of governmental institutions would require a separate, thorough treatment well beyond the scope of this chapter. The focus here is on the nonprofit hospital and the duties owed the patient or visitor in jurisdictions which have removed all charitable immunities. Most states have now adopted full liability with respect to the voluntary hospital.

The Nature and Role of the Community Hospital

Even after the abolishment of charitable immunity, many courts regarded a community hospital as a mere facility, or hotel, whose reason for existence was simply to provide a place where a licensed physician practiced medicine in his individual way of caring for his private patients. In other words, the hospital was no more than a "doctor's workshop" in the minds of many lawyers and judges as well as in the view of many physicians and hospital administrators. A relatively sharp distinction was drawn between hospital services and medical services. The corporate practice of medicine rule was frequently asserted as a valid reason for this distinction. The legal duties of the hospital to the patient were accordingly quite limited, since the respective roles of the hospital and the physician or medical professional were thought to be distinctly separable.

346

In the 1970s there is still considerable confusion in the minds of some lawyers and medical professionals concerning the respective roles of the doctor and the hospital in caring for hospitalized patients. Nevertheless it is abundantly evident that the role and nature of the modern community hospital have been changing and will continue to change rapidly. Forward-looking physicians and professionally trained hospital administrators have openly and energetically attacked the doctor's workshop concept of a hospital. In all respects medical practice has become increasingly institutionalized, the physician depending upon the hospital and the hospital depending upon the physician. It is not an overstatement to say that the practice of scientific medicine is impossible today unless the physician has access to a hospital. The practice of medicine is increasingly hospital-oriented; specialization of practice and the individual physician's increasing need for consultation with specialists lead inevitably to institutionalization. Meanwhile the medical profession has also developed techniques of auditing hospital care, whereby peer groups of physicians evaluate the medical performance of colleagues in the interest of raising the standards of patient care.

The services provided the community by the hospital and its medical staff have continually expanded. Instead of confining its role to the care of acutely ill patients, the modern community hospital now renders a wide range of services formerly provided by others or not provided at all. The public has become increasingly sophisticated in demanding excellent care and an increased range of services. The great growth in insurance coverage and third-party financing arrangements since World War II has contributed significantly to this aspect of the changing role of the hospital. The hospital's out-patient services and its role in the diagnosis of illness—as contrasted with acute care—are far more important today than a decade or two ago. Hospital emergency rooms render more and more services; indeed, the emergency room is often utilized by the public in place of a doctor's office. Hospitals are now developing home care and preventive health programs and are entering into contractual arrangements with nursing homes and other institutions for long-term care.

The institutionalization of medical practice and the increasing range of hospital services to the community have meant that salary arrangements between the hospital and professional persons have been increasing in number and importance. For example, it is not now unusual to find a chief of the medical staff, or a medical director, being paid a full- or part-time salary to compensate him for his institutional responsibilities. Formerly a licensed physician had few institutional responsibilities, but modern medical practice and the development of the hospital as a community health center have greatly increased the ties between the corporate hospital and the doctor.

Adequate medical administration has actually been lacking in many community hospitals despite the fact that the care of patients is the central function of a hospital. Medical administration cannot be accomplished by busy private practitioners devoting to administration only the little time that remains after attending their patients. A designated physician is clearly needed who will assume authority delegated by the hospital governing body for medical administration and who will report to and be accountable to the board of trustees through the hospital's chief executive officer.

This person, whether his title is chief of staff or medical director, has both overall authority for hospital-medical staff relationships and operational direction of all clinical departments. Specifically he coordinates the planning and development of health care programs for the hospital, provides administrative direction for heads of the clinical departments as well as staff support to the governing board and the organized medical staff, maintains professional liaison with the nursing staff and other professionals who support the practice of medicine, and participates actively in improving the hospital's relations with other organizations and professional associations. Thus professionals now recognize that a hospital does not consist of two organizations—one a business entity and the other a medical center. Rather, hospitals are single organizations whose purpose is to arrange for and to a large extent control the delivery of total patient care in accordance with recognized professional standards.

Licensure of medical and paramedical personnel is not a satisfactory legal vehicle for controlling the quality of medical care. In the first place licensure statutes specify only minimal qualifications for practice and cannot measure competence for medical and surgical specialization. Secondly, the statutes provide no satisfactory method of assuring the continuing competence of an individual over the years; periodic review of competence and educational qualifications is seldom conducted under the licensure statutes, and relicensure is not required. The enforcement and disciplinary powers of the governmental administrative agencies responsible for licensure are limited. Revocation or suspension of a license to practice are relatively rare events.

Since for these reasons licensure of professional individuals cannot be depended on to improve the quality of medical care and allied care, the American voluntary hospital system and the medical profession, to their great credit, have together assumed the burdens of raising standards and promoting excellence in the care of patients.

In their efforts to raise standards and to bring the best of American medicine to the public, the hospitals have been immeasurably aided by several national voluntary organizations which have promulgated and enforced standards. At the forefront has been the Joint Commission on Accreditation of Hospitals, whose member organizations are the American Medical Association, the American Hospital Association, the American College of Surgeons, and the American College of Physicians. In other words, the shortcomings of the licensure laws have been admirably made up for by the hospitals and voluntary professional organizations.

Neither this central role of the hospitals in establishing, maintaining, and improving standards of medical care nor the rapidly changing role of the community hospital have been overlooked by the courts. The law of hospital liability has expanded and developed because the role of the hospital in the community has changed in the past two decades and will continue to evolve. If a hospital is a single corporate organization responsible to the community for the delivery of total health care, the medical staff of a hospital is ethically and legally answerable to the corporate board of trustees in that the board becomes ultimately responsible for medical staff appointments and privileges, the rights and responsibilities provided for in the medical staff bylaws, and the discipline of staff. In other words, professionals in medicine and hospital administration, courts, and legislatures have now recognized that the corporate institution is ultimately responsible for standards of hospital medical care. This ultimate responsibility cannot be delegated by the governing body of the corporation to the medical staff. Accordingly, if the hospital fails to exercise adequate control over medical staff appointments and privileges, fails to "supervise" the attending physician in certain circumstances where the patient is in jeopardy, fails to require the attending doctor to seek consultation with specialists, or even fails to remove the doctor from a case in extreme situations, the result may be hospital liability. Such liability is avoided in the modern hospital by an organized system of peer group evaluation of medical staff performance.

The establishment and the maintenance of professional standards in the hospital consequently become a joint effort of lay hospital administration and medical staff. Lay administrators cannot ignore medical standards without great legal peril, as will be demonstrated. No longer can the business administration of a hospital be neatly separated from medical administration. The authority, as distinct from responsibility for direct and immediate control of medical standards, has to be delegated of course to the medical staff by the board of trustees. But the medical staff must then be held accountable for its delegated authority. In liability cases no real purpose is served—and certainly the quality of care is not improved—when the hospital blames the doctor, or the doctor blames the hospital and its employed personnel. As medical care becomes more institutionalized and the role of the hospital in controlling quality more central, the hospital's defenses grounded on the traditional legal doctrines of independent contractor and borrowed servant are more frequently circumvented by the courts in liability cases. The long-standing dichotomy between a community hospital's medical staff and its lay administration must be eliminated both in the interests of patients' care and to reduce the exposure of the institution to liability.

Sincere, diligent efforts are being made by hospital administrators and institutionally oriented physicians to minimize the traditional separation between hospital administration on the one hand and clinical medicine on the other.[1] The concept that the hospital as a corporate institution must establish, maintain, and be ultimately responsible for the standards of medical care practiced within its walls is recognized by the Joint Commission on Accreditation of Hospitals and by some public licensing authorities responsible for the licensure of hospitals. The jury may consider such standards to be evidence of expected performance by hospital personnel and medical staff.[2] This extension of corporate or institutional responsibility to the patient has also been forcefully recognized in several more recent judicial cases, by rules and regulations of federal programs for financing medical care, and by the statutory law of several jurisdictions. These developments will be thoroughly reviewed in the ensuing discussion.

Fault as the Basis for Liability

As a matter of substantive tort law, the hospital is not an insurer of patients' safety or a guarantor of satisfactory results from medical care and treatment. The usual basis for hospital liability is some theory of the law of negligence, or fault, in the sense that either

[1] See, for example, C. W. Eisele, M.D. (ed.), *The Medical Staff in the Modern Hospital* (New York: McGraw Hill Co., 1967).
[2] *Darling v. Charleston Community Hospital*, 33 Ill. 2d 326, 211 N.E. 2d 253 (1965), *cert. denied*, 383 U.S. 946, *aff'g*, 50 Ill. App 2d 253, 200 N.E. 2d 149 (1964).

an employee of the institution or the institution itself has deviated from professionally recognized standards and that such a breach of standards has been the proximate cause of plaintiff's injuries.

Occasionally attempts have been made to assert that the hospital is liable on a theory of strict liability in tort or breach of implied warranty. The essence of liability founded upon breach of warranty or strict liability in tort is that the plaintiff need not allege or prove a negligent act or omission. Some of these attempts to assert liability without negligence have been successful in the courts, especially in cases where the patient contracted serum hepatitis as a result of a blood transfusion; others, such as the cases asserting liability due to malfunction of or the use of allegedly defective hospital equipment, have failed. Efforts to establish liability without negligence in the courts have also failed in factual situations involving staphylococcal infections. Both warranty and strict liability apply primarily to the sale or the furnishing of goods or products.

Insofar as personal injury law generally is concerned, the basis for liability for breach of implied warranty is found in the Uniform Commercial Code, Sections 2-314 and 2-315. The code is statutory law enacted in all jurisdictions except Louisiana. The relevant warranty sections pertain to the sale of goods and in general provide that a merchant selling goods impliedly warrants or promises that the goods shall be "merchantable," which means that they shall be fit for the usual and customary purposes for which they are sold. In particular circumstances also a seller who knows that the buyer is purchasing goods for a specific purpose impliedly warrants that the goods he sells are fit for that purpose. Since a hospital does not normally sell goods to its patients, but rather provides services, these warranty sections of the Uniform Commercial Code are not relevant or applicable to the typical or usual hospital liability case. Some leading case decisions in the field of products liability, however, have extended the protection of warranty to consumers of services when a defective or unmerchantable product was involved. For example, it has been said in several cases that warranties attach to a lease of an automobile or other similar equipment as well as to a sale.

Such an extension of warranty liability was applied to a hospital in which blood infected with hepatitis virus was administered to a patient. Pennsylvania's court held in *Hoffman*, a leading case, that warranty liability could attach to a transfusion of blood even if it were a service.[3]

---

[3] *Hoffman v. Misericordia Hospital of Philadelphia,* 439 Pa. 501, 267 A. 2d 867 (1970).

Strict liability in tort in the field of products liability is a further extension or liberalization of implied warranty liability. Stated most simply, warranty liability is basically contractual in nature while tort liability does not necessarily depend upon a contractual relationship between the parties. Strict liability in tort is a judicial doctrine founded upon the provisions of the *Restatement (Second) of Torts,* Section 402 (A) 1965. The *Restatement* provides that one who sells a product which is unreasonably dangerous to a consumer or user, or to his property, is liable for physical harm caused by the defective item if the seller is engaged in the business of selling a product, and if it reaches the user without substantial change in the condition existing at the time of sale. As in the warranty cases, in the general field of products liability law the courts have extended the theory of strict liability to one furnishing goods or products and have not confined the concept to a sale.

In 1970 the Illinois Supreme Court applied this concept of strict liability in tort to a hospital where a patient named Cunningham became ill with hepatitis following a blood transfusion. The court held that all of the foregoing requirements of the *Restatement* were present in the situation: the hospital had "sold" an "unreasonably dangerous product" to the patient.[4] The fact that there was no known means of discovering the hepatitis virus in the blood prior to the transfusion was, of course, no defense.

Following the *Cunningham* and *Hoffman* decisions, nearly all of the states enacted statutes intended to reverse the result of these cases. Some of the statutes provide only that the furnishing of blood by a hospital or a blood bank is a service and not the sale of a product. By so providing, these statutes may fall short of the intended result, because a court could still hold that liability without negligence is applicable to the rendition of a service. In other words, what may still be needed in some states is a forthright statute providing that the theories of implied warranty and strict liability in tort do not

---

[4] *Cunningham v. MacNeal Memorial Hospital,* 47 Ill. 2d 443, 266 N.E. 2d 897 (1970). See also: *Community Blood Bank, Inc. v. Russell,* 196 So. 2d 115 (Fla. 1967): (Warranties of sale possibly apply against both blood bank and hospital); *Jackson v. Muhlenberg Hospital,* 53 N.J. 138, 249 A. 2d 65 (1969): (Warranties of sale possibly apply against both a blood bank and a hospital); *Reilly v. King County Central Blood Bank, Inc.,* 6 Wash. App. 172, 492 P. 2d 246 (1971): (Strict liability applies to blood bank). Prior to these decisions in Illinois, New Jersey, Florida, Pennsylvania, and Washington applying products liability law to the hepatitis virus cases, the leading decision was *Perlmutter v. Beth David Hospital,* 308 N.Y. 100, 123 N.E. 2d 792 (1954), which had held that the administration of a blood transfusion was a service and not a sale. See generally: "Torts—Strict Liability—A Hospital is Strictly Liable for Transfusions of Hepatitis-Infected Blood," 69 *Michigan L. Rev.* 1173–89 (1971).

apply to the provider of hospital or medical services. The Louisiana statute, for example, is more comprehensive than others in that it says specifically that blood banks and hospitals supplying whole blood or its components are immune from liability in all causes of action except negligence. Such an immunity statute is constitutional and does not violate due process or equal protection.[5]

Even without a protective immunity statute a court is, of course, free to reject the theory of implied warranty or strict liability in tort as applicable to blood transfusions or other factual situations where liability without negligence is asserted. This was the result in a 1973 California case, where the court held that a blood transfusion was a service, that a hospital was not in the business of distributing blood in commerce for profit, and that solely as a matter of public policy hospitals should not be liable without proof of negligence or an intentional wrong.[6] Moreover, to apply strict liability there must be a defective or unreasonably dangerous product that caused the injury. Strict liability could therefore not apply to the administration of blood containing Kidd B antigen which was incompatible with antibodies already existing in the patient's blood as a result of previous transfusions.[7] Such blood was pure and not defective. Even in products liability law generally, the seller of a product is not liable for breach of warranty or strict liability when the allegedly injured person is allergic to the product.

In those jurisdictions which have an immunity statute but whose courts are prone to accept a theory of liability without negligence, the immunity statutes do not, of course, apply to incidents in which blood transfusions caused serum hepatitis prior to the passage of the statute.[8]

Accordingly, in most jurisdictions liability of the hospital in the blood transfusion cases must be based upon a theory of negligence. The negligence can consist of various possible factual patterns: for

---

[5] *McDaniel v. Baptist Memorial Hospital*, 469 F. 2d 230 (6th Cir. 1972): (Tennessee statute); *Heirs of Fruge v. Blood Services*, 506 F. 2d 841 (5th Cir. 1975): (Louisiana statute).

[6] *Shepard v. Alexian Brothers Hospital*, 33 Cal. App. 3d 606, 109 Cal. Rptr. 132 (1973). See also: *Brody v. Overlook Hospital*, 127 N.J. Super. 331, 317 A. 2d 392 (1974): (Strict liability was not applicable to a blood transfusion), *reversing*, 121 N.J. Super. 299, 296 A. 2d 668 (1972). Accord: *Foster v. Memorial Hospital Association of Charleston*, 219 S.E. 2d 916 (W. Va. 1975): (As a matter of common law, implied warranty does not apply to blood transfusions since a hospital does not sell blood); *St. Luke's Hospital v. Schmaltz*, 534 P. 2d 781 (Colo. 1975): (Neither implied warranty nor strict liability applies to blood transfusions).

[7] *Evans v. Northern Illinois Blood Banks, Inc.*, 13 Ill. App. 3d 19, 298 N.E. 2d 732 (1973).

[8] *Mercy Hospital, Inc. v. Benites*, 257 So. 2d 51 (Fla. App. 1972).

example, lack of reasonable care in administering the transfusion or processing the blood, careless selection of the blood bank or other source of supply, mistyping or mismatching the patient's blood type, or mislabeling the blood.

As an example of negligent administration of a blood transfusion, in *Sherman v. Hartman* a hospital nurse failed to supervise adequately the administration of blood; the needle slipped out of the patient's vein and blood infiltrated the tissues causing injury to the plaintiff's arm.[9] Nurses who fail to discover adverse reactions early in the course of the transfusion may be found negligent, and in such cases the hospital can be liable.[10]

If there is adequate proof of an error in typing or matching a patient's blood, a clear case of liability exists. A leading example is *Berg v. New York Society for the Relief of Ruptured and Crippled,* where an incorrect testing of the patient's Rh blood factor occurred.[11] Similarly, when a hospital technician inadvertently interchanged samples of blood from two patients there was liability.[12] A third example is *Smith v. McComb Infirmary,* where a pregnant patient's blood was misgrouped as Rh-positive when in actuality her Rh factor was negative.[13] The illness of the baby at birth was not recognized as the result of Rh factor incompatibility, and the baby died a year later.

Violation of known professional standards with respect to the processing, storage, or care of blood or blood products clearly indicates negligence. For example, because chilling of blood effectively destroys any syphilitic agents that may be present, a failure to chill could be negligent.[14] By the same token, when it is known to medicine that storing blood plasma at room temperature for six months destroys virtually all hepatitis virus, failure to follow this standard of care could lead to liability.

A hospital has the duty to exercise reasonable care in procuring blood from a blood bank or other source of supply, including a duty to ascertain that the supplier is in fact screening donors of

---

[9] 137 Cal. App. 2d 589, 290 P. 2d 894 (1955).
[10] *Joseph v. W. H. Groves Latter Day Saints Hospital,* 10 Utah 2d 94, 348 P. 2d 935 (1960). (Jury verdict on facts for defendant.)
[11] 1 N.Y. 2d 499, 154 N.Y.S. 2d 455, 136 N.E. 2d 523 (1956).
[12] *Mississippi Baptist Hospital v. Holmes,* 214 Miss. 906, 55 So. 2d 142 (1951). Moreover, the doctrine of res ipsa loquitur may apply in the case of a proven error in the typing of blood. *Redding v. United States,* 196 F. Supp. 871 (W. D. Ark. 1961).
[13] 196 So. 2d 91 (Miss. 1967).
[14] *Giarnboze v. Peters,* 127 Conn. 380, 16 A. 2d 833 (1940).

blood in accordance with professional standards.[15] For example, donors must be asked whether they have any history of hepatitis. As it becomes better known to the medical sciences that with paid blood donors as a group there is a high risk that whole blood from this source will be infected with serum hepatitis virus, some future court might hold that obtaining blood from a paid source could be negligence. Up to this time, however, the mere fact that a donor was paid a fee for blood which caused hepatitis was not proof of negligence. The donor in this case was a known person without a history of hepatitis at the time the blood was taken, and the blood bank promptly notified the patient's physician that the donor had developed hepatitis three weeks after giving the blood. The Montana Supreme Court held that the blood bank was not chargeable with negligence.[16] This court also held in the same case that the failure of the blood bank to use the serum glutamic oxaloacetic transaminase test on donated blood was not negligence, since no blood bank in the country was using the test at the time. Note, however, that if such a test for the presence of serum hepatitis virus becomes scientifically reliable then the failure to test could be negligence, especially if blood banks adopt the test as a routine precaution in accordance with recommendations of professionals. Of course, if testimony at trial is simply to the effect that the plaintiff contracted hepatitis following a blood transfusion, this is not proof of negligence in the processing, distribution, or administration of blood.[17]

Also illustrating the fundamental proposition that hospital liability is based upon concepts of negligence law and not of warranty or strict liability in tort are the cases in which a hospital patient developed a staphylococcal infection. Since a hospital is not an insurer or guarantor of a patient's safety, as a general rule there is no liability upon mere proof that the plaintiff developed an infection. Moreover, the doctrine of res ipsa loquitur would not apply to raise an inference or a presumption of negligence. To put the matter another way, in order to present a question for the jury, the plaintiff must show by expert testimony that the hospital in some way breached prevailing standards of care. Several leading cases establish these general rules.[18]

[15] *Hoder v. Sayet*, 196 So. 2d 205 (Fla. App. 1967); *Bowman v. American National Red Cross*, 39 Misc. 2d 799, 241 N.Y.S. 2d 971 (1963).
[16] *Hutchins v. Blood Services of Montana*, 161 Mont. 359, 506 P. 2d 449 (1973).
[17] *St. Martin v. Doty*, 493 S.W. 2d 95 (Tenn. App. 1972).
[18] *Thompson v. Methodist Hospital*, 211 Tenn. 650, 367 S.W. 2d 134 (1962); *Aetna Casualty and Surety Co. v. Pilcher*, 244 Ark. 11, 424 S.W. 2d 181 (1968); *McCall v. St. Joseph's Hospital*, 184 Neb. 1, 165 N.W. 2d 85 (1969); *LeFort v. Massachusetts Bonding and Insurance Company*, 358 F. 2d 741 (5th Cir. 1966).

They recognize that staphylococcal infections are very difficult to control and that they may occur despite reasonable care. Such an infection may be unforeseen and unpredictable, and when this is so there can be no liability.

On the other hand, of course, liability can be placed upon the hospital if the plaintiff establishes that the hospital staff deviated from accepted standards in its sterilizing techniques and that this breach of standards was the proximate cause of the infection. A major case illustrating such negligence was *Helman v. Sacred Heart Hospital*, decided in 1963, in the state of Washington. In this litigation the plaintiff was placed in a hospital room with a patient who had developed a boil that soon began to drain. Plaintiff had undergone hip surgery. During the three-day interval between discovery of the roommate's boil and the laboratory report that the drainage was an S. aureus infection, nurses and other hospital personnel attended both patients, administering baths, changing dressings, and giving backrubs without washing their hands or following other precautionary measures while awaiting the laboratory report. Although the originally infected patient was placed in isolation immediately following the diagnosis of an S. aureus infection, the plaintiff contracted the same strain of staphylococcal infection at the site of his hip surgery. On these facts a question of negligence was presented for the jury, and the Supreme Court of Washington upheld a verdict for the plaintiff.[19]

Another case which succeeded for the plaintiff was *Kapuschinsky v. United States*. A naval hospital had assigned a Medical Corps Wave aide to attend newborn infants in the hospital nursery. She had been recently attached to this particular hospital and was not given a physical examination before going to work in the nursery. Although she exhibited no symptoms of staphylococcal infection, she was indeed so infected. This was discovered after one of the patients, a premature infant, developed a severe and serious infection. Under the Federal Tort Claims Act the government was liable on the basis that it had permitted an infected nurse's aide to attend patients in the nursery without an appropriate physical examination.[20] This should have included laboratory tests, especially since it is known that premature babies are particularly susceptible to infection. It had to be established at the trial, of course, that the employee and the infant were infected with the same strain of staphylococcus.

---

[19] 62 Wash. 2d 136, 381 P. 2d 605 (1963).
[20] 248 F. Supp. 732 (S.C. 1966).

In a few cases the plaintiff has asserted that there should be strict liability in tort when hospital equipment which has malfunctioned or been defective has caused injury. So far the courts called upon to rule on the matter have rejected this theory. In *Silverhart v. Mount Zion Hospital*, the California intermediate appellate court held that strict liability would not apply when a surgical needle broke during a hysterectomy.[21] The court's reason for refusing the cause of action based upon strict liability was simply that the hospital was not in the business of supplying or furnishing the equipment to the patient. Rather the hospital itself and not the patient was the user or consumer of the product as contemplated by Section 402 (A) of the *Restatement (Second) of Torts.* In short, the hospital was using the needle in the course of rendering its services to the patient, and its liability would have to be based on negligence. Quite possibly, however, the patient could succeed in a products liability lawsuit on strict liability against the manufacturer of the defective equipment, if the proof required by the *Restatement of Torts* were sufficient.

By the same token a hospital is not at present strictly liable for the quality of the drugs it administers to the patient. Accordingly, when a plaintiff alleged that he was given a contaminated drug and based the cause of action on warranty liability, it was proper to dismiss the action.[22] When the wrong drug is administered to the patient, or generally in cases of errors in administering medication, there can be no implied warranty liability, and the cause of action must be based upon negligence. Hence the statute of limitations applicable to the relevant tort would apply to the action, rather than the longer limitation period applicable to actions for breach of contract.[23]

In the final analysis the extent to which some theory of liability without negligence is applicable to the hospital rests upon legislative and judicial views of public policy. Plaintiffs and their attorneys will make continued efforts to assert the law of implied warranty or strict liability, or both of these, against providers of medical care, including hospitals as well as physicians. At the present time, however, the defendants have been successful more often than not in maintain-

[21] 20 Cal. App. 3d 1022, 98 Cal. Rptr. 187 (1971).
[22] *Shivers v. Good Shepherd Hospital,* 427 S.W. 2d 104 (Tex. Ct. Civ. App. 1968).
[23] *Mauran v. Mary Fletcher Hospital,* 318 F. Supp. 297 (D. Vt. 1970). (The court, however, specifically reserved for future decision the issue of whether or not a hospital could be liable for the quality of drugs it dispenses to the patient on a theory of warranty of merchantability.) See also: *Carmichael v. Reitz,* 17 Cal. App. 3d 958, 95 Cal. Rptr. 381 (1971). (A physician cannot be held strictly liable as a "retailer" of drugs.)

ing their position that institutional and individual liability must be based upon some kind of negligence.

Liability for Injuries to Patients:
Two Theories

Hospital liability is fundamentally based on either corporate (institutional) negligence or vicarious liability. The latter, of course, is the doctrine of respondeat superior, which literally translated means "let the master answer." Both theories of liability have been expanded by judicial decision during recent years and each will be discussed separately.

Historically these two theories of hospital liability are separate and distinct from each other. Corporate or institutional negligence is the breach of a duty owed directly to the patient by the hospital. On the other hand, liability founded upon respondeat superior is imposed upon the hospital when an agent or servant (an employee) has been negligent within the scope of his or her employment and thereby caused injuries to a third person. The employer has not been negligent or at fault; accordingly it is sometimes said that vicarious liability is "nonfault" liability, an accurate statement in the sense that the employer has not directly or personally violated any duty owed to the third person.

As will be demonstrated throughout the ensuing discussion, courts and commentators have sometimes so confused or misapplied these two separate doctrines that they have become nearly merged or even indistinguishable in relation to a given set of facts involving multiple corporate or individual professional defendants. At least one can say that liability to the patient on the part of the hospital is likely, regardless of the theory argued by the plaintiff, as long as the trial establishes that either institutional standards or professional standards articulated by medical or other professional practitioners were breached and that the breach of standards was the proximate cause of injury to the patient. Nevertheless, for a proper understanding of each of the two theories they must be discussed separately.

One should always remember that even if an employer is found to be liable under the doctrine of respondeat superior the employee who committed the tort can also be held individually and personally liable for the injuries caused by his or her wrongful act or omission. Hospital employees are more and more often joined as defendants in liability suits along with their employer. When vicarious liability applies, the liability of the employer and employee is joint and several.

This means that the aggrieved plaintiff may sue any one or more of the parties separately or all of them together at his option, obtain a court judgment against all the defendants, and collect the judgment in whole from one or in part from each of the defendants. The plaintiff is not, of course, permitted to collect each judgment in full from two or more defendants; in other words he may not collect double (or more) damages to compensate for his injuries. If the plaintiff collects the judgment in whole or in part from the employer, in theory the employer in turn has a right of indemnification from the negligent employee. Sometimes this right is asserted when the employer and employee are insured against liability by different insurance carriers.

Standards of Care

Regarding the standard of care owed by a hospital to its patients, the Alabama case of *Doctors Hospital of Mobile, Inc. v. Kirksey* is informative.[24] In this litigation, the trial court had instructed the jury as follows:

> The court charges the jury that a hospital such as Doctors Hospital of Mobile, Inc., is directly responsible to its patients for providing competent medical care.[25]

It was further stated:

> The court charges the jury that a hospital is under a duty to furnish competent medical care to the patients entrusted to its care, and if you are reasonably satisfied from the evidence in these cases that Doctors Hospital of Mobile, Inc., failed to furnish competent medical care to Mrs. Kirksey while she was a patient at such hospital and as a proximate result thereof, Mrs. Kirksey suffered injuries complained of, then the hospital is liable.[26]

These instructions constituted reversible error because they implied that the hospital's duty was that of an insurer or guarantor of the competence of hospital personnel. Rather, the standard required is that of reasonable and ordinary care, diligence, and skill; and in Alabama this is measured by the standards used by hospitals

---

[24] 290 Ala. 220, 275 So. 2d 651 (1973).
[25] *Id.* at 222, 275 So. 2d at 652.
[26] *Id.* at 223, 275 So. 2d at 653.

generally in the community. The instructions, in other words, failed to define for the jury either the hospital's duty or what constitutes reasonable and ordinary care, diligence, and skill. Questions of law are not to be submitted to the jury, and the effect of the instructions given by the trial court violated that rule.

With respect to the general standard of care owed by a hospital to its patients, a leading decision is *Foley v. Bishop Clarkson Memorial Hospital*, decided by the Supreme Court of Nebraska in 1970.[27] During the later stages of pregnancy, Mrs. Foley had suffered from a cold and sore throat. Upon admission to the hospital for delivery no medical history was taken. This omission was contrary to hospital rules that required a written history within twenty-four hours of admission as well as a report to the attending physician of any suspected infection. The staff also failed to take a blood count which the physician had ordered to be taken within twenty-four hours of admission. The baby was delivered the day of admission and the mother expired approximately thirty-one hours after giving birth to the child. The cause of death was a severe beta hemolytic streptococcus infection. Following the birth of the baby, Mrs. Foley's vital signs of temperature, pulse, and respiration had deteriorated, but no report was made by the hospital or the nursing staff to the attending physician—again contrary to hospital rules. Codeine and ice had been administered against the doctor's orders.

The trial court directed a verdict for the defendant hospital based on the rule "that the proper measure of the duty of a hospital to the patient is the exercise of that degree of care, skill, and diligence used by hospitals generally in the community where the hospital is located or in similar communities," and on the further rule "that a patient is entitled to such reasonable care and attention as her *known* mental and physical condition may require." On the basis of the evidence, the trial judge felt that there was insufficient proof of a *known* infection to raise a question for the jury.

In reversing the directed verdict for the hospital, the Nebraska court rejected case precedent establishing the rule that a hospital must exercise reasonable care only with respect to known conditions. Observing that this standard of care promotes carelessness, since one could reason that the less the hospital staff knows about a patient's condition, the better its legal position, the court adopted the rule that a hospital must also guard against conditions that it should

---

[27] 185 Neb. 89, 173 N.W. 2d 881 (1970).

have discovered by the exercise of reasonable care.[28] Hence, whether or not this standard had been met on the facts and evidence was a question for the jury. Plaintiff had offered expert medical testimony to the effect that if an adequate medical history had been promptly taken or if the attending doctor had been notified promptly of changes in the patient's vital signs following the birth of her baby and more than twenty-four hours prior to her death, Mrs. Foley's life might have been saved.

A further point should be made with respect to the *Foley* case. The rules and regulations of the defendant hospital standing alone are not sufficient to establish community standards. This means that the plaintiff is entitled to introduce expert testimony simply to the effect that all hospitals make a general practice of obtaining medical histories from newly admitted patients, and that good nursing practice requires notification to the attending doctor when the patient's vital signs change significantly.

In sum, then, as stated by a leading treatise, when a patient seeks redress for injury incurred in a hospital the usual standard of care for patients is "that degree of care, skill, and diligence used by hospitals generally in the community" (not necessarily the local community) and "such reasonable care and attention for their safety as their mental and physical condition, if known, may require."[29] As noted above, the *Foley* case extended the latter rule to cover conditions that ought to have been known.

In *Kastler v. Iowa Methodist Hospital* the court emphasized that, although standard treatises appear to lump these two rules together, they are actually separate and distinct, depending upon the facts and circumstances giving rise to the litigation.[30] The first rule, speaking of the care and diligence generally exercised by hospitals, relates to the conduct of the hospital's professional staff. Hence to prove a breach of duty the plaintiff must normally introduce expert

---

[28] The Nebraska court acknowledged that this is a minority rule in the hospital liability cases, although it is a general rule in the law of negligence. Hence, the *Foley* case has simply applied the general law of negligence to the hospital.

[29] 40 Am. Jur. 2d *Hospitals and Asylums*, sec. 26, at 869. Since many local communities have but one hospital, a strict interpretation of the traditional community rule would allow a single hospital to be measured solely by standards set by itself. Clearly most courts are recognizing that this is not justifiable and that hospitals, like physicians, should be judged by standards and practices prevailing generally in like or similar communities in like circumstances. In a given case the jury may consider the customs and practices of the particular local community as an element in expected performance, but local practice should not be conclusive. See text discussion and case citations below, especially notes 40 through 45.

[30] 193 N.W. 2d 98 (Iowa 1971). See also: *Dickinson v. Mailliard*, 175 N.W. 2d 588 (Iowa 1970).

testimony relative to the practices of hospitals generally. On the other hand, when the conduct involves "nonmedical administrative, ministerial, or routine care" the second rule, which speaks simply of "reasonable care," applies. In such a case a question for the jury is presented, and there is no necessity to offer evidence of the standards of hospitals generally or to introduce expert testimony.

In *Kastler* a psychiatric patient, who was known to be subject to fainting, was permitted to take a shower without direct and immediate assistance. She became faint, fell, and was injured. In the opinion of a psychiatrist, Mrs. Kastler was an epileptic. The Supreme Court of Iowa reinstated a jury's verdict for the plaintiff, reversing the trial court which had granted a motion for a directed verdict for the hospital notwithstanding the jury's verdict. Thus the jury was permitted to use its own knowledge and good sense with respect to the hospital's conduct. The fact that the standing orders of the physician attending the patient had not prohibited showers did not insulate the hospital from liability, since subsequent circumstances showed the need for a change of action. Two dissenting judges wrote that the majority opinion had in effect adopted a fictional "reasonable man" concept, thus permitting the jury to engage in speculation, and this minority opinion would have required plaintiff to introduce evidence of customary practice and care exercised by hospitals generally.

In general, by the prevailing view, there is no duty to exercise reasonable care with respect to an unforeseeable plaintiff.[31] Further, even if the plaintiff is clearly foreseeable, there is no breach of duty or negligence unless the injury or death of the plaintiff was foreseeable or should have been anticipated. Negligence is conduct inconsistent with standards of behavior required by law for the protection of others. If the defendant could not have anticipated or foreseen that his conduct constituted an unreasonable risk to another, then there was no negligence. Some courts have from time to time inserted the requirement of foreseeability of harm as an element in the issue of proximate cause. The prevailing and better view, however, would seem to be that if action is taken that entails a foreseeable risk to the plaintiff the duty to exercise care has been breached; and so far as proximate cause is concerned the defendant should be liable for all directly caused consequences of his negligence,

[31] *Palsgraf v. Long Island Railroad Company*, 248 N.Y. 339, 162 N.E. 99 (1928). See also: 59 A.L.R. 1253; *Restatement (Second) of Torts*, sec. 281, comment *C* (1965). Also see the discussion below with respect to the recovery of damages for emotional and mental distress.

even if such consequences were not anticipated. Directly caused consequences can be defined as those which sequentially follow from failure to exercise reasonable care, not those caused by independent intervening events or forces.

The element of foreseeability of harm or injury to the patient may be illustrated by the cases asserting liability for suicide of the patient and by litigation alleging that hospital staff failed to restrain adequately a confused, disoriented, or incapacitated patient. A hospital can be liable for suicide of the patient if the patient's known emotional and mental condition was such that a reasonably prudent person could have anticipated the attempt. If the suicide attempt could have been anticipated, then the question is whether the hospital staff exercised reasonable care in guarding the patient under the circumstances and, if not, whether the failure was the proximate cause of the death.[32]

These principles of law as applied to a particular set of facts are illustrated in the 1972 case of *Johnson v. Grant Hospital,* in which the result in the Ohio Supreme Court contrasted strikingly with the decision of the intermediate court of appeals.[33] Mrs. Johnson, a patient in a general hospital, was provisionally diagnosed as a "schizophrenic reaction, schizo-affective type." Her attending physician was a specialist in neurology and psychiatry. Knowing that she had spoken of suicide, her husband gave notice to the hospital nurses to watch her closely. Four days after her admission she was discovered attempting to jump from a window. The attending doctor then ordered that she be moved to a security room, but with instructions to leave the door open. An hour later the patient left the security room and again attempted to take her life by jumping from a window. The physician then modified his order, so that the door to the security room would be locked at night. After the door was unlocked the next morning (and after both the patient and her family had complained by telephone to the doctor about the locked door), the patient succeeded in leaving the room and jumped from the ninth floor of the hospital to her death. On the morning of her death, the patient was in the sole care of a nurse's aide, who apparently

---

[32]A recent case illustrating these principles is *Harris Hospital v. Pope,* 520 S.W. 2d 813 (Tex. Ct. Civ. App. 1975). (A hospital was not liable for the suicide of the patient, since she had not exhibited signs of irrational behavior and appeared normal and not despondent, and since the hospital had no knowledge that she had attempted to take her own life on two previous occasions.)

[33]32 Ohio St. 2d 169, 291 N.E. 2d 440, (1972), rev'g, 31 Ohio App. 2d 118, 286 N.E. 2d 308 (1972).

was neither informed of the events of the night before nor given instructions to attend and supervise the patient personally and continually. The physician had in fact not ordered continuous supervision.

In the subsequent suit, the trial court directed a verdict for the hospital on the grounds that the nursing staff had followed the orders of the attending doctor and that the patient's death was her own voluntary act and not the result of negligence of the hospital staff.

The Ohio Court of Appeals reversed and sent the case back for a jury trial. First of all, this court ruled, the fact that the staff of the hospital followed the physician's orders does not necessarily show that reasonable care was exercised. Moreover, according to the court, no expert testimony had to be offered by the plaintiff relative to the standard of care required, since the patient's two attempts at suicide the night preceding her death permitted the jury to determine the matter of reasonable care simply on the basis of common general experience and knowledge. Thus, whether the hospital had exercised reasonable care under the circumstances and whether negligence of staff was the proximate cause of the death were questions for a jury, since reasonable minds could differ with respect to these issues.

The facts of the *Johnson* case raised directly the issue of the relation between hospital staff and the attending physician. The majority court of appeals opinion seemed to say that the hospital staff should have anticipated another attempt at suicide in view of the two on the preceding evening, even if the attending physician did not foresee the third attempt and did not countermand his orders for the patient's door to be unlocked during the day. In short, according to the majority, the nursing staff should have intervened, though against the professional judgment of the doctor, since the fact that the staff was following the doctor's orders would not necessarily relieve the hospital from being found negligent. Perhaps what influenced the majority opinion of the court of appeals most of all was that neither the nurse's aide nor the charge nurse on duty on the morning of the patient's suicide was aware of her attempts at suicide the night before. All they knew was that the door could be unlocked during the day, as stated in the physician's orders. This failure of night staff to communicate relevant information to day staff was treated as negligence.

On appeal to the Supreme Court of Ohio the ruling of the court of appeals for the plaintiff was reversed, and the judgment of the trial court granting a directed verdict for the defendant hospital was deemed proper. Although the court did not dispute the general rule that a hospital owes a duty to the patient to exercise such reasonable care as the patient's known mental and physical condition may require, it observed that the defendant was a general hospital not equipped or staffed to care for mental patients, and that accordingly it should not be held to the same standard of care as a hospital for the mentally ill. In the circumstances the hospital fulfilled its duty by following precisely the orders of the attending physician, and hospital staff need not have intervened to anticipate an act of self-destruction when the doctor had not ordered restraint of the patient.[34] The death was the voluntary act of the patient.

One of the judges concurred in this opinion on the basis that the court of appeals had, in effect, cast a duty on hospital personnel to disobey the orders of the attending physician and that the factual pattern of this case would not have justified such action. He stressed, however, that in other instances the duty to exercise reasonable care for the safety of the patient would indeed require the nursing staff to exert a judgment different from that of the physician in order to protect the patient.[35]

Even though generally the hospital will have fulfilled its duty of reasonable care by following the orders of the attending physician, situations may thus arise where the orders are clearly erroneous or contrary to usual practice, and hospital staff will then have the duty at least to question the phsyician. Moreover, there may be crises or emergencies in which nurses or other staff members must intervene directly to protect the patient, perhaps acting in contravention of physician's orders or at least acting independently in the absence of orders.

For example, in *Burks v. Christ Hospital* the attending physician had not specifically ordered that siderails on the patient's bed be raised, nor had he issued orders against their use. The patient, an obese person under heavy sedation and exhibiting restlessness, fell from a bed with rollers and without siderails. Good and customary

---

[34] Accord: *Clements v. Swedish Hospital,* 252 Minn. 1, 89 N.W. 2d 162 (1958). See also: *Nelson v. Salem Hospital,* 551 P. 2d 476 (Ore. 1976). (A hospital is entitled to have a jury consider evidence that a deceased patient voluntarily jumped from a window.)

[35] See: *Toth v. Community Hospital at Glen Cove,* 22 N.Y. 2d 255, 239 N.E. 2d 368 (1968). (A hospital's nursing staff generally has a duty to follow the orders of an attending physician, unless they know them to be contrary to acceptable practice.) Further, nurses have a duty to observe patients and report damaging effects of medication or treatments to physicians. See below in the text.

nursing practice, as evidenced by a hospital teaching manual for nurses, indicated that for such patients siderails were to be raised unless the physician had specifically ordered otherwise. In addition, the manual provided that the rollers were to be removed from the bed if the patient was not protected by rails and if he was likely to arise from the bed unassisted. When the case reached court it was held that the issue of negligence was a question for the jury, and if the jury should find negligence it must also determine whether that negligence was the proximate cause of the patient's injury.[36] Further, the teaching manual was ruled admissible in evidence to help establish the standard of care expected under the circumstances. To be contrasted with *Burks* is the case of *Killgore v. Argonaut-Southwest Insurance Company*. In *Killgore* no liability followed when a patient fell from bed without siderails and when all orders and rules relative to the use of restraints had been observed.[37]

Another case, however, is consistent with *Burks* insofar as it held that the attending physician's failure to issue orders regarding the use of siderails or other form of restraint did not necessarily protect the hospital from liability. This is the recent Louisiana case of *Hunt v. Bogalusa Community Medical Center*. A 73-year-old postsurgical patient under heavy sedation and with a medical history of stroke and dizziness fell from bed while protected by only partial siderails. Even though the attending physician had not ordered the use of full guardrails, and even though the use of partial rails was in accordance with customary and standard hospital practice in the local community (at trial of the case, administrators from two neighboring hospitals had testified that their hospitals used partial rails unless a physician ordered full rails), the court ruled that the hospital's duty was to exercise the amount of care that the patient's condition required.[38] By reinstating the trial court's decision awarding damages to the patient and reversing the decision of the Louisiana appellate court, the supreme court in effect held that the community standard of care was too low in the circumstances. There were two dissenting opinions. One judge would have held for the hospital because the physician had not ordered the use of full guardrails and any negligence was the physician's. The other dissent observed

---

[36] 19 Ohio St. 2d 128, 249 N.E. 2d 829 (1969). See also: *Haber v. Cross County Hospital*, 378 N.Y.S. 2d 369 (1975). (A violation of a hospital rule that bed rails are to be raised for all patients over the age of fifty is evidence of negligence, even though the attending physician had not specifically ordered the rails to be raised.)
[37] 216 So. 2d 108 (La. App. 1968). See also: *Thompson v. Hospital Authority of Upson County*, 114 Ga. App. 324, 151 S.E. 2d 183 (1966).
[38] 303 So. 2d 745 (La. 1974), rev'g, 289 So. 2d 219 (La. App. 1973).

that the patient was under the care of a private duty nurse as ordered by the attending doctor, and the nurse had left the room for a few minutes. Accordingly, in his view, her absence was the proximate cause of the patient's injuries.

Despite such judicial opinions as the majority in *Hunt*, the mere occurrence of an injurious accident does not create liability. Foreseeability of harm to the patient is still generally a necessary requisite in establishing that a defendant was negligent.[39]

As noted above, medical standards of care are becoming nationally uniform and comprehensive for both physicians and hospitals. The "local community" rule is being demolished in hospital liability and malpractice cases. This is a natural development in an era of readily available communication systems and in a society which is employing great resources in continuing educational programs for physicians and other professional persons. The courts are measuring existing standards and procedures at individual hospitals against standards prevailing at institutions in similar communities, and even against standards employed in the great medical centers. The "community" becomes nationwide, at least with respect to the practice of medical specialties.

This was so in *Darling v. Charleston Community Memorial Hospital*, where it was said in the course of the appeal that conformity with the standard of care observed by other hospitals in the local community cannot necessarily, in itself, be a defense in a negligence action.[40] The Illinois court was not the first to recognize that the standards of the local community should not be conclusive. In *Leonard v. Watsonville Community Hospital* it was held that a jury could reasonably find that failure to count instruments before and after surgery was negligence, even if it was the practice of local community hospitals not to count them.[41] Likewise the court held in both *Kolesar v. United States*[42] and *Kapuschinsky v. United States*[43] that no defense was possible on the basis that the accepted standard of care is measured by prevailing practices within the local community. In *Favalora v. Aetna Casualty and Surety Company* the Louisiana court ruled the practice of a radiologist not to check the medical history of patients to be

---

[39] *Doctor's Hospital, Inc. v. Kovats*, 16 Ariz. App. 489, 494 P. 2d 389 (1972). (A hospital was liable when a confused and hostile patient, who had frequently escaped from a restraining belt, attacked another patient. Such an event was a foreseeable consequence of the failure to use a more secure restraint.)

[40] 33 Ill. 2d 326, 211 N.E. 2d 253 (1965).

[41] 47 Cal. 2d 509, 305 P. 2d 36 (1957).

[42] 198 F. Supp. 517 (S.D. Fla. 1961).

[43] 248 F. Supp. 732 (D.S.C. 1966).

unreasonable, even though it was not customary for radiologists in that locality to make such a review.[44] He was considered especially at fault because medical school training recognizes that the practice of the community in question was inadequate.

A significant 1967 Washington case accelerated this trend in the liability of both hospitals and physicians. The victim of an accident had to undergo dental surgery during his hospitalization. Anesthesia was administered by a nurse, and the dental surgeon, according to his own admission, had no knowledge regarding the use or administration of general anesthesia. Because of inadequate ventilation the patient suffered convulsions and cerebral anoxia or hypoxia. He remained unconscious for almost a month and suffered permanent disabilities. No medical doctor was present in the hospital at the time, and more than an hour had passed before a physician could be found to attend him. The rule of the institution was that dental patients were to be coadmitted by a physician who was then "responsible for the patient's medical care." In this instance the admitting physician had left the hospital.

At the trial level the court instructed the jury in accordance with the traditional local community rule regarding standards of care, and the jury returned verdicts for the defendants. The Washington Supreme Court in reversing this finding removed the locality limitations with respect to standards and held that the hospital was negligent as a matter of law in these circumstances for permitting dental surgery without the presence and supervision of a medical doctor in the operating room.[45] Neither the violation of the hospital rule nor the standards of hospital accreditation were relied upon as the basis for liability, but undoubtedly such evidence was influential in the reasoning of the court. The breach of the hospital rule regarding medical standards at the very least fortified the court's conclusion. With respect to the standards of the local community, the court indicated that such standards were only one of several elements to determine the degree of skill and care expected. In the same vein, the 1968 case of *Brune v. Belinkoff* in Massachusetts held New Bedford physicians to the same standard of care with respect to the dosage level of an anesthetic as prevailed in New York and Boston.[46]

---

[44] 144 So. 2d 544 (La. App. 1962).
[45] *Pederson v. Dumouchel,* 72 Wash. 2d 73, 431 P. 2d 973 (1967).
[46] 354 Mass. 102, 235 N.E. 2d 793 (1968). See also the following typical cases rejecting the notion that prevailing standards of the local community are conclusive: *Riley v. Layton,* 329 F. 2d 53 (10th Cir. 1964); *Hundley v. Martinez,* 151 W. Va. 977, 158

The greatest immediate impact of the cases which have overturned the local community rule is that plaintiff may introduce expert witness testimony from geographically remote areas. The expert witness testifying for the plaintiff and against a physician or a hospital may come from another part of the country, not merely across town or across the hall in a physicians' office building. Needless to say, this judicial development has greatly extended a plaintiff's ability to obtain expert testimony and has required physicians and hospitals to be aware of standards in force or recommended elsewhere.

As noted above in regard to the *Kastler*[47] and the *Hunt*[48] cases, sometimes the standard of care to be applied is simply that of the reasonably prudent person, and the plaintiff will be entitled to have his case decided by a jury without having to present expert witness testimony. A case which further emphasizes this—and which illustrates the respective roles of the hospital and the doctor—is *Washington Hospital Center v. Butler*. The medical chart of a hospitalized diabetic person indicated that the patient was subject to weakness and dizziness. When x-rays were ordered, the requisition form showed only that the patient suffered from diabetes with complications, no reference being made to specific symptoms. During the x-ray procedure the plaintiff became dizzy and fell. At trial, in suit against both the hospital and the radiologists, there was no expert testimony regarding standards of practice governing the kind and extent of information customarily supplied on hospital x-ray requisition forms. Nevertheless it was held proper to instruct the jury to measure the conduct of the defendants simply by standards of the reasonably prudent man, with the actual standards of practice having evidentiary value only.[49] The jury was told that it could justifiably find the hospital negligent in failing to supply the radiologists with complete information concerning the patient's condition. In other words, reasonably prudent conduct by those preparing the x-ray requisition form would have been to furnish more information. As to the liability of the radiologists, the jury could find them negligent, since the doctors had been placed on notice that the patient was a diabetic, and no

---

S.E. 2d 159 (1967); *Naccarato v. Grob*, 384 Mich. 248, 180 N.W. 2d 788 (1970); *Avey v. St. Francis Hospital and School of Nursing, Inc.*, 201 Kansas 687, 442 P. 2d 1013 (1968); *Carrigan v. Roman Catholic Bishop*, 104 N.H. 73, 178 A. 2d 502 (1962).
[47]See n. 30.
[48]See n. 38.
[49]384 F. 2d 331 (D.C. Cir. 1967). See also: *Newhall v. Central Vermont Hospital, Inc.*, 349 A. 2d 890 (Vt. 1975). (Expert testimony was not required to prove a hospital negligent in making a patient wait an unreasonable length of time for a bedpan, with the result that she fell attempting to walk to the lavatory while under sedation. Common knowledge and experience is sufficient to guide the jury.)

prudent person would have failed to furnish aid for such a patient standing upright at the x-ray machine.

In summary, the leading decisions have established that a hospital has a duty to the patient to exercise that degree of care, skill, and diligence used by hospitals generally in the community or in similar communities in like circumstances.

The second major rule of a hospital's duty is that staff must exercise all the reasonable care and attention that the known physical or mental condition of the patient requires. This rule of duty has been enlarged by a growing minority of courts to impose liability when hospital staff members fail to guard against conditions that should have been discovered by the exercise of reasonable care. Sometimes, depending upon the facts and circumstances of a particular case, the plaintiff is entitled to have his case decided by the jury without presenting expert witness testimony. This result is probable whenever the facts show that the jury is competent simply from its own experience to determine and apply such a standard of reasonable care.

The standards and practices prevailing locally are no longer conclusive with respect to the issue of negligence, and when expert testimony is required plaintiff may present evidence of standards in effect elsewhere, including in some instances standards promulgated by teaching institutions. In short, the courts in recent years have extended the duty of a hospital to "similar communities" and have then in effect broadened the definitions of "similar" and "like circumstances" to require of a local community hospital and its medical staff the same degree of knowledge, skill, and diligence found in professional colleagues practicing in larger hospitals geographically remote from the defendant hospital or defendant physician. Moreover, standards promulgated by state hospital licensure authority, by the federal government through Medicare and other programs which finance hospital care, by private accreditation agencies such as the Joint Commission on Accreditation of Hospitals, and by the defendant hospital's own administrative or medical staff rules and regulations are all admissible in court for the jury to consider in determining negligence.[50] Violation of a hospital's own rules and

---

[50]There are many case decisions to this effect. Leading cases are *Darling v. Charleston Community Memorial Hospital*, 33 Ill. 2d 326, 211 N.E. 2d 253 (1965); *Purcell and Tucson General Hospital v. Zimbelman*, 18 Ariz. App. 75, 500 P. 2d 335 (1972), discussed below; *Suburban Hospital Association, Inc. v. Hadary*, 22 Md. App. 186, 322 A. 2d 258 (1974): (Regulations of Maryland State Department of Health relative to storage of sterile supply and equipment were admissible in evidence, and no further expert witness testimony was required for jury determination of negligence).

regulations regarding the care and treatment of patients, adopted in the interest of patients' safety, is especially likely to lead to a jury's determination of liability or even liability as a matter of law.[51] Once the plaintiff has presented sufficient evidence of breach of duty, the factual questions of whether there was negligence and whether the negligence was the proximate cause of the injury are frequently for the jury to determine. One may generally test whether a jury question is presented by asking whether or not reasonable men could differ on the basis of the evidence presented.

Damages for Mental Anguish

One essential element of a cause of action in negligence is actual loss or damage to the legally protected interests of the plaintiff. As is amply demonstrated throughout this chapter, the law of negligence protects interests in personal security and tangible property when a duty to exercise care exists, when the duty is breached, and when proximate cause is established. If the plaintiff asserts that his damage was mental disturbance, emotional shock, or fright, however, the courts have considerable difficulty in determining whether or not compensation is due.

As a general rule, mental or emotional disturbance is compensable when it accompanies or is the result of actual physical injury. In the opposite sequence of events, when physical harm results from mental or emotional shock the traditional view until recently had been that there can be no recovery of damages unless there was an "impact" upon the person of the plaintiff. An impact has generally been construed as a physical touching of some sort, however slight. Presumably it was required to test whether the mental or emotional injury was genuinely a cause of the subsequent physical harm. Most courts, however, have abandoned the requirement of an impact and do allow recovery in cases where emotional or mental shock leads to physical injury, as long as a duty is owed to the plaintiff and sufficient proof of proximate cause is established. One major problem confronting the courts is to determine under what facts and circumstances a duty to exercise reasonable care is owed.

Whether a cause of action exists for emotional or mental shock followed by physical harm is a frequent issue when the plaintiff is involved in or witnesses a negligent act of defendant which causes

---

[51] See *Pederson v. Dumouchel*, 72 Wash. 2d 73, 431 P. 2d 973 (1967). See also: *Hunt v. King County*, 4 Wash. App. 14, 481 P. 2d 593 (1971). (This case involved violation of a rule by the staff of a psychiatric hospital that a utility room door be locked.)

injury or death to another person, although the issue is not necessarily limited to such a factual situation. In the situation described, most courts have now abandoned the requirement that there be a physical impact upon the plaintiff in order to give him or her a right of action and damages. Some courts, in eliminating the impact rule, adopted in its place the "zone-of-danger" test; that is, if the plaintiff himself was in the zone of danger and was personally threatened with physical harm by the negligent act of the defendant, then recovery of damages for mental anguish will be permitted.[52] The zone-of-danger test is employed to establish a duty owed to the plaintiff; in other words, no duty is owed by the negligent defendant to the plaintiff unless harm to the plaintiff was foreseeable or anticipated.

Other courts have further liberalized the criteria for the recovery of damages for emotional shock arising from a negligent act of the defendant. They now require only that the plaintiff be in reasonably close physical proximity to the negligent act, that he be closely related to the victim of the negligence, and that he establish by sufficient proof that his emotional shock was a direct result of the accident, occurring contemporaneously with his observance of it. To illustrate this liberalized and minority view, in *Dillon v. Legg* a mother who saw an automobile strike her child could recover damages for an emotional shock which in turn caused physical symptoms.[53] On such facts, even though there was no physical impact upon the plaintiff and even though she was not in the zone of danger, the defendant owed a duty to the plaintiff because harm to her was foreseeable.

When courts determine whether a cause of action exists for emotional or mental shock, even one followed by such physical injury as a miscarriage or a heart attack, they are of course concerned with many related matters: the need to establish sufficient proof of proximate cause of the alleged injury; the difficulty of determining the plaintiff's actual damage or of placing a monetary value on mental

[52] *Neiderman v. Brodsky*, 436 Pa. 401, 261 A. 2d 84 (1970). See also: *Scarf v. Koltoff*, 363 A. 2d 1276 (Pa. Super. Ct. 1976). (No recovery was granted in an action for wrongful death on behalf of a wife who suffered a heart attack and died after seeing her husband struck by automobile, the reason being that she was not in the "zone of danger.")
[53] 68 Cal. 2d 728, 69 Cal. Rptr. 72, 441 P. 2d 912, 29 A.L.R 3d 1316 (1968). Accord: *D'Ambra v. United States*, 338 A. 2d 524 (R.I. 1975): (A mother could maintain action for serious emotional distress accompanied by physical symptoms resulting from witnessing the death of her child caused by negligent defendant, even though no impact upon mother occurred and despite the fact that she herself was never in physical danger); *Husserl v. Swiss Air Transport Company, Ltd.*, 388 F. Supp. 1238 (S.D. N.Y. 1975): (An international airline passenger recovered damages for mental trauma and psychosomatic injuries involving "demonstrable physiological manifestations," even though no "impact" upon her person occurred when an airliner was hijacked).

anguish; the prospect of being confronted with a large number of frivolous and unmeritorious suits; and the risk of making negligent defendants liable to an unlimited number of persons. Hence, in attempting to resolve these difficulties a court will use either the zone-of-danger test or the liberalized view in the *Dillon* case to determine and identify plaintiffs to whom a duty is owed.

The guidelines set forth by the California Supreme Court in *Dillon* are illustrated by subsequent California cases. In *Archibald v. Braverman*, a mother heard an explosion and immediately thereafter discovered the battered body of her son. Recovery of damages for her emotional anguish was permitted.[54] In contrast, a wife was denied damages for the emotional injury suffered when she arrived at a hospital emergency room and found her husband paralyzed as a result of an automobile accident.[55] On these facts the criteria for recognizing a duty owed by the defendant to the plaintiff, as outlined by *Dillon*, were not met.

A leading decision in the hospital field, more conservative than *Dillon v. Legg* and representing what is probably the modern majority rule, was handed down in the North Dakota litigation entitled *Whetham v. Bismarck Hospital.* An employee of the hospital, who was carrying a newborn infant to the mother's bedside, dropped the baby in the presence of the mother. The fall to a tiled floor caused the infant grievous injuries, including a fractured skull. The infant, of course, would have a cause of action against both the negligent employee and the hospital as the employer; further, the parents could recover damages not only for the additional medical expenses of caring for the baby but for the expenses of the mother, whose hospitalization was prolonged by the injury to her child. However, the North Dakota court denied the mother damages for the suffering caused by the emotional and mental shock of observing the accident.[56] The basis for the decision was that the negligent act of the hospital employee had not threatened physical harm to the plaintiff or placed plaintiff within the zone of danger.

---

[54] 275 Cal. App. 2d 253, 79 Cal. Rptr. 723 (1969).
[55] *Deboe v. Horn,* 16 Cal. App. 3d 221, 94 Cal. Rptr. 77 (1971). Similarly, a mother could not recover for the emotional trauma from observing the gradual deterioration in health and subsequent death of her 5-year-old son, allegedly caused by malpractice. *Jansen v. Children's Hospital Medical Center of East Bay,* 31 Cal. App. 3d 22, 106 Cal. Rptr. 883 (1973). See also: *Justus v. Atchison,* 53 Cal. App. 3d 556 (1976). (Two fathers who were present in the delivery room and saw their sons delivered stillborn could not recover for emotional shock. They were voluntary witnesses, and their emotional distress occurred later, not contemporaneously with the event.)
[56] 197 N.W. 2d 678 (No. Dak. 1972).

The Supreme Court of Hawaii would undoubtedly have reached a different conclusion on the facts of the *Whetham* case, for it has recognized a duty to exercise reasonable care to avoid negligent infliction of serious mental distress upon another, even when no physical impact occurs and when no close blood relationship exists between the victim and the plaintiff. Moreover, Hawaii has held that damages can be recovered for serious mental distress that results in no physical injury to the person of the plaintiff. In *Rodrigues v. State*, the plaintiff's home was damaged as a result of flooding attributed to the defendant's negligence. Plaintiff was awarded damages for mental distress.[57] The same result was reached in *Leong v. Takasaki*, where the plaintiff, a ten-year-old child, witnessed the death of an elderly woman who was not a relative but whom he lived with and loved dearly.[58] The two were crossing a street together when the woman was struck and killed by an automobile. In both cases the court held that the mental distress was a reasonably foreseeable consequence of the defendant's negligence.

However, there is a limit to those to whom a duty is owed, even in Hawaii. In *Kelley v. Kokua Sales and Supply Company*, the plaintiff, Mr. Kelley, was residing in California when he learned by telephone that his daughter and granddaughter had been killed in an automobile accident in Hawaii as a result of the defendant's negligence. The accident also critically injured another granddaughter. Shocked and grieved, Mr. Kelley died the same evening of a heart attack. Although the Hawaiian court had previously recognized a duty on the part of defendants to refrain from negligent infliction of serious mental distress upon a plaintiff, even when there had been no physical impact or family relationship and indeed not even any resulting physical injury, on the facts of the *Kelley* case there could be no recovery.[59] The court held that the duty of the defendant extended only to those located within a reasonable distance of the actual scene of the accident, since only then could the defendant reasonably foresee the consequences of his negligent conduct. A person in California was not considered to be within a reasonable distance of an accident in Hawaii.

The decision as a matter of law was based simply on public policy: to extend a duty of care to every relative, bystander, or friend of

[57] 52 Hawaii 156, 472 P. 2d 509 (1970).
[58] 55 Hawaii 398, 520 P. 2d 758 (1974).
[59] 532 P. 2d 673 (Hawaii 1975).

the victim of negligent conduct who suffered shock and grief as a result of his loss would lead to "unmanageable, unbearable, and totally unpredictable liability."[60] A strong dissent in *Kelley* would have recognized a duty of care to the plaintiff and would have permitted the jury to grant recovery for serious mental distress upon proper proof of injury, thus trusting the trier of fact to separate meritorious claims from those that may be feigned.

When a plaintiff claims injury or damage consisting solely of mental or emotional distress without resulting physical harm, the general and majority rule is that there can be no recovery of damages if the mental disturbance arises out of negligent conduct by the defendant. Cases do permit recovery for the intentional or willful and wanton infliction of emotional injury, as will be noted. But unless the conduct was intentional or unusually flagrant, the courts have hesitated to allow recovery. Various reasons may be cited: the difficulty of determining actual damage from mental anguish or of placing a monetary value on it, the prospect of being confronted with a large number of frivolous and unmeritorious suits, and the difficulties in deciding whether the plaintiff who claims injury was foreseeably within the ambit of defendant's duty to exercise care.

Although a few cases have permitted recovery for mental distress without resulting physical injury when it was caused by defendant's negligent conduct, as shown by the Hawaiian cases discussed previously,[61] the general rule can be illustrated by two cases. In each case the hospital discharged a mother who had recently given birth in the maternity department and sent her home with an infant not her own. Both times the mistake was soon discovered and corrected;

---

[60]*Id.* at 532 P. 2d 676.

[61]As further examples, some cases have awarded damages for the negligent mishandling of corpses: *Klumbach v. Silver Mount Cemetery Association,* 242 App. Div. 843, 275 N.Y.S. 180 (1934). A recent Louisiana case approved a $3,000 damage award for "anxiety." A patient suffering the symptoms of a heart attack was taken to a hospital emergency room. The EKG was abnormal, but the physician failed to compare this current EKG with previous ones, although they were available, and sent the patient home. The next day the patient was hospitalized. In a suit for damages, the appellate court concluded that the physician had been negligent in diagnosis and failure to hospitalize the patient immediately. The patient was not able to prove, however, that the delay in hospitalization caused additional heart damage. Indeed, expert testimony established that irreversible heart damage had occurred before the patient first appeared in the emergency room, and damages for the delayed diagnosis were denied. Nevertheless a $3,000 award was given for pain and anxiety, even though the negligence did not cause physical harm. *Fox v. Argonaut Southwest Insurance Company,* 288 So. 2d 102 (La. App. 1974). See also: *Johnson v. State,* 372 N.Y.S. 2d 638, 334 N.E. 2d 590 (1975). (Damages were awarded for expenses incurred in making funeral arrangements and for emotional distress when the hospital negligently and erroneously reported to plaintiff that her mother had died.)

and lawsuits by the parents seeking damages for mental anguish failed.[62]

On the other hand, courts do now recognize the intentional infliction of mental distress or suffering as a tort, and damages can be recovered. Willful and wanton conduct, or conduct that is outrageous and flagrant or is accompanied by malice, is tantamount to an intent to inflict emotional suffering. The factual situations illustrating this tort could be limitless: playing a cruel, heartless practical joke; sending a threatening letter; oppressive humiliation or insult of another; and flagrant misuse of authority. These have all been recognized as constituting tortious acts, and recovery of damages for the resulting mental distress has been permitted.

More relevant to hospital administration and medical care is the recent Oregon case of *Rockhill v. Pollard*. In this litigation, the plaintiff, her ten-month-old daughter, and her mother-in-law were injured in an automobile accident. The infant was unconscious at the scene of the accident. At a physician's office, where they were taken, the doctor was allegedly rude to them, saying there was nothing wrong with them, although they had suffered visible cuts and bruises and both were limping. Moreover in response to their requests that he examine and treat the unconscious child, the doctor refused to do more than place a stethoscope on her chest and test her reflexes with an instrument, even though the child had vomited in his presence. When the mother asked the doctor what to do with the baby, he simply shrugged his shoulders and said he did not know. The mother-in-law then informed the physician that someone would come to the office to take them elsewhere, and the doctor allegedly replied, "My God, woman, I can't stay here until somebody comes and gets you." He told them to wait outside in freezing weather and with the baby's clothing and blanket wet with vomit. When the child was

[62]*Carter v. Lake Wales Hospital Association*, 213 So. 2d 898 (1968); *Espinosa v. Beverly Hospital*, 114 Cal. App. 2d 232, 249 P. 2d 843 (1953): (Lack of sleep caused by mental distress was not considered physical harm). See also: *Pazo v. Upjohn Company*, 310 So. 2d 30 (Fla. App. 1975): (Parents have no claim for the mental pain and anguish they suffer from the birth of a deformed infant, the birth defects allegedly having been caused by a drug taken by the mother during pregnancy. They have, however, a claim against the drug manufacturer for negligence or breach of warranty). *Kraus v. Spielberg*, 37 Misc. 2d 519, 236 N.Y.S. 2d 143 (1962): (A patient had no claim for mental anguish unaccompanied by physical damage when a physician in good faith erroneously diagnosed her case as tuberculosis). *Brooks v. South Broward Hospital District*, 325 So. 2d 479 (Fla. Ct. App. 1975): (Parents had no cause of action for mental distress when a hospital negligently misplaced the body of their stillborn child. There was no evidence of physical injury to the parents, nor was there wanton or malicious behavior); *Conway v. Spitz*, 407 F. Supp. 536 (Pa. 1975); *White v. Diamond*, 390 F. Supp. 867 (Md. 1974).

later taken to a hospital, she was found to be suffering from shock and possibly to have incurred a head injury requiring medical treatments. In a suit which the child's mother brought against the physician for damages to compensate her for the emotional shock resulting from the defendant's allegedly outrageous and flagrant conduct, the Oregon court held that the facts were sufficient to be submitted to a jury.[63]

The intentional or willful and wanton infliction of mental distress and suffering can perhaps be termed the new "tort of outrage." The Supreme Court of Washington has spoken in such a vein in a case where the defendants were a physician and a hospital. A husband alleged that the defendants had abandoned and failed to care for and treat his wife. He further alleged that this conduct was willful and wanton, reckless, and outrageous. Before his wife expired, he said, he was present and observed the defendants' conduct in question, and he was forced helplessly to witness the suffering of his wife and her agonizing death. The plaintiff husband claimed damages for severe emotional distress and mental anguish which, according to his statement, resulted in physical injury. In reversing the decision of the trial court, which had dismissed the husband's action, the majority of the supreme court held that the allegations were sufficient to require a trial of the case on factual issues.[64] Three justices dissented on the basis that the conduct of the defendants was, at most, passive; for a cause of action to exist, they said, there must be evidence of active conduct exhibiting willful intent to inflict harm upon the plaintiff.

In summary, with respect to the recovery of damages for emotional and mental stress, whether or not it is followed by physical harm of any kind, the law is still very much in a state of development and case-by-case growth. Liability for mental distress is likely to be expanded and extended, especially as medical science recognizes more and more that mental stress can often be as real and as damaging as physical illness or injury. The major problem for the courts will then be to sort out, as a matter of law, the frivolous and feigned claims from the more meritorious ones. To reduce the possibility of suits alleging emotional damage, medical and hospital personnel must at the very least refrain from words and conduct that could

[63]259 Ore. 54, 485 P. 2d 28 (1971).
[64]*Grimsby v. Samson*, 85 Wash. 2d 52, 530 P. 2d 291 (1975). See also: *Johnson v. Woman's Hospital*, 527 S.W. 2d 133 (Tenn. App. 1975). (Compensatory and punitive damages were awarded for "outrageous conduct" by a hospital which attempted to dispose of the body of an infant as a surgical specimen and subsequently exhibited the body, preserved in formaldehyde, to its mother.)

possibly be construed as outrageous, flagrant, or willful and wanton when dealing with patients and their families.

Liability Based upon Respondeat Superior

The basis for applying the doctrine of respondeat superior is the right of the employer to control the activities of an employee. In the hospital setting this raises twin questions: first, the existence of an employment relationship; and second, the right of control with respect to an employee's responsibilities.

In general, a staff physician, with no closer relation to the hospital corporation than having the privilege of treating his private patients who are hospitalized there, is not an employee of the institution. Hence the traditional view has been that the hospital is not vicariously liable to the patient for the physician's professional negligence. The doctor is an independent contractor, and the hospital is not liable for the tort of an independent contractor unless the tort committed by the contractor occurs during the performance of a nondelegable corporate or institutional duty.[65] This is certainly sound doctrine when there is a genuine relationship of private physician to patient, with the patient selecting and paying the doctor for medical care.

Changing methods for the delivery of modern medical care, however, create more opportunities for the courts to circumvent the independent contractor doctrine. For example, salary arrangements between hospital and doctor are becoming more numerous. These open the door to applying respondeat superior and holding the hospital responsible.[66] An employment relationship then exists, and the professional status of the employee performing medical acts does not bar the application of vicarious liability. This is dramatically seen in the cases involving resident physicians, interns, and nurses.

Resident physicians and interns in training are considered employees when performing their normal duties, and thus the hospital is vicariously liable for their negligence or malpractice.[67] The courts

---

[65]For example: *Mayers v. Litow and Midway Hospital,* 154 Cal. App. 2d 413, 316 P. 2d 351 (1957); *Rosane v. Senger,* 112 Colo. 363, 149 P. 2d 372 (1944); *Black v. Fischer,* 30 Ga. App. 109, 117 S.E. 103 (1923); *Zelver v. Sequoia Hospital District,* 7 Cal. App. 3d 934, 87 Cal. Rptr. 79 (1970); *Dickinson v. Mailliard,* 175 N.W. 2d 588, 36 A.L.R. 3d 425 (Iowa 1970): (A hospital was not liable for the negligence of a staff radiologist, even when the patient did not select the physician); *Heins v. Synkonis,* 58 Mich. 119, 227 N.W. 2d 247 (1975).
[66]For example: *Gilstrap v. Osteopathic Sanitorium Company,* 224 Mo. App. 798, 24 S.W. 2d 249 (1929); *James v. Holder and City of New York,* 309 N.Y.S. 2d 385 (1970); *Newton County v. Nickolson,* 132 Ga. App. 164, 207 S.E. 2d 659 (1974).
[67]*Waynick v. Reardon,* 236 N.C. 116, 72 S.E. 2d 4 (1952); *City of Miami v. Oates,* 152 Fla. 21, 10 So. 2d 721 (1942).

have ignored their status as professional persons, and the clear trend in the cases is to acknowledge no distinction between a medical act and nonmedical act.[68] The patient has not employed these house physicians, who are usually compensated by the hospital. The strict application of the borrowed-servant and captain-of-the-ship doctrines on appropriate facts would change the foregoing conclusion with respect to the liability of the hospital, but as discussed below these doctrines have been substantially modified in recent years.

Moreoever, the increasingly important doctrine of apparent or ostensible agency provides an avenue for a court to circumvent the independent contractor rule and hold the hospital vicariously responsible for the tort of a physician. Reliance on this doctrine will grow, as specialization in medicine increases and as hospitals turn more to various types of contractual arrangements with medical specialists. A modern community hospital finds the services of specialists indispensable in providing patients with proper care. Sometimes the contractual arrangement between a hospital and a specialist emerges as a contract of service, with the specialist compensated by salary; sometimes the contract is a lease of space; frequently a contract for services provides that the specialist is compensated by a stated percentage of either gross or net departmental income. In any case, the patient as a rule does not voluntarily select the hospital-based specialist whose services are procured or to whom he is referred; and frequently the patient is led to believe that the doctor is a hospital employee, even though in fact he is not.

In such circumstances quite a number of courts, applying the apparent agency doctrine, have reached the conclusion that the hospital is liable for the negligence or malpractice of a doctor. In the leading California case of *Seneris v. Haas* an anesthesiologist's negligence led to hospital liability.[69] The physician worked at the defendant hospital only as one of six such specialists on call, and the hospital had requested that he render service to the patient. Although the anesthesiologist billed the patient directly, the question of whether or not the patient was led to believe that an employment relationship existed was one for a jury to determine.

An Ohio hospital was held liable for the professional negligence of an independent pathologist. Representations to the patient estopped the hospital from asserting independent contractor as a defense.[70] In a Montana case, *Kober v. Stewart*, the hospital's x-ray

[68] *Klema v. St. Elizabeth's Hospital*, 170 Ohio St. 519, 166 N.E. 2d 765 (1960).
[69] 45 Cal. 2d 811, 291 P. 2d 915, 53 A.L.R. 2d 124 (1955).
[70] *Lundberg v. Bay View Hospital*, 175 Ohio St. 133, 191 N.E. 2d 821 (1963).

department was operated under contract with a private clinic. The clinic supplied the department's director and a qualified radiologist to read the patients' films. As is typical, the hospital employed all of the x-ray technicians, owned the equipment, billed the patients, and compensated the clinic by paying it 35 percent of the department's gross receipts. The Montana court held that the trial judge erred in giving a summary judgment for the hospital on the theory of independent contractor, and that it should have been an issue of fact for the jury to determine whether or not the doctor was an agent or servant of the hospital.[71]

Similar reasoning has been applied in Delaware and North Carolina to hospitals which staff their emergency rooms with full-time physicians on a contractual basis through a landlord-tenant arrangement, or a percentage of revenue, and even to those institutions utilizing a rotating on-call system of coverage.[72] As medical care and practice inevitably become more institutionally oriented, vicarious liability is certain to expand.

A very recent judicial pronouncement on the doctrine of respondeat superior in hospital liability is Beeck v. Tucson General Hospital.[73] Plaintiff's physician, an orthopedic consultant, ordered a diagnostic lumbar myelogram, which consisted of a fluoroscopic x-ray procedure to be conducted in the radiology department of Tucson General Hospital. The x-ray screen struck a needle which had been placed in the patient's spine, injuring the plaintiff, who subsequently contracted pneumonia. At issue was whether the hospital was liable for the negligence of the radiologist.

The radiologist and his partner had an exclusive contract with the hospital for professional services. The physicians were compen-

---

[71] 148 Mont. 117, 417 P. 2d 476 (1966).
[72] Rucker v. High Point Memorial Hospital, 20 N.C. App. 650, 202 S.E. 2d 610 (1974), aff'd, 285 N.C. 519, 206 S.E. 2d 196 (1974). Schagrin v. Wilmington Medical Center, 304 A. 2d 61 (Delaware Super. Ct. 1973); Vanaman v. Milford Memorial Hospital, 272 A. 2d 718 (Delaware 1970): (The jury was to determine whether a staff physician on assigned, rotating emergency-room duty treated the patient in his "private" capacity or in the capacity of one performing a hospital function); Mduba v. Benedictine Hospital, 384 N.Y.S. 2d 527, 52 A.D. 2d 450 (1976): (A hospital was liable for the negligence of physicians staffing its emergency-room coverage, notwithstanding contractual language to the effect that physicians were independent contractors, since the defendant hospital held itself out to the public as providing emergency services). See also: Restatement (Second) of Torts, sec. 429. One who employs an independent contractor to perform services for another which are accepted in the reasonable belief they are being rendered by the employer is liable for physical harm caused by negligence of the contractor. Contra: Pogue v. Hospital Authority of DeKalb County, 120 Ga. App. 230, 170 S.E. 2d 53 (1969): (A member of a medical partnership under contract with a hospital to staff the emergency room was ruled an independent contractor).
[73] 18 Ariz. App. 165, 500 P. 2d 1153 (1972).

sated, as is frequently the case, by a percentage of the departmental income. Undoubtedly both the hospital and the physicians considered their relationship to be that of employer and independent contractor.

Nevertheless the Arizona appellate court found the relationship to be one of employment and reversed the summary judgment for the hospital.[74] The hospital could thus be vicariously liable for the physician's negligence. The result, said the court, was justified by the following factors: the patient had not personally selected the radiologist, and she had no choice of physician; the hospital had the legal right to control standards of professional performance; the contract was an exclusive arrangement for radiological services which are an essential function of the hospital; the doctors did not practice privately; and, finally, the hospital owned the space, bought the supplies and equipment, employed the department technicians, controlled the billing to patients, provided vacations, and controlled the hours of work.[75]

Furthermore, according to the court, a form headed "Conditions of Admissions," which the patient signed, thereby purportedly agreeing to such an independent contractor relationship and acknowledging that the radiologist was not an employee of the hospital, was of no legal effect.[76] To be sure, in *Beeck* the patient, a native of Germany, was handicapped in her understanding of English, this being one reason why the court disregarded the contractual language.[77] The result would probably be the same, however, even without any language barrier, chiefly because the bargaining power of the parties in the hospital setting is so grossly unequal.

It seems perfectly clear that hospital nurses are employees of the institution when performing their routine nursing functions, including carrying out medical orders. In 1957, New York led the way by abolishing any distinction between medical and administrative nursing acts in the landmark case of *Bing v. Thunig.*[78]

One of the most recent cases to follow *Bing* is *Bernardi v. Community Hospital* in Colorado. A seven-year-old patient suffered permanent injury to his foot after an injection of tetracycline into an adjacent nerve. The injection, ordered by the attending physician, had been given by a hospital nurse. In the suit against the hospital the defendant contended that this negligence, if any, occurred during the course

---

[74] 500 P. 2d at 1159.
[75] 500 P. 2d at 1158.
[76] 500 P. 2d at 1159.
[77] *Id.*
[78] 2 N.Y. 2d 656, 163 N.Y.S. 2d 3, 143 N.E. 2d 3 (1957).

of a medical act for which the hospital could not be held vicariously liable. The Colorado Supreme Court held, however, in accordance with *Bing v. Thunig*, that the doctrine of respondeat superior did apply to the hospital.[79] On the other hand, the physician who gave the order could not be held liable vicariously because he was not the master of the nurse. He was not present at the time the nurse gave the injection and thus possessed no control over her action; the mere giving of a medical order does not create a master-servant relationship between the physician and the hospital nurse. Nor could the doctor be held liable for personal fault, since there was no negligence in his giving the order. In a nursing situation similar to that in *Bernardi*, a hospital was liable when a nurse conducting a gastric analysis negligently administered a solution of 10-percent sodium hydroxide instead of the prescribed 85-percent saline solution.[80]

Another significant aspect of *Bernardi v. Community Hospital* should be noted. The Colorado court held that the hospital's incident report was available to the plaintiff and admissible into evidence.[81] Argument on behalf of the hospital contended that the report of the incident was prepared for the hospital attorney and thus fell within the attorney-client privilege. In ruling against the hospital the court observed that a copy of the report was filed in the patient's medical record with copies to both the hospital administrator and the director of nurses. The hospital's counsel acknowledged that he had not seen this particular report until after suit was filed. In view of the report's distribution throughout the hospital and the attorney's testimony regarding his understanding of the purpose of the report, the court concluded that the report was prepared for the hospital's administration as a management aid and thus was not protected by the attorney-client privilege. In other words, the report was not prepared for the attorney, even though his general advice was to use incident reports and even though the reports were from time to time made available to him.

The danger—as a potential result of this ruling—is that hospitals will now hesitate to prepare incident reports of accidents. Such a result would be extremely unfortunate because the analysis of incidents by hospital administration, medical staff, and counsel is neces-

---

[79] 166 Colo. 280, 443 P. 2d 708 (1968).
[80] *Gault v. Poor Sisters, d/b/a St. Joseph's Hospital*, 375 F. 2d 539 (6th Cir. 1967).
[81] Note 79 above. *Contra: Picker X-Ray Corporation v. Frerker*, 405 F. 2d 916 (8th Cir. 1969). (A hospital incident report was ruled not admissible in evidence because it was prepared by persons not available as witnesses or subject to cross-examination.)

sary to improve standards of patient care and prevent future mistakes. Moreover, the provisions of most hospital malpractice insurance policies require the reporting of incidents. This Colorado decision should not become an excuse to discontinue systems of incident reporting. Rather, hospital counsel should carefully analyze the case and use it to strengthen systems of incident reporting, stressing that the primary purpose of a report is to enable the attorney and insurance carrier to evaluate potential hospital liability arising from an incident. Copies can still be forwarded to the hospital administrator and supervisory professional personnel, for they too need to know the possible legal implications of an event. A copy of the report should not, however, be filed in the patient's medical record. As attorneys know, the medical chart is generally admissible in evidence, and the filing of the incident report in the chart is inconsistent with the primary purpose of a reporting system.

Incident reports should be strictly factual, describing when and how the accident occurred, the condition of the patient before, during, and after the accident, and what was done by way of remedial action. They should include supporting statements of witnesses. Never should an incident report contain either accusations of fault directed toward particular hospital employees or physicians, or opinions, conclusions, and assumptions with respect to the cause of the accident or injury to the patient.

In most instances the hospital employer is liable for nurses' errors in administering medication and for other manifestations of negligence in nursing. The duty of the nurse includes the obligation to notify the hospital administration if she knows, or in her professional judgment should know, that the attending physician is not caring properly for the patient.[82] Therefore nurses have a responsibility to challenge physicians and to inquire about prescriptions of medications, whenever they as professional persons know or should know that the physician's judgment is not right or that his prescription is erroneous or incomplete.

In *Norton v. Argonaut Insurance Company* a nurse received a prescription of Lanoxin for an infant patient. It read simply: "Give 3 cc Lanoxin today for one dose only." Apparently the physician intended the medication to be administered orally, and the evidence

---

[82] *Goff v. Doctor's General Hospital*, 166 Cal. App. 2d 314, 333 P. 2d 29 (1958). (When the attending physician was unavailable and the nurse knew that an obstetrical patient's life was threatened by profuse bleeding, it was negligence to fail to take action through the hospital administration to procure medical attention for the patient.)

showed that the patient had previously been receiving the drug orally. But this nurse was not aware that the drug was available in oral form, and the prescription seemed to her a large dose to be given by injection, the mode of administration familiar to her. Instead of calling the prescribing physician for clarification, she asked two other doctors present in the hospital about the prescription. They apparently told her, in effect, that if the attending physician wrote the order, then she should administer the prescription. She gave the medication by injection, and it proved to be a fatal overdose. A jury verdict against the prescribing physician was affirmed, since testimony indicated that the better practice is to specify the mode of administering such a drug. Judgment against the nurse was likewise affirmed; she was negligent in giving a drug with which she was not familiar. Finally, the hospital was vicariously liable on the doctrine of respondeat superior because the nurse was acting as an employee within the scope of her employment at the time of her negligence.[83]

The interrelation between hospital nurses and an attending physician with respect to the latter's orders has frequently been the subject of litigation. If the order is clearly incomplete or inconsistent with acceptable standards of practice, and if the nurse knows or should have known of this lack of clarity or inconsistency, then the nurse, as noted in the *Norton* case, must challenge the order or at least try to clarify it. In short, nurses must not blindly follow the physician's order. They have their own professional responsibility for the safety and protection of the patient.

A recent case possibly in point is *Variety Children's Hospital v. Osle*, in which a surgeon removed a cyst from each of plaintiff's breasts. The two cysts were commingled and placed in the same container for transport to the pathology department. A nurse assisting the surgeon inquired about this procedure, and although the factual evidence was conflicting, the physician allegedly replied that she should use a single container since the cysts were not likely to be malignant. Because of the commingling, the pathologist was unable to determine which specimen of tissue had been removed from which breast, although even then he might have been able to obtain proper identification of each portion of tissue. After the examination revealed that one of the cysts was malignant, however, there was by that time no alternative but to remove both breasts. Testimony at trial established clearly that placing the two sections of tissue in the same

---

[83] 144 So. 2d 249 (La. Ct. App. 1962).

container was a violation of acceptable standards of practice, whether the doctor had issued an order or not; and the court rejected the hospital's argument that it was not responsible when its employees were simply carrying out the direct order of a physician.[84] The surgeon was also held liable. Possibly, also, the pathologist could have been found legally responsible for his failure to attempt to reestablish the identity of the two specimens of tissue prior to dissection, but his negligence was not raised as an issue in this particular litigation.

On the other hand, of course, failure on the part of a hospital's nursing staff to execute an order by the attending physician can lead to the hospital's liability when the failure is the proximate cause of injury or death. There are numerous cases to this effect.[85] A leading New York case, Toth v. Community Hospital at Glen Cove, establishes the general proposition that nurses have a duty to follow the orders of the physician unless such orders are contrary to acceptable standards of practice.[86] Accordingly in Toth the plaintiff was entitled to a jury trial against the hospital on the factual question of whether nurses had properly followed the physician's orders or had deviated from them in administering oxygen to prematurely born twins.

Nursing personnel and other staff responsible for using or operating hospital equipment must, of course, be constantly aware of the characteristics of such equipment and continually alert ot malfunction or improper operation. Never should hospital staff be responsible for using sophisticated equipment without thorough training. In Webb v. Jorns, one of the factors leading to possible liability for the death of a patient from cardiac arrest was evidence that the arrest was caused either by an overdose of Halothane, an anesthetic agent, or by a lack of proper oxygenation of the patient. The nurse anesthetist had set the machine for a flow rate of gas mixture at two liters per minute instead of the proper rate of four liters per minute. This setting was not in conformance with the manufacturer's instructions, and hence a jury question was presented on the issue of liability of the hospital.[87]

It is not possible to identify or categorize by factual situation all

---

[84]292 So. 2d 382 (Fla. Dist. Ct. App. 1974).

[85]For example: Cline v. Lund, 31 Cal. App. 3d 755, 107 Cal. Rptr. 629 (1973). (Among other factual evidence that a hospital's negligence caused the death of a postsurgical patient were the following: the nurse failed to monitor the patient's vital signs every half-hour, as ordered by the attending physician, and when she did discover a life-threatening situation she did not promptly and immediately notify the doctor.)

[86]22 N.Y. 2d 255, 292 N.Y.S. 2d 440, 239 N.E. 2d 368 (1968).

[87]488 S.W. 2d 407 (Texas 1972).

the instances of nursing negligence. In addition to the errors in administering medication, special mention has been made of failure to obtain medical care for a patient in obvious need of it, failure to challenge or inquire about a physician's order which was recognized or should have been recognized as not conforming with acceptable standards, failure to follow a physician's order that conforms with standards of practice, and improper use of hospital equipment. One should emphasize that certain other types of cases are particularly likely to cause litigation, and some of these are examined more fully elsewhere in this book. Court decisions involving nursing in the surgical suite, which carries a high risk, will be reviewed below in the discussion of the borrowed-servant rule. The use and misuse of restraining devices has previously been discussed. Failure to follow hospital, nursing, and medical staff rules and regulations is referred to frequently throughout this chapter. Emergency room nursing is considered in Chapter VII.

A "typical" case of nursing negligence that deserves emphasis is the lack of attention to the needs of a patient, sometimes amounting to outright abandonment of the patient. A critical and primary function of nursing is the exercise of reasonable care in observing patients and recording data and information in reports to attending physicians, to whatever extent is required by the condition and needs of each patient. Nursing negligence is doing something or failing to do something contrary to what a reasonably prudent nurse would do under all the facts and circumstances, in accordance with prevailing professional standards in the community or in similar communities under like circumstances.

A dramatic illustration of inattention to the needs of the patient is provided by the recent case of *Hiatt v. Groce.* After notice had been given to her physician, Mrs. Hiatt was admitted to Bethany Hospital for the birth of a child. She was placed in the labor room and spent an uneventful night. The next morning Nurse Groce came on duty and instructed Mr. Hiatt to time the length and interval of his wife's labor pains. He and the patient's mother, who herself had given birth to sixteen children, did so, and at least three times in approximately an hour and a half they reported the frequency and intensity of the pains to the nurse, who was in a room down the hallway reading a magazine. Instead of responding promptly and examining the patient, the nurse continued to read her magazine. Twice she did measure the dilation of the patient at seven and eight centimeters but then ignored information from Mr. Hiatt that his wife had given birth to their first child upon reaching eight centimeters

of dilation. The hospital nurse also disregarded the information that
Mrs. Hiatt's labor pains were occurring at intervals of about two
minutes, refused several requests to summon the patient's physician,
and repeatedly told Mr. Hiatt and his mother-in-law that she was
in charge and would do whatever was necessary, remarking at one
point to Mr. Hiatt, "This hospital has never lost a father yet, so
you just go back there and sit down."

Following that remark Nurse Groce returned to the nurses' office
and resumed the reading of her magazine. Mrs. Hiatt's doctor was
not summoned until birth had begun. The baby was then delivered
by the nurse while an unscrubbed physician, Dr. Sullivan, who was
hastily brought in from the hallway, simply observed. To make matters
worse, the hospital ordered Nurse Groce to record in the patient's
chart that Dr. Sullivan had delivered the infant, although in fact
he had not. As a result of the delivery, the patient suffered lacerations
that required extensive suturing and caused extreme pain and
discomfort. The Supreme Court of Kansas upheld a jury verdict
of $15,000 for the plaintiff, even in the absence of expert testimony
that the standard of nursing care had been violated and even after
experts for the defendants had testified that the standard had been
met.[88] In the words of the court:

> Expert medical testimony is ordinarily required to establish
> negligence on the part of either a physician or a hospital
> in their care and treatment of a patient, unless the medical
> procedures employed are so patently bad that negligence
> or lack of skill is manifest to a lay observer or other acts
> complained of' could be regarded as negligent by applying
> the common knowledge and experience of mankind.[89]

A nurse to whom a medical task is delegated must exercise the
same care required of a physician. Hence, in *Thompson v. Brent*
a nurse given the task of removing a cast with a Stryker saw was
held to the standards required of a doctor performing the same
act.[90] Similarly, in *McBride v. United States* a hospital resident physician
who misinterpreted an electrocardiogram was measured by the
standard of physicians generally in similar communities, rather than
by what could reasonably be expected from a young doctor without
special training or skill.[91] In contrast, a relatively old Ohio case held

[88] 215 Kan. 14, 523 P. 2d 320 (1974).
[89] 215 Kan. 14, 19, 523 P. 2d 320, 324 (1974).
[90] 245 So. 2d 751 (La. Ct. App. 1971).
[91] 462 F. 2d 72 (9th Cir. 1972).

that interns were required to possess such skill and to exercise such diligence as interns ordinarily possess and exercise under similar circumstances, having regard to the same or similar localities. According to the ruling, it would be unreasonable under the circumstances of this case (service in a hospital's emergency room) to hold an intern to the same degree of knowledge and skill as a practicing physician.[92] Nurses, resident physicians, and interns are developing more independence in their functions, and other cases will probably arise which will further specify the standard of care required of these professional persons.

Attention should be addressed to still another development of personal injury law as articulated by the courts, one that has created significantly greater exposure to liability in tort. It relates to the ability of an unborn child to maintain a cause of action in tort for injuries or for death inflicted by a tort-feasor prior to birth.

At common law an infant in the womb of the mother had no separate legal existence. Hence if it was subsequently born alive but with injuries resulting from a tort before birth the infant had no cause of action.[93] Because there could be no recovery of damages by the injured infant for prenatal injuries, any damages had to be sought by the mother for her own injuries. Moreover, if an unborn fetus was killed or suffered death as the result of a tort, there was no cause of action in the estate of the deceased infant or in the survivors, since at common law no tort cause of action could be based upon the death of any person.

Both of these rules have been changed, the former in the vast majority of states, and the latter in nearly half the jurisdictions. With respect to a cause of action for prenatal injuries the modern rule, accepted in nearly all states, is clearly that an infant born alive with injuries resulting from a tort committed at a time when it was viable in the womb of the mother may maintain an action for personal damages.[94] This judicial development recognizes that a viable unborn infant is capable of life separate from the mother and accordingly should have legal rights in addition to and independent of the mother's. Some jurisdictions have even extended the right to recover

---

[92] *Rush v. Akron Hospital,* 84 Ohio L. Abs. 292, 171 N.E. 2d 378 (Ct. App. 1957).
[93] *Dietrich v. Inhabitants of Northampton,* 138 Mass. 14, 52 A.L.R. 242, (1884); *Drobner v. Peters,* 232 N.Y. 220, 133 N.E. 567, 20 A.L.R. 1503 (1921).
[94] *Woods v. Lancet,* 303 N.Y. 349, 102 N.E. 2d 691, 27 A.L.R. 2d 1250 (1951). *Sylvia v. Gobeille,* 101 R.I. 176, 220 A. 2d 222 (1966): (A mother's physician did not administer gamma globulin for exposure during pregnancy to german measles. The child, born deformed, could recover damages); *Womark v. Buckhorn,* 384 Mich. 718, 187 N.W. 2d 218 (1971); *Bonbrest v. Kotz,* 65 F. Supp. 138 (D.C. 1946).

for prenatal injuries to fetuses not viable in the legal sense. Pennsylvania, for example, has recognized a right of action in a person born deformed, when the tort causing injury occurred at one month of pregnancy.[95] To put the matter concisely, in the context of cases raising the issue of the right to recover for prenatal injuries the courts now recognize that modern concepts of justice require recognition of a child's legal right to begin life with a sound mind and body.

Consistent with this recognition of a cause of action for prenatal injuries are the recent cases in which a cause of action against a tort-feasor is granted to the estate of or to the survivors of a viable unborn fetus that is stillborn or loses life as the result of the tort. As mentioned above, the common law took the view that no cause of action could be based upon the death of any person. In other words, tort causes of action died with the death of the victim. Hence the estate of the victim had no cause of action, nor had the survivors who lost the services and companionship of the deceased.[96]

In both England and the United States this ancient doctrine was changed by statute to provide for the survival of causes of action based upon tort. Every state has some type of statutory remedy for wrongful death. Most of the statutes create a new cause of action for death and permit the estate of the decedent to recover damages. Some states, however, provide merely that the decedent's cause of action "survives" his death and that damages resulting from the death can be recovered. Under either type of statute the proper plaintiff is the executor or the administrator of the decedent's estate. In still other states the statutes permit a new cause of action for the benefit of particularly named surviving relatives, who may maintain the action for damages in their names.

Whatever type of statute exists in a particular state, an issue still remains: does the statute apply when the death of an unborn fetus results from a tort? Since most of the statutes do not precisely answer this question the matter is one for judicial decision. The clear trend of judicial decisions is in the affirmative. Approximately half the states now recognize that an action may be maintained for the death of a viable unborn child. Others have expressly forbidden such actions. Illustrating the concept that a viable fetus is a "person," thus entitling the estate or the surviving relatives to maintain an action in tort

---

[95] *Sinkler v. Kneale*, 401 Pa. 267, 164 A. 2d 93 (1960).
[96] *Baker v. Bolton*, 1 Camp. 493, 170 Eng. Rep. 1033 (1808).

under the local statute, are recent decisions in Michigan, Illinois, and Oregon.[97]

This brief overview of liability based on respondeat superior reveals a strong tendency to place liability on the institution for the negligent acts of professional persons working or performing services inside or near the hospital's "walls." Liability, like medical practice, has been institutionalized.

These expanding concepts of the doctrine of respondeat superior were readily predictable as early as 1960, when it had become apparent that charitable hospitals were no longer protected by immunity from tort liability. In that year this observation seemed pertinent:

> The third trend in the law of hospital liability is the most significant. It is the increasing tendency . . . to impose vicarious liability on facts where none would have been imposed heretofore. By some leading decisions it no longer follows that a professional person using his own skill, judgment and discretion in regard to the means and methods of his work is an independent contractor. . . . Gradually, the test of hospital liability for another's act is becoming simply a question of whether or not the actor causing injury was a part of the medical care organization.[98]

Borrowed-Servant and Captain-of-the-Ship Doctrines

The doctrine of the borrowed or loaned servant holds that a resident physician, a nurse, or some other person usually in the employ of the hospital may temporarily become an employee under the direct control and supervision of another. When the doctrine applies, the new temporary master is liable for the negligence of the employee under the doctrine of respondeat superior. The determining factor in the application of the borrowed-servant doctrine is, in theory, the right to control and direct the means and methods of the servant's work.

Most of the cases which have applied the borrowed-servant doctrine have involved negligent acts during obstetrical delivery or surgery, although application of the notion is not necessarily limited to such

---

[97] *O'Neill v. Morse*, 385 Mich. 130, 188 N.W. 2d 785 (1971): (The estate of a stillborn infant had a cause of action for wrongful death); *Maniates v. Grant Hospital*, 15 Ill. App. 3d 907, 305 N.E. 2d 422 (1973): (A father might maintain action for negligence in treating a viable fetus born dead); *Libbee v. Permanente Clinic*, 268 Ore. 258, 518 P. 2d 636 (1974): (Cause of action exists for alleged negligence by hospital staff in failing to monitor frequently enough a fetal heartbeat, with the result that the infant was stillborn).
[98] Southwick, "Vicarious Liability of Hospitals," 44 *Marq. L. Rev.* 153, 182 (1960).

factual situations. The fundamental idea of the doctrine is that the temporary employer or master has not himself been personally negligent in any way but is vicariously liable for the tort of another on the basis of his right to control that person's negligent acts or omissions. The concept is also frequently referred to as the captain-of-the-ship doctrine, meaning that the head surgeon, who is often the central figure in surgery or childbirth, is captain of all those assisting him and hence liable for any negligent act committed by a member of the surgical team.

The doctrine is illustrated by the Vermont case of *Minogue v. Rutland Hospital.* A nurse generally in the employ of the hospital was assisting a private physician during obstetric delivery. When she applied pressure to the patient's chest, as the doctor had requested, she fractured the patient's rib. The physician was liable for her negligence.[99] An often cited case, now substantially modified as we shall see, is *McConnell v. Williams,* decided in 1949 by the Supreme Court of Pennsylvania. A surgeon completing a Caesarean section was liable for the negligent act of an intern who introduced an excessive amount of silver nitrate into the eyes of the newborn infant.[100] In actuality the surgeon had no physical control over the intern's act, but it was said that he had the ultimate right of control over the surgical suite and over every person, whether a hospital employee or an independent contractor employed by the patient, who assisted in the surgery. Hence the surgeon was vicariously liable for the intern's act. In *Aderheld v. Bishop,* a surgeon was liable for the negligence of nurses assisting him, and in another Oklahoma case a radiologist was liable for the act of a hospital x-ray technician.[101] In an extreme instance, a physician was liable for the negligence of a hospital intern who had taken a medical history and failed to note that the patient was allergic to penicillin.[102]

These borrowed-servant, captain-of-the-ship cases, one should note, were decided in an era when the hospital was judicially immune from liability as a charitable institution, and at a time when medical-surgical practice was less specialized than at present—in other words, before the professional development and the consequent recognition of independent functions and responsibilities on the part of nurses,

---

[99]119 Vt. 336, 125 A. 2d 796 (1956).
[100]361 Pa. 355, 65 A. 2d 243 (1949). *McConnell* has been substantially modified by *Tonsic v. Wagner,* 458 Pa. 246, 329 A. 2d 497 (1974), discussed below.
[101]94 Okla. 203, 221 P. 752, 60 A.L.R. 137 (1923); *Hull v. Enid General Hospital Foundation,* 194 Okla. 446, 152 P. 2d 693 (1944).
[102]*Yorston v. Pennell,* 397 Pa. 28, 153 A. 2d 255, 85 A.L.R. 2d 872 (1956).

interns, and resident physicians employed by the hospital. The abolition of charitable immunity and the recognition of specialized, independent functions as the responsibility of nursing personnel and others are two factors that have led to recent decisions to abolish or substantially modify the captain-of-the-ship doctrine, a point that will be emphasized in the ensuing discussion.

In regard to hospitals a recurrent assumption has been that a given individual can have only one master or employer at a time. Hence in some cases it has been suggested that if the hospital employee temporarily becomes an employee of the attending physician, who himself is an independent contractor, then the hospital is insulated from liability.[103] This, however, seems an erroneous assumption. The *Restatement of the Law of Agency*, Section 226, indicates that under proper circumstances a given employee can have two masters simultaneously. An employee can thus serve both masters, or at least serve the mutual interests of two employers, and both employers can be liable for the employee's negligence.[104] A recent hospital case has followed this dual-master concept by holding that a hospital employee participating in a surgical operation was under the concurrent control of the hospital and an independent anesthesiologist.[105] The patient was entitled to go to jury in his suit against the hospital for nerve injuries that he sustained under anesthesia.

Recent cases illustrate that a physician who orders or prescribes treatment or medication does not become a temporary employer of the nurse carrying out the order. Normally, of course, the physician is not physically present at the time drugs are administered or treatment given, and he has no real ability to control the course of events. To illustrate, in *Honeywell v. Rogers* an infant patient suffered paralysis of the left leg. It was claimed that the injury resulted from a hypodermic injection ordered by a physician and given by a nurse. The physician had sketched instructions for administering the injection, although the technique of the administration was known to the nurse and practiced in the hospital, and he was held not responsible.[106] There was no evidence that he was himself negligent

[103] *Minogue v. Rutland Hospital*, 119 Vt. 336, 125 A. 2d 796 (1956); *Norland v. Washington General Hospital*, 461 F. 2d 694 (8th Cir. 1972): (It was ruled proper for the trial court to dismiss a case against the hospital and its insurance carrier when allegedly negligent acts of a hospital nurse assisting an obstetrician caused injury to an infant. Under Arkansas law, the hospital is not liable when the borrowed-servant doctrine is applicable); *McConnell v. Williams*, n. 100, was frequently interpreted as so holding.
[104] *Dickerson v. American Sugar Refining Company*, 211 F. 2d 200 (3d Cir. 1954).
[105] *Matlick v. Long Island Jewish Hospital*, 267 N.Y.S. 2d 631, 25 App. Div. 538 (1966). See also: *Tonsic v. Wagner*, 458 Pa. 246, 329 A. 2d 497 (1974), discussed below, reaching the same conclusion.
[106] 251 Fed. Supp. 841 (W. D. Pa. 1966).

in writing the prescription or issuing instructions. Moreover, the nurse was not a borrowed servant of the doctor, because he did not control the administration of the medication and therefore he could not be vicariously liable.

A similar case was *Bria v. St. Joseph's Hospital.* Here the trial court, it was said on appeal, should have instructed the jury that the doctor was not liable under the doctrine of respondeat superior when he ordered a certain postsurgical injection and when injury to the patient resulted because the hypodermic needle penetrated the sciatic nerve.[107]

In other words, according to these cases, the borrowed-servant rule does not apply to nonsurgical medication where negligence occurs in administering drugs. The hospital is liable for a nurse's error, but the attending physician is not responsible unless he was personally negligent in preparing the prescription or order, or in allowing the nurse to give the drug.

There is ample evidence that the courts are abandoning the borrowed-servant rule and the captain-of-the-ship doctrines, thereby removing potential liability from the physician and placing it upon the hospital, or that they are modifying the doctrines by finding the hospital and the doctor to be in concurrent control. As noted earlier, the substantive law of tort now permits the charitable hospital to be held liable. Even more significant is judicial recognition that nurses and other paramedical personnel possess independent professional responsibility and that in many situations the chief surgeon or attending physician has no real ability to control or direct the activities of those who carry out his orders regarding a patient's care.

Perhaps the first evidence of the decline of the borrowed-servant rule occurred in the cases where surgical sponges were miscounted. Several decisions have held that a nurse assisting in surgery remains under the general control of the hospital while she is performing a sponge count and reporting the count to the surgeon.[108] Hence,

---

[107] 153 Conn. 626, 220 A. 2d 29 (1966). Accord: *Burns v. Owens,* 459 S.W. 2d 303 (Mo. 1970). (A physician who admitted a patient to the hospital and a physician who prescribed Demerol were not liable for a nurse's negligence in injecting the drug.)

[108] *French v. Fisher,* 50 Tenn. App. 587, 362 S.W. 2d 926 (1962); *Danks v. Maher,* 177 So. 2d 412 (La. Ct. App. 1965); *Grant v. Touro Infirmary,* 254 La. 204, 223 So. 2d 148 (1969); *Buzan v. Mercy Hospital,* 203 So. 2d 11, 29 A.L.R. 3d 1059 (Fla. Dist. Ct. App. 1967): (Summary judgment for a hospital should not have been given in a case of a mistaken sponge count. Rather it was a question of fact for the jury whether the nurse at the time of the negligence was the hospital's servant or the surgeon's borrowed servant); *Sparger v. Worley Hospital,* 547 S.W. 2d 582 (Tex. 1977): (A hospital was liable for a nurse's mistaken sponge count, and the surgeon not vicariously liable for her negligence. The captain-of-ship doctrine was expressly rejected).

if an error is made in the count and damage to the patient results, the surgeon would not be liable to the patient. In reaching this conclusion some courts have attempted to distinguish between "administrative acts" and "medical acts" by nurses or other paramedical personnel, refusing to apply the borrowed-servant rule for administrative acts. But such a distinction is quite unsatisfactory and cannot be equitably applied. Instead, the inquiry on a case-by-case basis should be whether or not the physician against whom liability is asserted actually had the right and the power to control the activities of the negligent person. Consistent with the trend in cases involving surgical sponge counts is *Nichter v. Edmiston,* which held that a surgeon was not liable for the negligence of a nurse who had applied an excessive amount of disinfectant to a patient's arm, causing a burn when it made contact with an electrical surgical needle.[109]

In *Salgo v. Leland Stanford, Jr., University Board of Trustees,* the head surgeon was not liable for the negligence of an anesthesiologist;[110] and in *Thompson v. Liliehei* the surgeon was not liable for the acts of other physicians on the surgical team.[111] In the latter case all members of the surgical team were on salary from the hospital and were assigned to their separate roles by the head of the department of surgery. In a different medical situation, the hospital was liable for the negligence of personnel in permitting a weak patient in the x-ray department to stand until the patient fainted and fell. The hospital employees were not acting under the direct supervision and control of the doctor; therefore the hospital, not the doctor, was liable.[112]

The North Carolina court has held that even though a hospital-based salaried pathologist had general supervisory responsibility and control over the work of technologists who were also employed and paid by the hospital he was not the employer of the technologists. Thus he could not be held liable under the doctrine of respondeat superior when a technologist mislabeled a bottle of blood and the incompatible blood caused the death of a patient.[113] In New Jersey a private surgeon was ruled not vicariously responsible for the

---

[109]81 Nev. 606, 407 P. 2d 721 (1965).
[110]154 Cal. App. 2d 560, 317 P. 2d 170 (Dist. Ct. App. 1957). Accord: *Dohr v. Smith,* 104 So. 2d 29 (Fla. 1958). (Even though the surgeon is generally in command of surgery from beginning to end, the anesthetist performs his or her expert service independently.)
[111]164 F. Supp. 716 (D. Minn. 1958), *aff'd,* 273 F. 2d 376 (8th Cir. 1959).
[112]*Hillcrest Medical Center v. Wier,* 373 P. 2d 45 (Okla. 1962).
[113]*Davis v. Wilson,* 265 N.C. 139, 143 S.E. 2d 107 (1965).

negligence of a hospital resident physician who was carrying out postoperative orders of the surgeon.[114]

Two matters must be stressed, however, with respect to this strong judicial trend away from the borrowed-servant and captain-of-the-ship doctrines. First, since liability imposed by the doctrines is vicarious and rests upon the right of control over another's acts or omissions, the issue of control may on a case-by-case basis be a question of fact for the jury to decide. For example, a Virginia court in *Whitfield v. Whitaker Memorial Hospital* so held when liability was asserted against a surgeon for the negligent act of a nurse anesthetist.[115] In *Whitfield* there was evidence that the surgeon had chosen the anesthetic and had told the nurse when to begin and to stop administering it. In the absence of factual evidence showing real ability to control the activities of another who is assisting the doctor or carrying out his orders, the matter becomes one for the court to decide as a matter of law, as is amply demonstrated by many of the previous citations.

The second point is that a privately employed physician or surgeon, or indeed even a physician on salary from the hospital, can be personally liable for his own negligence in writing a prescription or giving an order to a nurse or to another, such as an intern or resident. Moreover the attending doctor can be liable for delegating a task to one whom he knows or should have known to be incapable of executing it or untrained for the task. In both of these situations the liability is direct and not vicarious. Hence attending physicians and surgeons must be certain that their orders to others are consistent with the qualifications and training of the persons to whom they delegate the task and that they accord with accepted standards of practice as well. Furthermore an attending physician or surgeon who retains or possesses a degree of control over any person assisting him always has his own responsibility to exercise reasonable care with respect to this right of supervision and control.

The foregoing statement is illustrated in the 1974 case of *Foster v. Englewood Hospital Association.* The patient, who had undergone surgery for a shoulder separation, expired from a lack of oxygen. When the defendant surgeon left the operating suite immediately after the surgery, the patient needed assistance in breathing, and oxygen was being given by the nurse anesthetist using a hand-con-

---

[114] *Stumper v. Kimel,* 108 N.J. Super. 209, 260 A. 2d 526 (App. Div. 1970).

[115] 210 Va. 176, 169 S.E. 2d 563 (1969); *Synott v. Midway Hospital,* 287 Minn. 270, 178 N.W. 2d 211 (1970): (It was a jury question whether on the facts an x-ray technician was a servant of the hospital or a servant of the surgeon).

trolled bag. The anesthetist then removed the patient to the recovery
room and connected a Bennett resuscitating machine. By this time
the patient's blood pressure was dangerously low and he was without
a detectable pulse. For the first time the nurse anesthetist realized
that the patient was in serious difficulty. Other physicians were called
in but were unable to resuscitate the patient, and death was pro-
nounced an hour later. In a suit against the estate of the defendant
surgeon, who had died just prior to the suit, the trial court directed
a verdict for the estate notwithstanding a jury's award of damages.
The appellate court of Illinois reversed.

The reversal was not, however, based upon the borrowed-servant
doctrine. Indeed, the court expressly rejected this doctrine and wrote
that employees of the hospital, including nurse anesthetists, remain
employees when assisting a surgeon. Nevertheless the surgeon does
retain elements of control and supervision over other persons participating in the operation, and he must exercise that control with
reasonable care. Since it is usual and customary medical practice
for the surgeon to remain in the operating room until the patient
is breathing without assistance, and since the patient should not
have been moved until that time, the surgeon could be found to
have breached his duty of reasonable supervision. It was therefore
proper to submit the issue of the surgeon's liability to the jury,
and the trial court's judgment was in error. In addition, both the
nurse anesthetist and the hospital were liable in damages.[116]

When a hospital furnishes an employee to assist a privately engaged
surgeon, the hospital has its own duty to the patient to exercise
reasonable care in assigning the employee to perform his or her
responsibilities as a member of the surgical team. Thus a hospital
was found liable by a jury when it employed a physician on salary
who was not licensed to practice medicine in Florida, and who had
never performed surgery at the time of his employment, and when
it nevertheless assigned him to assist in surgery. Such a hospital
could be found solely liable by a jury as long as there was no evidence
of negligence on the part of the private surgeon on any of the
theories discussed above.[117] In that situation the surgeon would be
entitled to full indemnification from the hospital and its employee
should a jury award damages to the patient against him.

If hospital-owned equipment in the surgical suite or elsewhere
injures a patient because it is defective, malfunctioning, or improperly

[116] 19 Ill. App. 3d 1055, 313 N.E. 2d 255 (1974).
[117] *Maybarduk v. Bustamante*, 294 So. 2d 374 (Fla. Dist. Ct. App. 1974).

operated by a hospital employee, the attending doctor or surgeon would not normally be liable to the patient unless he knew or should have known from the facts of the particular case that the equipment was unfit for the intended purpose or that the operator was incompetent. To put the matter another way, negligence on the part of the hospital in maintaining the equipment, or negligence by a hospital employee in operating the equipment, would not impose vicarious liability on the physician. The borrowed-servant and captain-of-the-ship doctrines would not apply. For example, an electrical cauterizing tool malfunctioned or was improperly operated by a hospital nurse during a hemorrhoidectomy and the patient suffered burns as a result. The surgeon was not liable for the injury on an assertion of the borrowed-servant rule, since he lacked the requisite amount of control over the machine and its operator.[118]

Two cases provide a sharp contrast in judicial policy—and a good illustration of how law or the interpretation of law changes as time brings changing circumstances and philosophies. These are the Pennsylvania case in 1974 of *Tonsic v. Wagner and Pittsburgh Hospital Association,*[119] which has substantially modified the captain-of-the-ship doctrine, and *McConnell v. Williams,* in which the doctrine was articulated in 1949.[120] At the conclusion of a colectomy operation performed by a Dr. Wagner, a Kelly clamp was not removed from Mrs. Tonsic's abdomen. The surgeon had been assisted by hospital nurses and an intern, as well as by Dr. Weitzel, an associate of Dr. Wagner. No member of the surgical team counted the surgical instruments or in any way kept a record of the instruments to be certain that all were removed from the patient. No one called Dr. Wagner's attention to the lost clamp when he closed the incision. The hospital did not have any rules or regulations requiring an instrument count.

The trial court judge, following literally the language and the apparent holding of *McConnell v. Williams,* ruled that the head surgeon, Dr. Wagner, was captain of the ship and instructed the jury that he could be vicariously liable for the negligence, if any, of a member of the surgical team. But the hospital could not be liable under the doctrine of respondeat superior, in his judgment, even though it was the general employer of the nurses and intern. The judge refused the request of plaintiff to rule that a jury must

---

[118] *May v. Broun,* 261 Ore. 28, 492 P. 2d 776 (1972).
[119] 458 Pa. 246, 329 A. 2d 497 (1974).
[120] 361 Pa. 355, 65 A. 2d 243 (1949), n. 100 and text above.

determine whether the hospital employees at the time of the event were under the control of the surgeon, the hospital, or both. The jury returned a verdict against Dr. Wagner amounting to $37,000.

The precise question on appeal to the Supreme Court of Pennsylvania was whether the trial court erred in ruling as a matter of law that the hospital could not be vicariously liable for the negligence of its personnel during the surgery. Noting that *McConnell* really did not specifically hold the hospital not liable—since charitable hospitals were then immune from tort liability, the hospital's liability was really not an issue—the court in *Tonsic* reversed the trial court, saying that the instructions to the jury referring to the captain-of-the-ship doctrine were erroneous.

As noted earlier in this discussion, a person may be a servant of two masters at one time as to one negligent act, even though the masters are not joint employers, provided that the service to one master does not involve an abandonment of the service to another.[121] Hence in *Tonsic* it became a question for the jury whether the surgeon or the hospital was the sole controlling master, or whether there was a joint control justifying the imposition of liability on both the surgeon and the hospital for the negligent act of a member of the surgical team. The plaintiff was accordingly entitled to a new trial in her suit against the hospital, the new trial to be solely on the issue of liability of the hospital; and the amount of the jury's verdict against the surgeon was permitted to stand.

Justice Pomeroy wrote a perceptive dissenting opinion in the *Tonsic* case, emphasizing in effect the difference between hospital liability based upon the doctrine of respondeat superior and the breach of a direct corporate duty owed to the patient. He agreed in principle with the law of agency as articulated by the majority of the court. But he stressed that the trial court's instructions to the jury with respect to the captain-of-the-ship doctrine, while perhaps overly broad, did not prevent the jury from finding the hospital liable on the basis of its failure to promulgate and enforce rules requiring a count of surgical instruments. The dissent pointed out that one of plaintiff's allegations of hospital negligence was the institution's failure to establish adequate safeguards against leaving clamps in a patient's body; that the trial judge had put this issue to the jury in his instructions; and that the jury had found in response to a

---

[121] *Restatement (Second) of Agency*, sec. 226 (1957); See: *Matlick v. Long Island Jewish Hospital*, 267 N.Y.S. 2d 631, 25 App. Div. 2d 538 (1966), cited in n. 105 and in the text above.

special question submitted for decision that the hospital was not negligent in failing to require a count of surgical instruments. In the view of the dissent, the jury and not the court had exonerated the hospital from liability and thus the jury verdict should stand.

The cases all indicate that the borrowed-servant doctrine is a dying defense so far as the hospital is concerned. The fundamental trends in the law of hospital liability clearly show that the institutionalization of medical care results in the institutionalization of liability. The courts are recognizing that a physician or surgeon in the hospital setting should not be held vicariously liable for the negligent act or omission of another professional person unless he has a genuine opportunity to control the other's activities. The rationale for the ancient doctrine of respondeat superior is simply public policy, and the gradual case-by-case transfer of vicarious responsibility from the operating room surgeon or some other professional to the hospital, or the recognition of dual responsibility, seems understandable because a corporate institution is better able to spread the risk of loss throughout the community.

Three Traditional Corporate or Institutional Duties

In corporate negligence, although human error or omission is involved, it is the hospital itself as an entity or a corporate institution that is negligent, and liability attaches directly to the hospital. The hospital owes a defined legal duty directly to the patient or visitor, and the duty is not delegable to the medical staff or other personnel. A Connecticut court once defined the corporate negligence of a hospital in these words: "Corporate negligence is the failure of those entrusted with the task of providing accommodations and facilities necessary to carry out the charitable purpose of the corporation to follow in a given situation the established standard of conduct to which the corporation should conform."[122]

Accordingly, the legal question is this: what duties does the hospital owe directly to the patient or visitor? To answer this query, we must consider the corporate purposes of a community hospital. Does a hospital—or should a hospital—restrict its function and role to furnishing physical facilities and accommodations wherein private physicians care for and treat their patients? In other words, is a hospital nothing more than a "doctor's workshop"? If so, the duties owed directly to the patient by the hospital can justifiably be quite

---

[122] *Bader v. United Orthodox Synagogue*, 148 Conn. 449, 453, 172 A. 2d 192, 194 (1961).

narrow and limited. Historically this has been the general attitude of the courts in corporate negligence cases.

On the other hand, if a hospital has broader purposes its corporate duties can be expected to be broader. As we noted at the outset of this discussion, the nature and role of the hospital vis-a-vis the community has indeed been broadening in recent years. Hospitals are doing more than providing physical facilities for the practice of medicine. In response to public demand, and encouraged by leaders in the medical-health care professions, hospitals are gradually becoming true community health centers. These developments will continue and accelerate in the decades ahead. In time, hospitals will become the focus for providing the community with the entire range of medical care—preventive as well as curative, out-patient care as well as care for acute illnesses demanding hospitalization. Hospitals are, and for the foreseeable future will continue to be, the primary vehicle for controlling and raising standards of quality of care. Hence court decisions in liability cases are likely to recognize the changing and central role of the hospital and gradually expand judicial concepts of corporate negligence.

MAINTENANCE OF BUILDINGS AND GROUNDS

Traditionally and historically, the situations illustrating corporate negligence were limited to three. The first is the well-recognized duty owed to all patients and invited visitors to exercise reasonable care in the maintenance of buildings and grounds. Local statutes may prescribe standards, and a violation of the statutory standards can be negligence per se. In the absence of a statutory standard the hospital must exercise reasonable care, and generally the plaintiff must prove that the defendant corporation through its employees knew or should have known of a defective or dangerous condition likely to cause injury.

Frequently these issues become jury questions, as in *Ackerberg v. Muskegon Osteopathic Hospital*[123] and *Wheeler v. Monadnock Hospital.*[124] In *Ackerberg* the Michigan Supreme Court said that the issue of negligence was for the jury to determine. In this case a father who had taken his daughter to the hospital emergency room became dizzy and stepped outside through an unmarked door. The door led to an unguarded platform, and the man fell two and a half to three feet to the ground. In the *Wheeler* case a six-year-old child

[123] 366 Mich. 596, 115 N.W. 2d 290 (1962).
[124] 103 N.H. 306, 171 A. 2d 23 (1961). See also: *Dowd v. Portsmouth Hospital,* 105 N.H. 53, 193 A. 2d 788, 95 A.L.R. 2d 986 (1963).

visitor fell from an unprotected retaining wall seven to nine feet high, and the evidence at trial tended to show that the hospital knew the wall was dangerous.

One should take special note that the mere occurrence of an accident, such as a slip or a fall, on hospital premises does not create liability to the injured person. The plaintiff must establish negligence with respect to the maintenance of premises. This requires the injured person to prove that the hospital either created a dangerous condition or that it knew or should have known of a dangerous condition and had failed to correct it. This duty to exercise reasonable care is the same as that applicable to landowners or occupiers generally with respect to those who enter upon their land. Moreover, there would not normally be liability to a person injured on the land of another if the dangerous condition had been readily apparent, open, and visible, since the plaintiff has a duty to exercise care for his own safety. Thus there was no liability when a hospital patient fell on an icy porch, because she knew the condition existed.[125]

Also worthy of emphasis is that the courts have traditionally drawn a sharp distinction between trespassers, licensees, and invitees in cases involving the liability of a landowner or occupier to those injured upon the land. The only duty owed to the trespasser is to refrain from active, willful, and wanton conduct causing injury. The traditional rule about licensees has been that they take the premises as they find them and that the only duty of the landowner or occupier is to warn them of dangerous conditions actually known to the owner or occupier and not readily apparent to the licensees. Courts have defined a licensee as one who enters upon land for his own benefit and with the owner's permission but without the owner's having any business purpose or potential economic benefit. In contrast, an invitee is a business visitor or at least one who enters land for the mutual benefit of himself and the landowner. Traditionally, only an invitee may expect the premises to be reasonably safe and free from hazard. Illustrating this historical approach is the Wisconsin case of *Voeltzke v. Kehosha Memorial Hospital* in which a visitor to a hospital fell as a result of an allegedly poorly maintained parking lot. She was considered to be a mere licensee and thus could not recover damages for her injury.[126] The clear trend of the law, however,

---

[125] *Gulfway General Hospital, Inc. v. Pursley*, 397 S.W. 2d 93, 16 A.L.R. 3d 1232 (Tex. Ct. Civ. App. 1965). See also: *Charrin v. Methodist Hospital*, 432 S.W. 2d 572 (Tex. Ct. Civ. App. 1968). (There was no liability to a patient who tripped on a television antenna wire running across the floor of her room, because she was aware of the wire.)
[126] 45 Wis. 2d 271, 172 N.W. 2d 673 (1969).

is to treat hospital visitors as invitees, thereby extending to them the same standard of care that is applicable to patients.[127] Even more significant, several courts have abolished the historical distinction between licensees and invitees (and perhaps even trespassers). Although they are not yet in the majority, they have developed a rule of law that landowners and occupiers owe to all who enter their premises a duty to exercise reasonable care in maintaining the land.[128] In determining "reasonable care," courts will consider all the facts and circumstances of each case. The principles would clearly apply to hospitals and all other medical care facilities, including of course the office premises of physicians.

MAINTENANCE OF EQUIPMENT.

The second direct corporate duty of the hospital to the patient concerns inadequate or defective equipment. This duty seems to have at least two aspects: the hospital is said to have a duty to exercise reasonable care under all the facts and circumstances in selecting equipment; and the hospital must exercise reasonable care in maintaining the equipment. An example of the first is *Milner v. Huntsville Memorial Hospital.* A heavily sedated patient was given a heating pad with three manual settings and suffered severe burns while using it during the night. Nobody knew how the control was changed to "high," but attendants could have prevented the burns by covering the pad with a towel regardless of the setting, or could have assured a particular setting by covering the control button. Consequently the trial court erred in giving a summary judgment for the hospital.[129] Rather, the question was one of fact for the jury: had the hospital failed in its duty to provide reasonably safe equipment for a sedated patient? Evidence that the same type of heating pad was used in other hospitals, and also that pads with more secure heat control mechanisms were available, could be considered by the jury.

The duty of maintaining equipment was in question in *South Highlands Infirmary v. Camp.* The hospital was ruled liable to the patient when it furnished a defective instrument used by a surgeon to remove skin.[130] Hospital personnel had not examined the instru-

[127] *Lesyk v. Park Avenue Hospital, Inc.,* 289 N.Y.S. 2d 873, 29 App. Div. 2d 1043 (1968). See also cases cited in n. 123 and 124.
[128] *Rowland v. Christian,* 70 Cal. Rptr. 97, 443 P. 2d 561, 32 A.L.R. 3d 496, (1968); *Pickard v. City and County of Honolulu,* 51 Hawaii 134, 452 P. 2d 445 (1969); *Gibo v. City and County of Honolulu,* 51 Hawaii 299, 459 P. 2d 198 (1969); *Mile High Fence Company v. Radovich,* 175 Colo. 537, 489 P. 2d 308 (1971).
[129] 398 S.W. 2d 647 (Tex. Ct. Civ. App. 1966).
[130] 279 Ala. 1, 180 So. 2d 904, 14 A.L.R. 3d 1245 (1965); *Weeks v. Latter Day Saints Hospital,* 418 F. 2d 1035 (10th Cir. 1969); *Nelson v. Swedish Hospital,* 241 Minn.

ment before it was given to the doctor, and the defendant argued that there was no duty to do so. The court rejected this argument, saying that there can be liability for failure to exercise reasonable care when equipment is furnished that is unfit for the intended uses and purposes. Similarly there was liability in a case where a footstool being used properly by the patient slipped because the rubber pads covering the four legs were very worn.[131] Liability cases involving equipment failures thus arise either because equipment was not properly selected to suit a given purpose and the patient's particular condition, as in *Milner,* or because of defective mechanical conditions which reasonably could have been discovered and corrected, as in *Camp* and *Clark.*

On the facts of the *Camp* case the physician who was using the defective instrument was not personally liable, since the defect was a "latent" one; that is, it was discoverable by proper maintenance but not by mere observation. Had the defect been obvious or clearly visible, then the user of the instrument might have been liable to the patient.

Of course, as long as the hospital has exercised reasonable care in selecting, maintaining, and operating its equipment there is no liability, even if the equipment should fail and injure the patient. To illustrate: because of an electrical power failure, a suction pump in use in the surgical suite stopped functioning, and in consequence a patient died. The death did not result in hospital liability. According to the evidence, an interruption of power, lasting from four to thirty seconds, occurred when a crane on a railroad struck a power line. A hospital employee telephoned the city's electrical department and learned that the hospital would be informed if further interruptions of power were expected, but a second failure occurred without warning. Although the hospital's emergency electrical generator had been immediately activated, the patient died during the second interruption of power. On these facts there was no negligence by the hospital, and a summary judgment for the defendant was proper.[132]

Likewise the hospital does not guarantee that all equipment will work perfectly. There was no liability when a glass thermometer broke while a nurse was shaking it down. The court observed that the hospital had carried out its duties by furnishing standard equip-

---

551, 64 N.W. 2d 38 (1954): (There is a duty to inspect and maintain hospital equipment with reasonable care).
[131] *City of Okmulgee v. Clark,* 425 P. 2d 457 (Okla. 1967).
[132] *Williams v. Lewis,* 11 N.C. App. 306, 181 S.E. 2d 234 (1971).

ment, by making reasonable inspection, and by remedying any defects discoverable by such inspections.[133] But sometimes the doctrine of res ipsa loquitur will apply to cases of faulty equipment. For example, the doctrine was held applicable in a Florida case in which a chair holding a bedpan broke, throwing a patient to the floor.[134] Similarly the court permitted res ipsa when a pivot shaft of an x-ray machine broke, injuring the patient.[135] The hospital had failed to make periodic inspections to determine whether parts had become worn, and the issue of negligence became a question of fact.

A hospital may not delegate its duties with respect to the maintenance of equipment by means of a service agreement with an independent contractor, thereby avoiding liability for a failure of equipment. Corporate duties are nondelegable. Accordingly, if such a service contract were entered into and the contractor were negligent in performing his service, the hospital would nevertheless remain liable to the patient.[136]

Failure on the part of the hospital to follow the rules and regulations of licensure authorities, the accreditation standards, and the instructional manuals supplied by the manufacturer for proper maintenance can be introduced at trial as evidence of negligence.[137] The same is probably true for the safety standards relating to equipment which are promulgated under the Federal Occupational Safety and Health Act and similar state acts. Hospital management must therefore make certain that all existing information on the maintenance and operation of hospital equipment is available and that the standards set forth in the various sources are met.

There is no duty on the part of a hospital to possess the newest, most modern equipment available on the market. In Georgia it was proper to dismiss a case in which an infant was allegedly burned by an unshielded light bulb in an incubator not equipped with a thermostatic heat control. Similar older models of such equipment were still in general use by similarly situated hospitals. The plaintiffs did not allege that the incubator was defective or unfit for the purposes intended; and the mere fact that newer equipment with automatic

---

[133] *Payne v. Garvey*, 264 N.C. 593, 142 S.E. 2d 159 (1965).
[134] *Williams v. Orange Memorial Hospital Association*, 202 So. 2d 859 (Fla. Dist. Ct. App. 1967).
[135] *Tucson General Hospital v. Russell*, 7 Ariz. App. 193, 437 P. 2d 677 (1968).
[136] *Hill v. James Walker Memorial Hospital*, 407 F. 2d 1036 (4th Cir. 1969).
[137] *Darling v. Charleston Community Memorial Hospital*, 33 Ill. 2d 326, 211 N.E. 2d 253, 14 A.L.R. 3d 860 (1965), *cert. denied*, 383 U.S. 946 (1966): (Licensure regulations and accreditation standards); *Monk v. Doctors Hospital*, 403 F. 2d 580 (D.C. Cir. 1968): (Manufacturer's instructional manual).

heat control was available on the market did not create liability.[138] More recently, a hospital's failure to equip its pathology department with a cryostat to cut tissue to be used in tests for malignancy could not be construed as negligence.[139] In place of the allegedly more sophisticated cryostat, which could cut thinner sections of tissue for more accurate diagnosis, the hospital utilized a freezing microtome process. Tissue cut by this method was examined by the hospital's pathologist and diagnosed as cancerous. In fact, there was no malignancy, and the removal of the patient's breast was unnecessary. Since plaintiff produced no expert testimony to the effect that the microtome was an unsatisfactory instrument, and since the pathologist was free from personal negligence in his mistaken diagnosis, there was no liability on either the hospital or the pathologist. There is a duty, however, to have available the customary and usual equipment for any purpose, procedure, or service that the hospital undertakes to render. Hence sterilization of hypodermic needles by boiling them in water in the open air—instead of using an appliance to sterilize them by steam under pressure—could be the basis for liability.[140]

Recent cases have expanded corporate duties regarding equipment and facilities, so that liability exists if a hospital does not have the equipment, facilities, and personnel necessary to treat the patient's case adequately. For example, there was liability in *Carrasco,* a California case in which a patient with third-degree burns was retained for 53 days in a hospital that did not have facilities for the "open method" of treating burns and for skin grafting. The court said the hospital failed to have the equipment reasonably necessary for the treatment required by the patient, and under these circumstances there was a duty to transfer the patient to another hospital.[141]

In *Ball Memorial Hospital v. Freeman* a paying out-patient was injected with a fluid labeled "Novocaine." The label had been affixed by a hospital employee and was inaccurate. In this case of a wrong medication, the plaintiff alleged that his injuries were caused by the institution's negligence in using an improper system of preparing and dispensing Novocaine. A jury verdict for the plaintiff was upheld upon appeal, the Indiana court saying that the failure to employ proper instrumentalities and facilities in preparing, bottling, and

[138] *Emory University v. Porter,* 103 Ga. App. 752, 120 S.E. 2d 668 (1961).
[139] *Lauro v. Travelers Insurance Company,* 261 So. 2d 261, 50 A.L.R. 3d 1130 (La. Ct. App. 1972).
[140] *Peck v. Charles B. Towns Hospital,* 275 App. Div. 302, 89 N.Y.S. 2d 190 (1949).
[141] *Carrasco v. Bankoff,* 220 Cal. App. 2d 230, 33 Cal. Rptr. 673, 97 A.L.R. 2d 464 (Dist. Ct. App. 1963).

dispensing medications constituted negligence on the part of the hospital.[142]

In *Ball* the doctrine of res ipsa loquitur applied, because the hospital had complete control and dominion over the instrumentality causing the injury. The surgeon had done nothing to change the character of the solution, and the crystals used in mixing the preparation were not defective in any way. The dissent held the case to be one of vicarious liability, or liability for the negligence of servants of the hospital, and maintained that charitable immunity applied. The majority of the court, however, seemed to extend the idea of corporate negligence. Now that charitable immunity for vicarious liability has been removed in Indiana by a subsequent decision, the same result could be reached on the doctrine of respondeat superior.[143] In another case involving inadequate facilities and personnel, a Texas hospital was liable when it failed to employ a licensed pharmacist and thus violated standards established by the Joint Commission on Accreditation of Hospitals and the American Hospital Association.[144]

More recently a Pennsylvania court has held that a basis of liability was created when a hospital had an inoperative electrocardiogram machine in its emergency room and no backup instrument. Because of this lack, an emergency patient had to be moved to another location, where he died while the electrocardiogram was being made.[145] The issue of proximate cause was for the jury to determine.

In *Bellaire General Hospital v. Campbell*, a Texas case, a postsurgical patient in a semiprivate room was experiencing cyanosis and receiving oxygen to aid her breathing. At the request of her husband and upon the order of her attending physicians, hospital personnel undertook to move Mrs. Campbell to a private room. Only then did they discover that the electrical outlet in the new room would not accommodate the oxygen machine. A portable oxygen unit was sent for, but during the delay of approximately five minutes the patient died from a lack of oxygen and cardiac arrest. The hospital was negligent in failing to have oxygen available in the room to which the patient had been moved, in failing to use a portable machine during the move, and in failing to have a cardiac stimulator at hand.[146]

---

[142] 245 Ind. 71, 196 N.E. 2d 274, 9 A.L.R. 3d 567 (1964).
[143] *Harris v. YWCA*, 250 Ind. 491, 237 N.E. 2d 242 (1968).
[144] *Sullivan v. Sisters of St. Francis of Texas*, 374 S.W. 2d 294 (Tex. Ct. Civ. App. 1963).
[145] *Hamil v. Bashline*, 224 Pa. Super. 407, 307 A. 2d 57 (1973).
[146] 510 S.W. 2d 94 (Tex. Ct. Civ. App. 1974).

Since these omissions established a reasonable probability of the cause of death, according to expert witnesses, the jury was justified in determining that the plaintiff had satisfactorily proved proximate cause.

Failure of hospital management and medical staff to communicate adequately can create liability on a theory of corporate neglect. Delays in communication are especially likely during holidays and weekends, a fact vividly demonstrated in *Keene v. Methodist Hospital.*[147] In this litigation a patient, who had been injured in a dispute on Christmas Eve, was x-rayed at the hospital's emergency room and sent home by a private doctor serving on rotating duty in the emergency room. Early Christmas morning the radiologist detected a possible skull fracture and suggested additional x-rays. This tentative diagnosis and recommendation was dictated into a mechanical recorder but not otherwise transmitted to the attending physician, the patient, or the hospital administration. The dictation was not transcribed for two days. In the meantime, on Christmas afternoon, the patient became unconscious and was returned to the hospital. There he underwent emergency surgery but died of a fractured skull and hemorrhage.

Even though the private physician on duty in the emergency room was negligent in his examination of the patient on Christmas Eve and in sending the patient home, this negligence could not be vicariously imposed upon the hospital. Nevertheless there was evidence that the patient's life could have been saved by timely and appropriate care, and the hospital was liable as a corporate institution for its failure to transmit immediately the radiologist's report to the treating physician or the hospital administration so that they could arrange for surgery or other treatment on Christmas morning. A hospital's failure to have and to implement adequate rules and regulations for communicating vital information to others can be costly in terms of human life.

The several foregoing cases do not mean, of course, that every community hospital, however limited in physical and human resources, must have available a complete range of equipment, facilities, and services. Specially equipped and staffed intensive care and cardiac units have recently been developed by many community hospitals.

---

[147]324 F. Supp. 233 (N.D. Ind. 1971). See also: *Ravenis v. Detroit General Hospital,* 63 Mich. App. 79, 234 N.W. 2d 411 (1975). (A hospital can be liable for negligence if it fails to establish adequate procedures to enable persons responsible for determining the suitability of a cornea for transplant to have access to the medical records of the donor.)

But there is no legal requirement that all hospitals be so equipped, and the mere absence of a cardiac care unit in a particular hospital should not lead to liability, even with statistical proof that such specially equipped units save lives. A judicial law of liability which required, in effect, that all hospitals provide a full range of facilities and specially trained personnel would be economically unsound, if not impossible, and certainly inconsistent with accepted principles of area-wide hospital planning.

What the judicial law can justifiably require in the interests of raising standards of care is to impose liability whenever a hospital holds itself out as being reasonably equipped and staffed to care for a particular patient's needs but in fact is not. The *Carrasco* case, mentioned above, can be explained and approved on this basis. Moreover it is justifiable to find liability whenever a hospital fails to employ reasonably its facilities, equipment, and staff in the face of need, or fails to implement explicit standards of accreditation or licensure. There is in general no judicial or statutory requirement that a hospital provide a fully equipped department for emergency care. When the hospital is in fact equipped for emergency care and refuses aid in an unmistakable emergency, different considerations, of course, prevail, and the refusal can lead to liability.[148] But no decision has yet been rendered—nor should one be—requiring every hospital to install all the sophisticated equipment and facilities known to modern medicine.

SELECTION AND SUPERVISION OF EMPLOYEES

The third type of corporate negligence is failure by the hospital to exercise reasonable care in selecting or retaining personnel, a matter that is often for the jury to determine.[149] This direct duty to the patient has relevance to the employment of pharmacists, medical technicians, nurses, and other professional persons in the hospital as well as to nonprofessional personnel. Certainly the administration must check the references, credentials, background, and training of all people employed. A valid current license to practice a given profession will not in and of itself establish that the hospital has met its duty of reasonable care. Furthermore the administration must make certain that its in-service training programs are up to date.

---

[148] See discussion and citations in Chapter VII.
[149] *Hipp v. Hospital Authority of Marietta, Georgia*, 104 Ga. App. 174, 121 S.E. 2d 273 (1961). (The question of liability was for the jury when a hospital employed an orderly with a criminal record for a sexual offense, and he molested a patient.) See also: *Garlington v. Kingsley*, 277 So. 183 (La. Ct. App. 1973), *rev'd on other grounds*, 289 So. 2d 88 (La. 1974).

Employees should be discharged or transferred when it has become apparent that they cannot do the assigned job. Professional individuals might also be liable for failure to supervise properly those for whom they are responsible. For example, directors of nursing or pharmacists could be individually liable for the failure to exercise reasonable care in assigning duties to subordinates, assessing qualifications, and supervising employees within their department or area of responsibility.

Negligence in Selecting and Retaining Medical Staff

The tendency to institutionalize liability, noted earlier in connection with the doctrine of respondeat superior, is even more apparent under the second of the two theories of hospital liability mentioned early in this chapter, namely, the violation of a duty owed directly by the institution to the patient. Application of this theory has constituted a direct attack upon the existing dichotomy between hospital management and medical staff. Prior to the landmark case of *Darling v. Charleston Community Memorial Hospital,* decided by the Supreme Court of Illinois in 1965,[150] the case law recognized only very limited direct duties owed by the hospital to the patient. The *Darling* decision was destined to change that. It gave impetus to a legal clarification of the respective roles of hospital trustees, administration, and medical staff.

A young man named Darling suffered a fractured leg while playing football and was brought to the Charleston Community Memorial Hospital's emergency room where he was attended by Dr. Alexander, the staff physician on call. He was thereafter admitted to the hospital as a patient of Dr. Alexander's. Then the grim series of events leading to the lawsuit occurred: the doctor's dilemmas regarding a constricted cast which was causing circulatory difficulties; the patient's continual pain and complaints; the nurses' knowledge of clinical difficulties and their failure to communicate them to hospital administration; Dr. Alexander's failure to call for a consultation, as arguably required by a medical staff bylaw; the failure of the chief of staff or the hospital administrator to seek enforcement of the bylaw; and, finally, the removal of the patient to Barnes Hospital in St. Louis, by which time it was too late to save the injured leg.

Suit was brought against both the physician and the hospital. The

---

[150] 33 Ill. 2d 326, 211 N.E. 2d 253, 14 A.L.R. 3d 860 (1965), *cert. denied*, 383 U.S. 946 (1966).

former settled the claim against him and was dismissed as a defendant
in the litigation. The case against the hospital was taken to trial,
and a jury found in favor of the plaintiff. Allegations against the
institution included claims that it had permitted an unqualified
physician to do orthopedic surgery, that the hospital failed to require
periodic reports from a medical staff tissue committee in order to
determine qualifications and privileges of individual physicians practicing within the hospital, and that the hospital administration knew
from the nurses' daily reports that the patient's case was difficult,
yet made no attempt to correct the situation. The administration
acknowledged that the hospital had done little or nothing to review
the doctor's qualifications for orthopedic practice since he obtained
his license to practice medicine in 1928; further, it appeared that
Dr. Alexander had not been responsible for the care of a major
leg fracture for several years.

   In support of the allegations, the plaintiff was permitted to
introduce into evidence the Standards of the Joint Commission on
the Accreditation of Hospitals to the effect that the hospital board
of trustees is ultimately responsible for the standards of patient care;
the Illinois Department of Public Health regulations under the
Hospital Licensing Act to the same effect; and the medical staff
bylaws of Charleston Community Hospital, which required attending
physicians to seek consultation with specialists in "problem cases."
The hospital defended on the general basis that it was prohibited
from practicing medicine under the law, that it was therefore
powerless to forbid or command any act of a licensed physician,
and that it could not be held liable for the conduct of a staff physician.
The hospital further relied on the prevailing standards, custom, and
practice of hospitals in the local community as a defense of its position.

   The Illinois Supreme Court ultimately upheld the jury verdict
against the hospital as supportable either because (1) the hospital
failed to have a sufficient number of trained nurses capable of
recognizing and bringing the patient's worsening condition to the
attention of hospital administration and medical staff, so that consultation could be secured, or because (2) the hospital failed to review
the treatment rendered to plaintiff and to require consultation as
needed.[151] Thus, the doctrine of respondeat superior was at most
an alternate basis for the court's holding;[152] the hospital's independent

[151]*Id.* at 333, 211 N.E. 2d at 258.
[152]See *Goff v. Doctor's General Hospital of San Jose,* 166 Cal. App. 2d 314, 333 P.
2d 29 (Dist. Ct. App. 1958). (A hospital was liable when nurses who knew a patient

negligence—alone—would be sufficient to impose liability.

The decision raises directly the issue of the respective roles of the hospital administration, the nursing staff, and the medical staff. The jury verdict against the hospital was permitted to stand even though plaintiff presented no precise, expert testimony that failure to review the qualifications of medical staff members or failure to require consultation actually caused plaintiff's injury. Thus some observers have contended that the case was unfortunate because it gave the jury an unwarranted opportunity to sympathize with the plaintiff and in the process to distort and further confuse the role of the hospital administration. Without doubt the facts and evidence at trial aroused considerable sympathy for young Darling's plight; in the language of lawyers the facts showed a "hard case."

However, the *Darling* decision should not be interpreted as meaning that lay individuals in hospital administration are now called upon to control the clinical practice of medicine on a case-by-case basis. Clearly the court does not require this; such lay control would be intolerable because only physicians can exercise clinical judgment. Rather, the court simply considered the "hospital" to be one organization—the administration and medical staff sharing jointly the responsibility for standards of care. The administration, represented by the board of trustees and the lay administrator, is now called upon to stimulate the medical staff of the institution to organize a means of reviewing the professional qualifications and performance of each individual staff physician. The physicians appointed to the hospital staff must have an established procedure for consultation, and lines of communication between clinical practice and lay administration must be open. The medical staff is held accountable to the corporate organization for standards of medical care. The chief of the medical staff must be a dedicated individual, essentially institutionally oriented, and devoted to implementing standards promulgated by responsible private and public agencies which accredit and license hospitals in

was suffering serious bleeding tried without success to reach her private physician and then failed to report to administration so that another physician could be called.) Accord with *Darling* that nurses have a duty to monitor a patient's condition with reasonable care, to recognize a deteriorating condition, to report to the attending physician, and if he is unavailable or unresponsive to report to the hospital administration so that appropriate action may be taken: *Collins v. Westlake Community Hospital*, 57 Ill. 2d 388, 312 N.E. 2d 614 (1974), and *Karrigan v. Nazareth Convent and Academy*, 212 Kan. 44, 510 P. 2d 190 (1973). See also: *Garfield Park Community Hospital v. Vitacco*, 327 N.E. 2d 408 (Ill App. 1975). (The hospital settled a claim alleging that nurses were negligent in failing to observe and report symptoms of impaired circulation. Even if the patient's attending physician was concurrently personally negligent, the hospital was not entitled to indemnity from the physician, since the nurses were employees and the physician not an employee of the hospital.)

the public interest. In other words, fragmentation and individualism within the walls of the hospital must be reduced insofar as is humanly possible. In this light, the case can be approved simply because it focuses on the obligation of the hospital through an organized medical staff to exercise control of standards of practice.

The case further indicates that legal doctrine should finally and forcefully reject the antiquated, rather meaningless notion that a corporation cannot practice medicine. To be sure, only a physician can exercise clinical judgment, but the realities of modern medical care clearly indicate that the doctor can practice adequately only with institutional affiliation and support. It can be asserted that the "corporate practice of medicine" rule as enunciated in the past in some cases and statutes has no relevance today to a nonprofit hospital striving for high standards of professional excellence.

The result of the *Darling* case is consistent with the views and attitudes of professionals concerned with the role of the modern hospital. It is consistent with the realities of modern clinical practice and the institutionalization of medical care. The welfare of hospitalized patients requires collective concern. The hospital is properly highlighted as the focal point for providing and coordinating medical care for the community and as the best available vehicle for controlling and improving standards of care. Hence, the real impact of the case is that it calls attention to the need for an organized medical staff willing and capable of accounting to itself and to the hospital for standards of care.

Darling was also a landmark decision in holding that promulgated Standards of the Joint Commission on the Accreditation of Hospitals, standards of governmental licensing authority, and provisions of medical staff bylaws are admissible for the jury to consider as evidence of negligence.[153] Violations of these standards and rules are not conclusive, of course; but proof that violation of a rule has caused an injury is certainly an important step toward a favorable verdict. Moreover the Illinois Supreme Court held that duties of the hospital are not to be determined solely by the standards of care in the local community.[154] This abolition of the "local community rule," as applied to both hospitals and physicians, has gained widespread acceptance.[155]

The hospital is not liable, however, for all lapses of a staff doctor.

[153] 33 Ill. 2d at 332, 211 N.E. 2d at 257.
[154] *Id.* at 331, 211 N.E. 2d at 257.
[155] See cases cited in n. 45 and 46. See also Hall, "The Locality Rule," 207 *J. Am. Med. Ass'n*, 627–28 (1969).

Corporate responsibility for standards of patient care and for medical staff privileges does not mean that all individual staff physicians are "agents" or "servants" for the purposes of the doctrine of respondeat superior in liability cases. As Jay Hedgepeth properly points out in a timely article, the *Darling* decision did not say that a hospital is liable for all negligent acts or omissions of individual staff physicians.[156] In view of the pretrial settlement with the attending doctor, his legal fault was never established, and therefore the hospital was not being held responsible for the negligence or malpractice of an actual or apparent employee. Rather, the hospital was liable for violation of direct duties owed the patient.

The view espoused in *Darling* has been embodied in the statutory law of several states. The 1968 Michigan statute, for example, states: "The governing body of each hospital shall be responsible for the operation of the hospital, the selection of the medical staff and for the quality of the care rendered in the hospital."[157] The 1971 Indiana statute recites that the governing board is the "supreme authority" in the hospital and makes the medical staff responsible to the board for the clinical work of the hospital and for reviewing professional practices.[158] Members of medical staff review committees are granted immunity from civil liability in their communications and reports.[159] Like Michigan and Indiana, Arizona requires the governing body of a licensed hospital to organize its medical staff into a committee structure to review both the necessity and the quality of professional care.[160]

The Montana Supreme Court, in *Hull v. North Valley Hospital*, recently dealt with the extent or the scope of institutional responsibility to monitor the current competence of staff physicians.[161] While some have argued that the case is contrary to *Darling*, or at least restricts in practical effect the concept of corporate responsibility for the quality of patient care, it is the writer's opinion that *Hull* is not an outright rejection of *Darling*, and that it can be adequately

---

[156]Hedgepeth, "Darling Revisited," 46 *J. Am. Hosp. Ass'n*, 58–60 (1972).
[157]Mich. Comp. Laws Ann., sec. 331.422 (1970); Mich. Stat. Ann., sec. 14.1179 (12) (1969). The statute further recites that the governing body shall ensure that the physicians admitted to practice in the hospital are granted hospital privileges consistent with their individual training, experience, and other qualifications; and that physicians admitted to practice in the hospital are organized into a medical staff in such a manner as to review effectively the professional practices of the hospital for the purposes of reducing morbidity and mortality and for the improvement of care of patients provided in the institution. *Id.*
[158]Burns Indiana Stat. Ann. (code edition), sec. 16–10–1–6.5 (1973).
[159]*Id.*
[160]Ariz. Rev. Stat. Ann., sec. 36–445 (1972).
[161]159 Mont. 375, 498 P. 2d 136 (1972).

distinguished. However, certain statements of the court indicate a tendency to limit the extent of the governing body's duty to make inquiry or require documented evidence concerning the current competence of members of medical staff.

The plaintiff in *Hull* alleged that a Dr. Kauffman had been negligent in the diagnosis of an orthopedic condition and in the conduct of surgery on the patient's knee. The physician was a private practitioner, selected and presumably paid by the patient. Suit against the doctor was settled, but it proceeded to trial against the hospital. The plaintiff did not claim the doctor to be a hospital employee, nor was there any claim that an institutional employee was negligent in the course of treatment.

Rather, the plaintiff in *Hull* argued and presented two issues for decision on appeal following a directed verdict for the hospital. First, was the hospital negligent in permitting Dr. Kauffman to use its facilities in ministering to his patients in the light of his previous record? Second, is the medical staff an arm of the hospital organization, and are the acts or omissions of the medical staff acts or omissions of the hospital? In presenting these issues the plaintiff relied on the *Darling* decision, and on the fact that the doctor's surgical privileges had at various times in the past been revoked or restricted and then reinstated. Full privileges had been restored in 1967, and the allegedly negligent surgery occurred in 1969. Both issues were decided in the negative. The court held that the hospital simply was not negligent in this instance in permitting Dr. Kauffman full surgical privileges.[162]

The court apparently recognized that the Montana Medical Practice Act did not give a licensed doctor the right to an unlimited hospital practice.[163] Neither did a state antidiscrimination statute, known in Montana as the "Thompson Act."[164] Significantly, the court recognized that standards of accreditation, licensing regulations, and the bylaws "regard it as both desirable and feasible that a hospital assume certain responsibilities for the care of the patient."[165] It "assumed" that the board had "a duty to 'act' when *put on notice* or *advised by the medical section* that a doctor is incompetent to continue to practice medicine."[166] (Emphasis added.)

---

[162] *Id.* at 390–91, 498 P. 2d at 144.
[163] *Id.* at 384, 498 P. 2d at 140–41.
[164] Mont. Rev. Codes Ann., sec. 94–3557, 94–3558 (1947), since repealed and superseded by Mont. Rev. Codes Ann., sec. 69–5217, 69–5221 (1947).
[165] 159 Mont. at 389, 498 P. 2d at 143.
[166] *Id.*

The Montana court then reviewed the record, which showed an effort by the hospital to supervise the quality of medical practice within the hospital. The past disciplinary actions against Dr. Kauffman apparently related solely to his medical record-keeping, and full privileges were restored after he promised compliance with the rules. These past faults of the doctor were not particularly relevant, nor were they the proximate cause of plaintiff's alleged injuries.[167]

Two matters relative to this case are of concern, however. First the Montana court distinguished *Darling* on the basis that Dr. Alexander was an "employee" and that liability in the Illinois case was based upon respondeat superior. This is a misreading or misunderstanding of both the facts and the law of the Illinois case as discussed previously;[168] hence *Hull* cannot be a rejection of *Darling*. Also, the two cases could perhaps be distinguished simply on the basis that the medical staff and administration in *Hull* had made an effort to follow accreditation standards and bylaw provisions and to conduct peer review, whereas no such effort was apparent in the record of the *Darling* case. Further, as the Montana court acknowledged, although it indicated that the failure was not necessary to sustain its opinion, plaintiff had failed in his direct negligence suit to carry the burden of proof on proximate cause.[169]

The second matter of concern in *Hull* relates to the court's assertion, as noted above, that the hospital board does have a "duty to 'act' when put on notice or advised by the medical section that a doctor is incompetent to practice medicine," and that "the law recognizes that this determination must be made by medical personnel skilled in medical sciences and competent to make this determination."[170] With this the writer can fundamentally agree. As previously pointed out, the board would normally seek professional advice on clinical matters and support its decisions with evidence. There may be situations, however, where incompetence is so gross as to be generally evident even to a layman, and then the board should have an obligation to discipline a physician or correct the situation without a formal recommendation or report from medical staff. Moreover the court in *Hull* rejected the testimony of two physicians who offered opinions

---

[167] *Id.* at 390–91, 498 P. 2d at 144.
[168] This is acknowledged in the defendant's petition for rehearing in *Darling*, Supreme Court of Illinois, September 1965. On this crucial point of an employment relationship between Dr. Alexander and Charleston Hospital, the Montana court in *Hull* quoted *Lundahl v. Rockford Memorial Hospital*, 93 Ill. App. 2d 461, 464, 235 N.E. 2d 671, 674 (1968), which contained an erroneous statement of fact in discussing *Darling*.
[169] 159 Mont. at 391, 498 P. 2d at 144.
[170] *Id.* at 389, 498 P. 2d at 143.

with respect to the doctor's current competence to practice surgery, saying that such testimony was relevant only to the doctor's ability and not the hospital's.[171] The court went on to say: "Knowledge within these doctors' minds uncommunicated to the board is not a demonstration of knowledge of the board as a matter of law, only a matter of conscience of the individual doctors."[172]

This judicial statement can be severely criticized as inconsistent both with standards of hospital accreditation and with the considered opinions of responsible leaders in the professions of medicine and hospital administration. It is also contrary to the hospital medical staff's fiduciary obligation. It seems to say that the less the board knows about the clinical competence of individual members of the medical staff, the better the hospital's position. The statement perpetuates the so-called "conspiracy of silence" among members of the medical profession, a leading reason for the widespread use of the doctrines of res ipsa loquitur in malpractice litigation. No professional person or medical staff committee holding a fiduciary status is privileged to remain silent before those to whom he owes loyalty and good faith.

Although to the writer's knowledge there is no precise judicial statement to the effect that a hospital medical staff is a "fiduciary" vis-a-vis the hospital, it is submitted that duly constituted medical staff committees do owe the institution duties at least akin to fiduciary duties. After all, staff committees on such matters as credentials, utilization, and medical audit derive their authority and responsibilities from the hospital's governing body. This authority is articulated in medical staff bylaws approved by the board. Accordingly, there is a duty in the committee to disclose to the board of trustees any documented incompetence of staff physicians. Revelation of known incompetence is not a matter of "conscience," at least with respect to the function of medical staff committees.[173]

Further, the Montana court said in *Hull* that the hospital board's duty to act when notified of a physician's incompetence would be satisfied by a formal complaint to the board of medical examiners.[174] This can be challenged, as a general proposition, on the basis of the well-known fact that medical boards in most jurisdictions are extremely handicapped either by a local medical practice act or by an unwillingness to suspend or revoke licenses to practice.

---

[171] *Id.* at 390, 498 P. 2d at 144.
[172] *Id.* at 391, 498 P. 2d at 144.
[173] Compare with text accompanying notes below.
[174] 159 Mont. at 390, 498 P. 2d at 144.

In sum, the writer can approve the result in *Hull* simply on the evidence that the medical staff of North Valley Hospital had apparently been exercising some form of peer review and had been enforcing medical staff bylaws. The plaintiff's case failed for lack of notice to the board of Dr. Kauffman's alleged current clinical incompetence. The reasons for the past disciplinary action against the physician were neither relevant nor the proximate cause of plaintiff's injury. But some of the court's statements to support its conclusions cannot be approved. Such statements only perpetuate the dichotomy between hospital management and medical staff.

The opinion illustrates well, as do many other liability cases, the great difficulty in distinguishing, in theory and in fact, between vicarious liability and corporate or independent institutional negligence. As previously noted, both doctor and hospital are sued more often than not, whatever the theory of alleged liability.[175] When patient care is a team matter—involving the attending doctor, perhaps a consultant or two, nurses, laboratory technicians, the hospital pharmacist, and others—it frequently becomes impossible to determine who did what, who failed to do something he or she was supposed to do, and who is responsible for whom.

Accordingly it makes good sense and would be sound economics to implement a program of joint hospital-medical staff insurance, as recently suggested by John Horty.[176] As he and others have frequently stressed, it is harmful in litigation for the hospital to blame the doctor, and the doctor to blame the hospital or its employees. If the same insurance carrier were involved, settlements prior to trial would be facilitated. The dichotomy dividing hospital and physician could be reduced. Such a program is in operation in England, in practical effect, where all hospital physicians are insured by one of only three defense unions, and the unions have an agreement with the hospital authorities to share jointly the cost of liability suits.[177] Since liability is a joint problem of hospital and medical staff, insurance protection should be similarly structured.

That liability claims are a joint problem of administration and medical staff is dramatically illustrated by the recent case of *Purcell and Tucson General Hospital v. Zimbelman*.[178] The case provides a

---

[175]See: Regan, "Why Sue Hospitals for Doctors' Errors?," 13 *Report on Hospital Law* 1 (May, 1972).

[176]Horty, "Why Not Joint Hospital-Medical Staff Insurance?" *Action Kit for Hospital Law* 1 (April, 1972).

[177]See generally: A. Southwick, *The Doctor, the Hospital, and the Patient in England—Rights and Responsibilities under the National Health Service*, 229–31 (1967).

[178]18 Ariz. App. 75, 500 P. 2d 335 (Ct. App. 1972). *Hull*, decided June 9, 1972, of course makes no reference to *Purcell*, decided July 20, 1972, and vice versa.

sharp contrast to the *Hull* litigation reviewed above, and is thoroughly consistent with the *Darling* philosophy.

A staff physician at Tucson General Hospital, Dr. Purcell, was asked by the general surgeon attending a patient named Zimbelman to consult with respect to the patient's intestinal condition. The doctor's tentative diagnostic opinion was that the patient was suffering from either intestinal cancer or diverticulitis. Upon surgery a lesion was found in the colon. A visual examination by a pathologist during surgery resulted in an opinion of cancer (no frozen section was obtained, although this could have been done during surgery), and Dr. Purcell thereupon performed a "pull-through" operation, technically known as a "Babcock-Bacon protosigmoidectomy." This surgical procedure resulted in serious, permanent disabilities to the plaintiff, who was subsequently found not to have had cancer.

Suit was brought against both Dr. Purcell and Tucson General Hospital. Expert witnesses were available to testify that customary surgical standards specify that the surgeon obtain a pathologist's report based upon a frozen section, and that the choice of procedure in this instance would have been an anterior resection and not a "pull-through" surgical procedure.[179]

Moreover plaintiff offered evidence that the doctor and the hospital had been sued four times previously, and at least two of these suits involved identical cases of diverticulitis where Dr. Purcell had failed to do an anterior resection. Still worse, at least two of these patients had recovered judgments against the physician. Since the hospital had been named as a defendant it certainly had notice of alleged prior malpractice by a staff doctor. The evidence of the prior lawsuits was held to be admissible against the hospital on the question of notice, not only as to the particular type of operation and ailment that was involved, but as to the general competency of Dr. Purcell.[180]

The Arizona Court of Appeals affirmed a verdict of $150,000 against both the physician and the hospital. The hospital was liable because accreditation Standards of the American Osteopathic Hospital Association require that the governing body assume responsibility for quality of medical care, that it carefully select professional staff, and that it have a means of assuring that physicians are competent.[181] Moreover there was evidence that the medical staffs of hospitals generally conduct medical audit and peer review for the purpose

[179] 500 P. 2d at 340.
[180] 500 P. 2d at 343–44.
[181] 500 P. 2d at 340–41.

of determining medical staff privileges. Most significantly, the court said:

> The Department of Surgery was acting for and on behalf of the hospital in fulfilling this duty and if the department was negligent in not taking any action against Purcell or recommending to the board of trustees that action be taken, then the hospital would also be negligent.[182]

Clearly, then, in contrast to the attitude of the Montana court in *Hull*, this court saw a clear, explicit, affirmative duty on the part of a hospital clinical department or duly constituted medical staff committee of disclosure of incompetence. Disclosure is not a matter of "conscience."

The Tucson General Hospital thus had a duty to control medical staff privileges. Its organized medical staff committees and departments acted on behalf of the institution. A breach of duty occurred when the surgical department knew, or should have known, that Dr. Purcell lacked the training and skill to treat the patient. Prior malpractice suits and claims were admissible as evidence of notice to the department of surgery—and hence to the hospital—of his incompetence. This information should at least have prompted a review of the physician's work and the extent of his privileges. Had this been done, the court concluded, it would have been reasonably probable that Mr. Zimbelman would not have been injured.[183] Accordingly, there was sufficient proof of proximate cause.[184]

In *Joiner v. Mitchell County Hospital Authority*, a Georgia case, Mrs. Joiner brought her husband to the hospital at 11:00 p.m. for treatment of chest pains. He was examined by Dr. Arturo Gonzalez, a member of the medical staff. According to later allegations, the doctor advised the patient that his condition was not serious, wrote a prescription, and sent him home. Less than two hours later the patient's distress had increased, and he and his wife started back to the hospital. Mr. Joiner expired before they arrived there. In bringing suit Mrs. Joiner alleged that the physician was professionally negligent, both in failing to make an adequate and proper examination and in failing

[182] 500 P. 2d at 341.
[183] 500 P. 2d at 343.
[184] *Id.* See also: *Tucson Medical Center, Inc. v. Misevch*, 113 Ariz. 34, 545 P. 2d 958 (1976): (A hospital has a duty to supervise the competence of staff physicians). *Cf.*: *Ferguson v. Gonyaw*, 64 Mich. App. 685, 236 N.W. 2d 543 (1975): (A hospital is not liable for failing to check the background and training of a physician while processing his application for surgical privileges, in the absence of proof that privileges would have been denied had an investigation been made).

to admit the deceased to the hospital. Against the hospital she alleged
independent negligence in failing to require satisfactory proof of
the physician's professional qualifications, character, and background.
The trial court rendered summary judgment for both defendants;
but the court of appeals reversed for a trial, and the decision was
affirmed by the Georgia Supreme Court.[185]

With respect to the doctor's liability the court ruled that there
were issues of fact regarding the professional care rendered and
the question of whether Mr. Joiner had rejected the doctor's invitation
to be admitted to the hospital as a bed patient.

More relevant to this discussion is the case against the hospital.
Was it independently negligent in appointing Dr. Gonzalez to the
staff and in permitting him to practice? Again, the court ruled that
a summary judgment for the hospital was improper. The evidence
may, in fact, show lack of competence or skill.[186] In other words,
the board is not absolved merely because staff recommended the
appointment. The intermediate appellate court had said:

> This [screening of candidates for staff appointment by
> existing staff] is not defensive, as these members of staff
> are agents of the Hospital Authority and it is responsible
> for any default or negligence *on its part* in properly selecting
> new members of the staff. Indeed, the law authorizes this
> duty to be delegated to staff. But even so the evidence is
> still insufficient to establish as a matter of law that the hospital
> is absolved of all blame. [A] hospital is not liable in the
> absence of allegations that it was negligent in the selection
> of an unskilled physician. . . . The hospital must act in *good
> faith* and with *reasonable care* in the selection of a physician,
> and it has fulfilled its obligation, and cannot be held liable
> when it "selects an authorized physician, in good standing
> in his profession."[187]

It would seem that the hospital board must not abdicate its
responsibilities for selecting and appointing staff physicians, and it
must be certain that recommendations of staff are documented with
evidence of current competence and skill. The governing body's
delegation to medical staff of the duty to recommend staff appointments does not relieve the hospital of responsibility. Further, aver-
ments that the hospital was negligent in granting an appointment

---

[185] 125 Ga. App. 1, 186 S.E. 2d 307, 51 A.L.R. 3d 976 (1971), *aff'd*, 229 Ga. 140,
189 S.E. 2d 412 (1972).
[186] *Id.* at 3, 186 S.E. 2d at 308.
[187] *Id.* at 2–3, 186 S.E. 2d at 308. (Citations omitted and emphasis added in part.)

to the doctor are not overcome simply because he holds a license to practice. Since it was not established beyond controversy that no issue of fact existed, a summary judgment for the hospital authority was therefore improper. Plaintiff was at least entitled to a trial.

A monumental trial court decision of nearly two hundred pages, written in late 1973 by a judge in Sacramento County, California, highlighted clearly the trend of the cases since *Darling* and emphasized the necessity of having an effective in-hospital peer review program. In *Gonzales v. Nork and Mercy Hospital*[188] the hospital and Dr. Nork, a surgeon, were liable for $1.7 million in damages to compensate the patient for his injuries; in addition, the physician was held liable for $2 million in punitive damages. Following this verdict of the court (a jury had been waived), the hospital reportedly settled with the plaintiff for $500,000 before final judgment of the trial court. Accordingly there was no appeal of the verdict against the hospital.

At the trial it was established that Dr. Nork, although not a board-certified orthopedic surgeon, conducted an unsuccessful laminectomy and spinal fusion on the patient, a 27-year-old man who had been injured in an automobile accident in 1967. Arachnoiditis developed and led to emotional problems which caused Mr. Gonzales to attempt suicide several times. He also became addicted to alcohol, and still later he developed cancer. Expert witnesses testified that the surgery was negligently performed as well as unnecessary and that the patient could have been treated successfully by far more conservative methods. His life expectancy had been reduced to an estimated 10 percent chance of surviving three years. Moreover evidence was introduced showing that Dr. Nork had performed more than three dozen other operations which were either unnecessary or negligently handled, or both of these, in the nine years from 1961 to 1970, that he persistently operated on the basis of false or inadequate diagnostic findings, that he refused to consult with his peers, that he failed to obtain an informed consent from his patients prior to surgery, and that he falsified his patients' progress reports. The doctor's own accountant testified that the surgeon needed money to avoid legal actions by various creditors. In an effort to reduce the punitive damages to be assessed against him, Dr. Nork himself testified that he was addicted to various drugs which affected his judgment.

The trial judge wrote in his opinion that the hospital was liable

---

[188]No. 228566, Sacramento Co. Super. Ct., Calif., 1973, *rev'd on other grounds*, 60 Cal. App. 3d 728 (1976).

for the breach of its duty to the patient to protect him from acts of malpractice by an independent or privately retained physician. The duty was breached if the hospital knew, had reason to know, or should have known of the surgeon's incompetence. Even if the hospital had no actual knowledge of Dr. Nork's acts of malpractice, it was negligent in not knowing, since at the time of these events the medical staff's peer review system for monitoring the performance of professional staff was casual, random, and uncritical. Cases selected for review were chosen haphazardly; reviews were infrequent; and even when they were carried out the medical staff was content to accept the personal judgment or standards of the reviewer, rather than to insist upon objective criteria. Moreover the review system then in effect at Mercy Hospital did not compare the physician's progress reports, which Dr. Nork falsified, with the nurses' notes.

Compliance with the then prevailing standards promulgated by the Joint Commission on the Accreditation of Hospitals did not fulfill the hospital's duty to the patient. The Joint Commission significantly strengthened its standards with respect to medical staff organization and medical audit, or peer review, in 1970, subsequent to the events which gave rise to the *Nork* litigation. In 1970 the hospital, upon learning that the physician's malpractice insurance had been canceled, acted promptly to place severe restrictions on his surgical privileges. Much earlier than that, however, in 1963, the hospital had learned that a malpractice suit had been filed against Dr. Nork and had done nothing at that time to review his professional competence to perform specialized surgery.

In summary, the trial judge's opinion represents a strong statement of the hospital's corporate or institutional responsibility to the patient. As in other cases, the hospital may not defend a suit such as this on the basis that its medical staff is independent and self-governing.[189]

Summary—Institutional Liability One Way or the Other

What the recent liability cases add up to in a final analysis is this: the historical distinction between the two presumably separate legal theories underlying hospital liability has been all but obliterated. Appellate courts are to an increasing extent failing to discriminate clearly between corporate or institutional negligence and respondeat

---

[189]See also: *Corleto v. Shore Memorial Hospital*, 350 A. 2d 534 (N.J. Super. Ct. 1975). (A hospital owes patients the duty to admit only competent physicians to its staff and to remove a known incompetent from the case when problems become obvious; a hospital could be liable for permitting a known incompetent to perform surgery.)

superior or vicarious liability. This is not for want of clear thinking or of scholarship, but simply the result of factual realities. The first of these realities is the increase in all sorts of malpractice and personal injury suits in a claims-conscious society. More significant to this discussion is the reality in the hospital-medical world that health care is increasingly delivered to the public through hospitals and similar institutions. There is an irresistible tendency to hold the institution responsible when things go wrong and when negligence can be established as the proximate cause of injury.

Accordingly, in litigation presenting genuine issues of an employment relationship, the doctrine of respondeat superior, the following legal developments have occurred. First, the doctrine has been applied to situations involving professional employees and their negligent acts, rather than being confined to "administrative" acts.[190] Second, the notion of apparent or ostensible agency was developed to allow a plaintiff to recover damages against a hospital which "held out" or made it appear that the negligent actor was an employee, when in fact he was not.[191] Third, the borrowed-servant doctrine is disappearing, thereby placing vicarious liability on the hospital and not on the physician alone for the negligent act of an intern, resident, or nurse.[192] And finally, as in *Beeck v. Tucson General Hospital*, there is a forthright finding of an employment relationship between hospital and doctor, even though the parties involved certainly considered their relationship to be otherwise.[193] The *Beeck* court did not find it necessary to speak in terms of "apparent agency" or a "holding out." The independent contractor defense can no longer be successfully raised by the hospital, except in limited circumstances where it is explicitly established that the negligent act which caused injury was performed solely by the doctor, and where a patient has expressly and voluntarily employed the physician privately.

In cases presenting issues of a hospital's negligence in failing to monitor the quality of care rendered by members of its medical staff—the *Darling, Hull, Purcell, Joiner,* and *Nork* decisions—the trend is clear. The organized medical staff and its committees act on behalf of the hospital. Their negligent omissions become the hospital's omissions. Institutional liability can thus be established in the hospital as long as adequate proof of proximate cause can be established.

---

[190] See n. 66, 67, 68, 73, 78.
[191] See cases cited in n. 69, 70, 71, 72.
[192] See cases cited in n. 100, 108, 119.
[193] See n. 73 and accompanying text.

The Hospital-Physician
Relationship

XIII

Medical Staff Appointments and Privileges

Aside from governmental regulation of the health care industry, the two most crucial legal matters currently occupying the minds of hospital trustees, administrators, physicians, and attorneys are hospitals' liability for negligence and the granting or withholding of medical staff privileges. These legal problems are inevitably related. Hospital liability has been reviewed in the preceding chapter, and this chapter will discuss some recent decisions concerning the rights of a physician to attain and retain medical staff privileges.

On one hand the liability decisions have recognized that failure on the part of the hospital as a corporate institution to exercise reasonable care in selecting and retaining medical staff, to delineate privileges of individual practitioners consistent with each person's current ability to perform particular tasks of medical and surgical practice, and to enforce standards of practice, as articulated by medical staff rules and regulations and by a host of other sources of standards, may occasion legal liability to the patient for corporate or institutional negligence, as long as the failure is established as the proximate cause of the plaintiff's loss or damage.[1] In other words, the ultimate responsibility for the quality of patient care rests squarely on the hospital as a corporation managed by the governing board. This responsibility for standards of medical practice cannot be delegated by the board to the medical staff.

The essential and primary purpose of a hospital is to furnish,

---

[1]See discussion and cases cited in chap. XII.

arrange for, and coordinate patient care consistent with professionally recognized standards of medical practice. To implement this duty of providing medical care to the patient, the corporate institution thus has the responsibility to create a workable system whereby the medical staff of a hospital continually reviews and evaluates the quality of care being rendered within the institution. The staff must be well organized with a proper committee structure to carry out this role delegated to it by the governing body. All powers of the medical staff flow from the board of trustees, and the staff must be held strictly accountable to the governing board for its control of quality.

A hospital, therefore, does not consist of two organizations— business administration and medical. Rather, a hospital is a single organization; the medical activities cannot be separated from the business side. All who serve the hospital must recognize this concept, especially the practicing attorney who advises the institution. Another absolute necessity is smooth and harmonious coordination between business administration and medical administration. Both business and medical administration report to the governing board through the chief executive officer of the hospital. The organizational structure of the medical staff, lines of communication among medical staff committees and between the board of trustees and medical staff, areas of delegated authority, and the site of ultimate responsibility must be well expressed in the medical staff and hospital bylaws. The hospital attorney should play a key role in making all this clear.

With respect to the hospital-physician relationship, two related issues emerge. The first is administrative or managerial: how can the physician best be integrated into the picture of hospital management so as to facilitate his institutional responsibility and loyalty? The second issue is more of a legal question: what are the rights of a licensed physician to attain and retain a hospital staff appointment?

Clearly the concept of institutional responsibility for selection and retention of medical staff, which in turn requires the governing board to make certain that medical staff is implementing effectively a continuing process of peer review, makes it highly advisable to have physicians on the board. Traditionally, in an era when business and medical administration were separated, it was thought that practicing physicians should not become voting members of a hospital's board of trustees. Sometimes it was said that conflicts of interest would exist if members of the medical staff were also members of the board. While it is true that conflicts of interest could occur whenever physicians are placed upon the governing body, the potential danger is no greater than the risk with many laymen who become members of the board. In any event, conflicts of interest in individual cases with respect to particular issues may be easily and readily resolved by full disclosure and by making certain that the interested trustee, whether a physician or not, takes no part in decisions before the board concerning matters in which he or she has a personal interest. In the light of the doctrine of institutional responsibility for the standards of medical practice, the reasons in favor of integrating physicians into the management of hospitals far outweigh the reasons in favor of a board of trustees consisting entirely of laymen. The medical staff of a particular hospital, however, should not be granted the privilege of electing their "representative" to the board. All trustees are to be appointed or selected as provided for by local corporate law and the corporate bylaws; and all must serve the institution, not represent a particular group of individuals or special interests.

It is clear that affiliation with a hospital is absolutely indispensable to the American doctor. Without staff privileges the physician is severely handicapped in practice and suffers an irreparable financial detriment. The legal issues relevant to a licensed physician's rights to attain and retain a hospital staff appointment with defined or delineated privileges are resolved in particular controversies by reference to constitutional law, statutory enactments, or simply the common law of judicial decision. The relevant law and the resolution of a particular case will, of course, depend upon the allegations made in the plaintiff's complaint, the facts of the case, and the philosophy of the court rendering the opinion.

In a sense,' both case and statutory law surrounding the related problems of hospital liability and medical staff privileges are attempts to resolve a dilemma. How should American legal doctrines balance the sometimes conflicting interests and public policies? On the one hand, as has been amply demonstrated in the preceding chapter, responsibility for adequate control over the quality of care is placed on the hospital. On the other, it is generally in the public interest to allow the licensed physician the greatest possible individual freedom to practice his profession. Are these propositions irreconcilable? Control of quality implies, perhaps, maximum discretion on the part of the hospital in selecting staff physicians and in regulating their professional practice. Individual freedom to practice implies the opposite—an absence of hospital control with respect to medical staff appointments and a minimum discretionary control over the scope of individual privileges, once a doctor has gained appointment.

This dilemma will be apparent throughout the ensuing discussion of some of the many recorded cases dealing with medical staff privileges. Since the courts have traditionally approached these controversies by first categorizing the hospital involved as either public or private—which in turn may determine the relevant rule or rules of law to apply—the discussion which follows will pursue a similar format.

Appointments in Public Hospitals

At the outset it can be noted that neither case nor statutory law of the United States has ever given a licensed physician an absolute legal right to attain or retain medical staff membership or privileges in either a public (governmental) hospital or a private, nonprofit (voluntary) hospital, although efforts have sometimes been made to create such a right by local state statute.[2] Such efforts have typically failed to gain legislative acceptance. State medical licensing laws certainly do not constitute a satisfactory vehicle for establishing and controlling professional standards. In the first place, licensing statutes are notorious for specifying only minimal qualifications for the practice of medicine. They often make no satisfactory distinctions between various schools of medicine. Moreover, the disciplinary powers of the state licensing board are often quite limited in law or in fact, although some states have recently been revising their medical practice acts to grant licensing boards more clearly defined authority to discipline errant physicians. Licensing furnishes no continuing control over an individual's professional competence; the statutes in no way recognize the demands placed upon the doctor by the ever-increasing specialization of medicine; accordingly they do not adequately protect the public from incompetence. Protection of the public must come from some other authority, usually the governing body of the individual hospital. The present licensing statutes for physicians, nurses, and other professional personnel also impede rather than facilitate improvements in the quality of health care by failing to clarify scope-of-practice problems.[3]

---

[2]There is no constitutional right to practice in a public hospital. *Hayman v. Galveston,* 273 U.S. 414 (1927); *Yeargin v. Hamilton Memorial Hosp.,* 225 Ga. 661, 171 S.E. 2d 136 (1969), *cert. denied,* 397 U.S. 963 (1970): (An applicant to a public hospital can be required to adhere to reasonable rules and regulations); *Moore v. Board of Trustees of Carson-Tahoe Hospital,* 88 Nev. 207, 495 P. 2d 605, *cert. denied,* 409 U.S. 879 (1972); *Rao v. Board of County Commissioners,* 80 Wash. 2d 695, 497 P. 2d 591 (1972), *cert. denied,* 409 U.S. 1017 (1972): (An applicant to a public or private hospital can be required to submit references); *Yeargin v. Hamilton Memorial Hospital,* 229

The general rule is that the governing body of a public hospital is always under a duty not to act arbitrarily, capriciously, or unreasonably in granting, withholding, or restricting medical staff privileges. According to the law, a publicly owned hospital must have well-stated, reasonable rules regarding staff appointments, and also fair procedures pertaining to enforcement of the rules. Without question the courts will inquire into the reasonableness of a given rule at issue, and they will also require that due process of law be extended in hospital enforcement proceedings. An individual physician may therefore succeed in court by attacking a given rule as unreasonable; or, even if the rule is reasonable, he may succeed on the grounds that he was denied procedural due process. These general principles have been derived on a case-by-case basis simply from notions of public policy, judicial interpretation of local statutes, application of federal or state civil rights statutes, or the guarantees of the Fourteenth Amendment to the U.S. Constitution.

By way of contrast, historically the courts have generally accorded the governing body of a private, voluntary hospital a far greater measure of discretion in selecting and retaining members of the medical staff. They have been slower to inquire into the reasonableness of a rule pertaining to staff privileges; and they have not in general required procedural fairness, unless the hospital bylaws provide affirmatively for procedural steps, such as a hearing upon failure to reappoint. The judicial attitude has traditionally recognized that a private hospital can select staff members and discipline physicians on any basis determined by the governing body, and the court will not interfere in the exercise of this discretion. Recent cases, however, as well as a few statutes, the Standards promulgated by the Joint Commission on Accreditation of Hospitals, and the conditions for participation in the federal Medicare program have cast grave doubt upon the permanence of this approach to the medical staff affairs of a private, nonprofit hospital. The clear trend of the law, statutory and case, reflects a narrowing of the line of distinction between public and private hospitals, as reviewed below.

Illustrative of the traditional distinction between governmental and voluntary hospitals is the case of *Group Health Co-operative v. King County Medical Society.*[4] In that case it was said to be unreasonable

Ga. 870, 195 S.E. 2d 8 (1972): (A public hospital may enforce a rule requiring a doctor to serve in the emergency room.)
[3] Forgotson and Cook, "Innovations and Experiments in Uses of Health Manpower—The Effect of Licensure Laws," 1967 *Law & Contemp. Prob.* 731.
[4] 39 Wash. 2d 586, 237 P.2d 737 (1951).

for a public hospital to declare a physician who practices "contract medicine" to be ineligible for staff membership, and the exclusionary action was enjoined. The court, however, refused to grant relief to the same doctor, who had also been excluded from a private hospital. The basis of this Washington decision seemed simply to be public policy.

Although a license to practice medicine does not grant an absolute or constitutional right to membership on the medical staff of a public hospital, the influence of licensure requirements and the role of other relevant local statutory law are illustrated by the 1972 Indiana case of *Porter Memorial Hospital v. Harvey*.[5] The hospital, a tax-supported institution, required that all staff applicants satisfactorily complete a one-year internship in an approved hospital. The rule, which had the effect of saying that *all* physicians lacking the qualification were automatically incompetent, was struck down as arbitrary, capricious, and unreasonable.[6] An internship was not necessary for licensure. The doctor involved had been practicing for twenty-five years, and there was no evidence that he was in fact incompetent. Moreover, Indiana statutes require that tax-supported hospitals permit the use of their facilities by all taxpayers and the personal physician of their choice.[7] Further, a 1971 statute placing responsibility for quality care on the hospital's governing body also provides that the board must consider the individual's medical education, his training, and his experience.[8] *Harvey* is likely to be applied, by way of one line of reasoning or another, to the private, voluntary hospital.

In a nutshell, what the courts and statutes are saying is this: individuals must be judged as individuals in the light of their training, experience, current demonstrated clinical and professional competence, ethical attitudes, and ability to function effectively with patients and colleagues. "Unreasonable, arbitrary, and capricious" can perhaps be defined as a failure to consider applicants for medical staff appointment on the merits and the facts of each situation.[9]

Over the years a number of cases involving controversies between

---

[5] 151 Ind. App. 299, 279 N.E. 2d 583 (1972).
[6] See also: *McCray Memorial Hospital v. Hall*, 141 Ind. App. 203, 226 N.E. 2d 915 (1967).
[7] Ind. Ann. Stat., sec. 22-3314 (Burns 1964).
[8] Ind. Ann. Stat., sec. 22-3141 (Burns 1971).
[9] The standards of both the Joint Commission on Accreditation of Hospitals and the "Conditions for Participation—Hospitals" contained in the federal Medicare program in essence support the above conclusions and reflect the host of judicial cases decided to date. *Accreditation Manual for Hospitals*, Joint Commission on Accreditation of Hospitals, Chicago, 1976, 103 *et seq.*, and *Second Supplement to Manual* (1977); and 20 C.F.R., sec. 405.1021 *et seq.* 1973.

governmental hospitals and physicians have accumulated. All the following rules and regulations have been held to be unreasonable, arbitrary, or too vague and incapable of objective enforcement, and hence have been struck down: a requirement that staff physicians be members of the local medical society;[10] a rule that the board of the hospital must be satisfied that patients will be given the best possible care before an individual is given staff privileges;[11] a rule requiring staff doctors to carry malpractice insurance;[12] a rule stating that the doctor who seeks admission to a public hospital staff must first obtain an appointment at a private hospital;[13] a staff bylaw which authorized the executive committee to reduce privileges "if in the opinion of such committee it appears that such a reduction would be in the best interests of the hospital and its patients."[14] The latter rule, contested in *Milford*, allowed the executive committee of the medical staff to reduce an individual's "privileges according to their whim or caprice, subject only to appeal to the staff and ultimately to the board, whose powers of review are equally arbitrary."[15]

Moreover, in *Milford* the Michigan court found that the suspended physician had been denied procedural due process of law, and held that he was entitled to a reasonably definite statement of the charges against him, notice of a hearing, the opportunity to be fully heard, the right to cross-examine witnesses, and the right to produce witnesses in his own behalf.[16] In the California case of *Rosner v. Eden Township Hospital District*,[17] the court invalidated a bylaw which required an applicant for staff membership to be "temperamentally and psychologically suited for cooperative staff hospital functions."[18]

Implicit in several of the foregoing cases is the proposition that the governing body of a public hospital—and indeed also a private

---

[10] *Foster v. Mobile County Hosp. Bd.*, 398 F. 2d 227 (5th Cir. 1968); *Ware v. Benedikt*, 225 Ark. 185, 280 S.W. 2d 234 (1955); *Hamilton County Hosp. v. Andrews*, 227 Ind. 217, 84 N.E. 2d 469 (1949), *cert. denied*, 338 U.S. 831 (1949).
[11] *Wyatt v. Tahoe Forest Hosp. Dist.*, 174 Cal. App. 2d 709, 345 P.2d 93 (1959). (The rule was judged to be too vague, thus inviting arbitrary action.)
[12] *Rosner v. Peninsula Hosp. Dist.*, 224 Cal. App. 2d 115, 36 Cal. Rptr. 332 (1964). This decision, however, has been repudiated by a recent California trial court case, *Utzinger v. Truck Insurance Exchange*, No. P28959 County Ct., Palo Alto, Calif., Sept. 26, 1975. Moreover, *Rosner* is not a precedent for litigation involving the validity of a private hospital's rule requiring staff physicians to carry malpractice insurance. See *infra*, n. 19.
[13] *Bronaugh v. City of Parkersburg*, 148 W. Va. 568, 136 S.E. 2d 783 (1964).
[14] *Milford v. People's Community Hosp. Authority*, 380 Mich. 49, 155 N.W. 2d 835 (1968).
[15] *Id.* at 62, 155 N.W. 2d at 841.
[16] *Supra*, n. 14.
[17] 58 Cal. 2d 592, 375 P.2d 431, 25 Cal. Rptr. 551 (1962).
[18] *Id.* at 596, 375 P.2d at 433, Cal. Rptr. at 552.

hospital—may not enforce rules which, in practical effect, delegate
responsibility for determining qualifications for staff appointment
to an outside group, such as for example a county or state medical
society or a malpractice insurance carrier.[19] In other words, the
governing board must not abdicate its responsibility to determine
a physician's qualifications for appointment to its staff.

Clearly no public hospital or private institution receiving federal
financial assistance (including funds pursuant to Medicare) can
discriminate in medical staff appointments on the basis of race, color,
or national origin.[20] Such discrimination violates not only specific
statutory prohibitions but also the equal protection clause of the
Fourteenth Amendment.[21] As is well known, the Fourteenth Amendment to the U.S. Constitution guarantees equal protection and due
process of law whenever governmental or state action is involved.
Without question, a governmental hospital acts in the name of the
state, and under certain circumstances so does a private or voluntary
hospital. The applicability of constitutional law to the private institution will be reviewed subsequently.

Moreover, the Fourteenth Amendment prohibits all forms of
arbitrary and unreasonable action—substantive and procedural—not
just discriminatory decisions on the basis of race or creed. What
specifically does equal protection and due process require? A leading
decision is *Sosa v. Board of Managers of Val Verde Hospital.*[22]

In *Sosa* the court upheld the hospital when it denied Dr. Sosa
admission to the medical staff. As a county institution, the defendant
hospital was clearly subject to the Fourteenth Amendment. The factors
considered by the Medical Staff Credentials Committee in recommending to the board the denial of the application—the character,
qualifications, and standing of the applicant in the community—were
deemed by the court to be reasonable and not arbitrary.[23] All standards

---

[19]Compare, however, reasonableness of a hospital rule requiring physicians to obtain
malpractice insurance, the *Rosner* case, *supra* n. 12, and *Pollock v. Methodist Hospital,*
392 F. Supp. 393 (E.D. La. 1975), which upheld such a rule of private hospital
as reasonable. *Pollock* is discussed *infra.*
[20]Civil Rights Act of 1964, 42 U.S.C.A. 2000 (d) (Supp. 1966); 42 U.S.C.A. 1395
et seq. (Supp. 1973).
[21]*Foster v. Mobile County Hosp. Bd.,* 398 F.2d 227 (5th Cir. 1968). *Meredith v. Allen
County War Memorial Hosp.,* 397 F.2d 33 (6th Cir. 1968); *Eaton v. Grubbs,* 329 F.
2d 710 (4th Cir. 1964); *Simkins v. Cone Memorial Hosp.,* 323 F. 2d 959 (4th Cir.
1963), *cert. denied,* 376 U.S. 938 (1964): (A private hospital receiving governmental
financial support is subject to the Fourteenth Amendment); *Birnbaum v. Trussell,*
371 F. 2d 672 (2d Cir. 1966).
[22]437 F.2d 173 (5th Cir. 1971).
[23]There was evidence at the hearing that the doctor had: (a) Abandoned obstetrical
patients in active labor because they could not pay his bill. (b) An unstable physical

and reasons for rejection need not be spelled out precisely and altogether objectively in the medical staff bylaws, itself a significant ruling.[24] The court discussed at length the application of the due process clause to the situation:

> [S]taff appointments may be constitutionally refused if the refusal is based upon "any reasonable basis such as the professional and ethical qualifications of the physicians or the common good of the public and the Hospital. Admittedly, standards such as "character, qualifications, and standing" are very general, but this court recognizes that in the area of personal fitness for medical staff privileges precise standards are difficult if not impossible to articulate. The subjectives of selection simply cannot be minutely codified. The governing board of a hospital must therefore be given great latitude in prescribing the necessary qualifications for potential applicants. So long as the hearing process gives notice of the particular charges of incompetency and ethical fallibilities, we need not exact a precis of the standard in codified form.
>
> On the other hand, it is clear that in exercising its broad discretion the board must refuse staff applicants only for those matters which are reasonably related to the operation of the hospital. Arbitrariness and false standards are to be eschewed. Moreover, procedural due process must be afforded the applicant so that he may explain or show to be untrue those matters which lead the board to reject his application.[25]

The court noted that there was considerable evidence regarding Dr. Sosa's lack of ethical and professional competency. It was reluctant to substitute its evaluation of such matters for that of the board, since the board, not the court, is charged with the responsibility of providing a competent staff of doctors.[26]

> The evaluation of professional proficiency of doctors is best left to the specialized expertise of their peers, subject only to limited judicial surveillance. The court is charged with the narrow responsibility of assuring that the qualifications imposed by the board are reasonably related to the operation

---

demeanor and visible nervousness which were likely to jeopardize surgical patients. (c) Failed to retain and utilize basic surgical techniques. (d) An unstable mental condition manifested by numerous examples of fits of anger and rage. (e) Unsatisfactory references. (f) Engaged in an itinerant medical practice over the years. (g) Plead guilty to two felony charges in criminal courts. (h) Suffered suspension of license to practice in both Michigan and Texas (since restored in Texas). *Id.* at 175.

[24] *Id.* at 176.

[25] *Id.* at 176–77 (citations omitted).

[26] *Id.*

of the hospital and fairly administered. In short, so long
as staff selections are administered with fairness, geared by
a rationale compatible with hospital responsibility, and unencumbered with irrelevant considerations, a court should not
interfere. Courts must not attempt to take on the escutcheon
of [the] Caduceus.[27]

Procedural due process means fundamental fairness under all the
facts and circumstances. New applicants to staff as well as current
appointees subject to discipline or nonrenewal of appointment are
entitled to due process. The concept has no fixed, ironclad definition.
It is related to the time, the place, and the circumstances of each
case. One of the most helpful statements here was delivered by the
unpublished opinion of the federal district court in the *Sosa* case:

> While the board is correct in its assertion that due process
> does not demand that they follow courtroom procedures,
> it is clear that due process requires that an applicant be
> afforded at least the following: (1) Notice of time and place
> of hearing; (2) A hearing before a properly authorized body;
> (3) A right to produce evidence and rebut that against him;
> (4) Consideration and findings as to specific qualifications
> based upon the evidence submitted; (5) Notification of where
> and why the applicant fell short, if refused; and (6) An appeal
> or final opportunity to rebut. While the details of fulfillment
> of these requirements may vary depending upon the unique
> problems presented in each case, the presence of each, in
> all cases, would seem the minimum demanded by fairness.
>   The court is aware that the requirements, substantive and
> procedural, set out above, are to be carried out by men
> untrained in the law, who serve on the board out of civic
> conscience as a public service. None of the requirements
> are beyond the capacity of such men. Others, especially the
> substantive requirements, require the aid of experts in con-
> nection with drawing bylaws, etc. When wielding the power
> of the government and applying it to the citizen, such
> inconvenience, if any, is small compared to the value of the
> basic rights protected.[28]

Charges of lacking surgical judgment, being without a surgical
assistant, and assisting another who had no surgical privileges, all

[27] *Id.* See also: *Schooler v. Navarro County Memorial Hospital,* 375 F. Supp. 841 (N.D.
Tex. 1973), *aff'd,* 515 F. 2d 509 (5th Cir. 1975). (When procedural due process
is followed, a hospital may deny staff appointment if there is evidence that the physician
had in the past displayed an inability to work harmoniously with other doctors and
hospital personnel and had charged patients excessive fees.)
[28] *Sosa v. Board of Managers of Val Verde Hosp.,* No. 29458 (W.D. Tex. Jan. 30, 1970),
rev'd, 425 F. 2d 44 (5th Cir. 1970), *aff'd,* 437 F. 2d 173 (5th Cir. 1971).

supported by medical records of specific instances, constituted "sufficient notice" for discipline in the case of *Woodbury v. McKinnon.*[29] The court also held that the hearing can be informal, the plaintiff's attorney need not be permitted to question the other doctors present, as long as the plaintiff could ask questions, and cross-examination need not be a part of every hearing to satisfy due process.[30]

A governmental hospital may thus exercise considerable discretion with respect to medical staff appointments and privileges when the motive is to enhance the quality of care. By way of further example, it has been held proper for a governmental hospital to have and enforce rules regarding the maintenance and completion of medical records.[31] Rules stating well-recognized professional qualifications as a prerequisite for defined privileges will be upheld by the courts as long as they are reasonable, definite, certain, and capable of objective application.[32] The key to validating a particular rule is apparently that it be related to individual qualifications for performing professionally the particular privileges sought or held by the physician. In the formulation of the rules, which should be stated in the hospital bylaws or the medical staff bylaws adopted by the governing board, the board may rely upon professional standards recommended by the medical staff. Thus in *Selden v. City of Sterling* the court approved a rule which stated that an associate medical staff member could not perform major surgery without having a full staff member in attendance.[33]

Similarly, in the interests of patient care, a governmental hospital may have a closed staff in the radiology department as long as the reasons for such a decision can be adequately documented.[34] Does

[29] 447 F. 2d 839 (5th Cir. 1971).
[30] *Id.* at 844. In the proper circumstances, a summary suspension of privileges will not violate due process as long as the physician is afforded an opportunity for a hearing within a reasonable time. *Citta v. Delaware Valley Hosp.,* 313 F. Supp. 301 (E.D. Pa. 1970). (The Fourteenth Amendment applied to the private hospital since it had received federal funds).
[31] *Board of Trustees of the Memorial Hosp. v. Pratt,* 72 Wyo., 120, 262 P. 2d 682 (1953). *Accord: Peterson v. Tucson General Hospital, Inc.,* 559 P. 2d 186 (Ariz. Ct. of App. 1976) (private hospital).
[32] *Green v. City of St. Petersburg,* 154 Fla., 399, 17 So. 2d 517 (1944); *Selden v. City of Sterling,* 316 Ill. App. 455, 45 N.E. 2d 329 (1942); *Jacobs v. Martin,* 20 N.J. Super. 531, 90 A. 2d 151 (1952). *Cf.: Armstrong v. Board of Directors of Fayette County General Hospital,* 553 S.W. 2d 77 (Tenn. 1977). (A public hospital could not require certification or eligibility for certification by the American Board of Surgery for the granting of specified surgical privileges when the physician was in fact competent.)
[33] 316 Ill. App. 455, 45 N.E. 2d 329 (1942).
[34] *Rush v. City of St. Petersburg,* 205 So. 2d 11 (Fla. App. 1967); *Benell v. City of Virginia,* 258 Minn. 559, 104 N.W. 2d 633 (1960). See also: *Letsch v. County Hosp.,* 246 Cal. App. 2d 673, 55 Cal. Rptr. 118 (1966); *Blank v. Palo Alto–Stanford Hosp. Center,* 234 Cal. App. 2d 377, 44 Cal. Rptr. 572 (1965).

a like philosophy prevail with respect to practitioners who do not
possess an M.D. degree? In most states at present the governing
body of a public hospital may deny privileges to licensed osteopathic
doctors and to members of other schools of the healing arts.[35] With
osteopathic physicians, however, local legislation is an important
consideration. If the licensing statutes and other legislation equate
doctors of medicine and of osteopathy, it is then recognized that
the osteopathic physician must be accorded equal substantive rights
and opportunities on the basis of his individual training and qualifications.[36] As the trend toward "merger" of the medical and osteopathic
professions continues, it is likely to be more difficult for the boards
of individual hospitals to exclude osteopathic physicians. Statutory
enactments are likewise crucial in determining the substantive rights
of chiropractors to practice in governmental institutions. For example,
the statutes of North Carolina and North Dakota extend to chiropractors the right to practice in public hospitals within the scope
of their licenses.[37] On the other hand, the statutes of Oklahoma
make a clear distinction between "physicians" and chiropractors, and
accordingly the latter can be excluded from the staff of a county
hospital.[38]

In any event, however, there is some authority that all licensed
practitioners of any school of the healing arts are entitled to procedural
due process when applying for privileges on the staff of a governmental hospital. A podiatrist must hence be granted a hearing upon
his application for privileges, including notice and a full opportunity
to be heard.[39]

A public hospital, again in the interests of its patients' care, may
discipline, suspend, or refuse to reappoint a staff physician if there
is sufficient evidence of incompetence or intolerable behavior.[40] In

[35] *Hayman v. City of Galveston*, 273 U.S. 414 (1927). (Exclusion does not violate the
equal protection clause of the Fourteenth Amendment.)
[36] *Stribling v. Jolley*, 241 Mo. App. 1123, 253 S.W. 2d 519 (Mo. 1952). A Wisconsin
statute, Wis. Stat. Ann., ch. 222, sec. 140.27 (2) (1967), prohibits denial of hospital
staff privileges to any licensed physician solely on the basis that he is an osteopath.
The crucial importance of statutory law with respect to the rights of osteopathic
physicians is also illustrated by *Taylor v. Horn*, 189 So. 2d 198 (Fla. App. 1966).
[37] N.C. Gen. Stat. sec. 90-153 (1965); N.D. Rev. Code, sec. 43-06-17, 43-14-23
(1960). These statutes also apply to private hospitals.
[38] *Boos v. Donnell*, 421 P. 2d 644 (Okla. 1966).
[39] *Shaw v. Hospital Authority of Cobb County*, 507 F. 2d 625 (5th Cir. 1975).
[40] See, e.g., *Mizell v. North Broward Hosp. Dist.*, 175 So. 2d 583 (Fla. App. 1965).
(Proof that the frequency of a physician's erroneous diagnosis was excessive is an
adequate basis for suspension of surgical privileges.)

Koelling v. Skiff Memorial Hospital[41] the Iowa court upheld an indefinite suspension of a staff physician charged with preparing deceptive and misleading medical records, giving fabricated, inconsistent explanations for his handling of a case, and rendering seriously inadequate medical care. The physician is entitled to, and was accorded in the *Koelling* case, a hearing, the right to present proof, and the right to cross-examine witnesses.

The disposition of the problem by the hospital authorities in the *Koelling* litigation should be carefully compared with the procedures followed in the *Milford* case.[42] The true issues in both cases would seem to be same: first, whether a reasonable, objective standard of medical practice in the genuine interests of quality care had been adopted by the governing body, and then whether the physician subject to disciplinary action had been accorded due process of law.

In short, a licensed physician cannot be charged with the violation of a nonexistent standard, nor can he be deprived of procedural safeguards. Having first adopted recognized professional standards capable of objective application for the control of medical practice and personal behavior within the hospital, the governing body of the governmental hospital must then be certain that in all situations involving medical staff appointments and privileges proper hearings are conducted on the merits of each individual situation. Both the standards and the procedural safeguards should be clearly defined in the medical staff bylaws adopted by the governing board.

The 1972 case of *Moore v. Carson-Tahoe Hospital*[43] is most instructive with respect to the hospital's duty on the one hand to exercise reasonable care in the selection and retention of medical staff, and on the other to extend both substantive and procedural rights of due process to the physician when disciplinary action is undertaken. *Moore* involved a medical staff appointment controversy at a Nevada public hospital. Dr. Moore was licensed to practice in Nevada, was certified by the board, and had specialized in obstetrics and gynecology. His privileges were terminated by action of the governing body on the grounds of unprofessional conduct as provided for in the

---

[41] 259 Iowa 1185, 146 N.W. 2d 284 (1966). See also: *Anderson v. Caro Community Hosp.*, 10 Mich. App. 348, 159 N.W. 2d 347 (1968). (The Michigan appellate court upheld the right of a public hospital to dismiss a staff physician who was extended the right of a hearing, when documented behavior clearly violated adequately defined standards of conduct.)
[42] *Supra* n. 14.
[43] 88 Nev. 207, 495 P. 2d 605 (1972), *cert. denied*, 409 U.S. 879 (1972).

medical staff bylaws. The specific acts precipitating the termination were not, however, expressly prohibited in the medical staff bylaws or rules and regulations. The doctor had allegedly attempted to administer a spinal anesthetic to an obstetrics patient but had failed to employ a proper, sterile technique: preparing the medication, performing a minimal skin preparation, and handling the spinal needle, all without the use of sterile gloves. Further, he was not successful in several attempts at spinal puncture. Two days later the chief of the medical staff, with the concurrence of another physician, canceled Dr. Moore's scheduled surgery for that day on the basis that he was "in no condition physically or mentally to perform surgery."

Dr. Moore brought suit to regain his hospital privileges. He did not allege any violation of his rights to procedural due process. Indeed, at the medical staff hearing of the charges against him he was permitted to have counsel present, to call friendly witnesses, and to cross-examine adverse witnesses. Rather, he maintained that he was denied *substantive* due process of law by reason of the uncertain meaning of "unprofessional conduct," the basis for revocation of his privileges.[44]

The Nevada Supreme Court disagreed, citing a Florida case which said: "Detailed description of prohibited conduct is concededly impossible, perhaps even undesirable in view of rapidly shifting standards of medical excellence and the fact that a human life may be and quite often is involved in the ultimate decision of the board."[45] To the same effect was an Oregon case, involving revocation of a license to practice medicine.[46] The *Moore* court held that the standard of "unprofessional conduct" was sufficiently objective, then went on to say:

> Today in response to demands of the public, the hospital is becoming a community health center. The purpose of the community hospital is to provide patient care of the highest possible quality. To implement this duty of providing competent medical care to the patients, it is the responsibility of the institution to create a workable system whereby the

---

[44]Nevada statutes authorize the board of trustees of a public hospital to adopt bylaws, rules, and regulations, governing admission of physicians to the staff, and they grant the board power to organize the staff. The bylaw of the medical staff authorized alteration or revocation of privileges on recommendation of medical staff for "unprofessional conduct." Nev. Rev. Stat. 450.160, 450.180, 450.440 (1971).
[45]*North Broward Hosp. Dist. v. Mizell,* 148 So. 2d 1, 5 (Fla. 1962).
[46]*In re Mintz,* 233 Ore. 441, 378 P. 2d 945 (1963).

medical staff of the hospital continually reviews and evaluates the quality of care being rendered within the institution. The staff must be organized with a proper structure to carry out the role delegated to it by the governing body. All powers of the medical staff flow from the board of trustees, and the staff must be held accountable for its control of quality. The concept of corporate responsibility for the quality of medical care was forcibly advanced in *Darling v. Charleston Community Memorial Hospital,* wherein the Illinois Supreme Court held that hospitals and their governing bodies may be held liable for injuries resulting from imprudent or careless supervision of members of their medical staffs.

The role of the hospital vis-a-vis the community is changing rapidly. The hospital's role is no longer limited to the furnishing of physical facilities and equipment where a physician treats his private patients and practices his profession in his own individualized manner.

The right to enjoy medical staff privileges in a community hospital is not an absolute right, but rather is subject to the reasonable rules and regulations of the hospital. Licensing, *per se,* furnishes no continuing control with respect to a physician's professional competence and therefore does not assure the public of quality patient care. The protection of the public must come from some other authority, and that in this case is the Hospital Board of Trustees. The Board, of course, may not act arbitrarily or unreasonably in such cases. The Board's actions must also be predicated upon a reasonable standard.[47]

In addition to the court's holding that the board had acted pursuant to sufficiently objective standards and rules and regulations, involving no denial of substantive due process, the court further held that the documented evidence at the hearing was sufficient to support the decision to terminate Dr. Moore's privileges.

The *Moore* case provides an excellent illustration of how the duly organized medical staff assumes its properly delegated function of recommending corrective action to the hospital's governing body in order to enforce reasonable rules and regulations *before* the fact of actual injury to the patient.[48] It further demonstrates how board,

---

[47] 88 Nev. at 211, 212, 495 P.2d at 608 (citations omitted). See also: Horty, "A Strong New Statement of Governing Board Responsibility for the Quality of Medical Care," *Action Kit for Hospital Law* 1 (Aug. 1972); Southwick, "Hospital Medical Staff Privileges," 18 *DePaul L. Rev.* 655 (1969).

[48] A dissent by two justices was based upon the following arguments: "Unprofessional conduct" is a vague and an ambiguous standard, not defined, even generally, in the medical staff bylaws. Hence, there is "substantial danger of arbitrary discrimination" and a grant to the board of "almost unlimited power, susceptible of abuse." Moreover,

medical staff, and hospital attorney can work together to guarantee procedural due process of law in connection with medical staff appointments and privileges. Working together is the way to eliminate discord.

Appointments in Private, Nonprofit Hospitals

The fundamental trends of the law in many jurisdictions point toward equating public (governmental) and private institutions, thus requiring the voluntary hospital also to act reasonably and not arbitrarily when determining medical staff appointment matters and to apply its rules and regulations with fundamentally fair procedures. There are at least four legal developments, or four sources of law, which lead to this result, depending upon the facts of the given case and the relevant statutory or judicial law.

These four developments are: relatively recent state statutory enactments which prohibit defined forms of discriminatory or arbitrary decisions by a hospital governing board; state judicial law which simply requires the hospital to act reasonably and with fairness as a matter of public policy; application of state laws prohibiting unlawful restraints of trade or malicious interference with a licensed physician's right to practice medicine; and finally the application of federal statutory civil rights legislation and of the Fourteenth Amendment to the private, voluntary hospital. All four of these fairly new developments reduce the range of freedom and discretion previously enjoyed by the voluntary hospital's board of trustees in appointing or reappointing staff physicians. Correspondingly the doctor's ability to gain appointment has been considerably improved.

Historically the state legislatures have been silent on the relation between a private hospital and the physician who seeks a medical staff appointment. This remains the situation in nearly all states, but statutes are now appearing which prohibit certain discriminatory action. For example, in Wisconsin private hospitals (as well as public) may not deny staff privileges solely on the basis that the individual is an osteopathic physician.[49] Similarly, in New Mexico a private hospital seeking to obtain a license must provide evidence that its

---

the dissent said that Dr. Moore's use of an anesthetic without sterile gloves was no more than an isolated instance of negligence which did not result in injury or damage to the patient, and thus was not a reasonable basis for revocation of privileges. Hence, since the hospital could not have been liable to the patient as a result of this occurrence, arbitrariness was indicated. 88 Nev. at 214, 495 P.2d at 610.

[49]Wis. Stat. Ann., ch. 222, sec. 140.27 (2) (1967).

bylaws or regulations apply equally to osteopathic and medical doctors.[50]

Louisiana provides that a voluntary hospital may not deny medical staff membership solely because of a physician's participation in a group medical practice or lack of membership in a specialty body or professional society.[51] New York hospitals, both public and private, may not reject an applicant on the basis of his participation in a group practice or a nonprofit health insurance plan.[52] Hospital counsel and professional staff must be alert to these local statutory provisions.

Historically and traditionally the posture of the courts has been that a voluntary hospital is a private institution, and hence the governing body could adopt and enforce whatever rules it wished in order to control medical staff appointments and the discipline of its staff, so long as the action was not capricious or with malice.[53] The range of discretion extended to the hospital board of trustees by this traditional judicial attitude is almost unlimited, since the courts have hesitated to inquire whether or not a rule concerning eligibility for a staff appointment or continuing appointment is arbitrary or unreasonable and thus have not intruded into the internal management of the hospital. Procedurally, an applicant for a staff appoint-

---

[50]N.M. Stat. Ann., sec. 12-5-10 (b) (1955), as amended (Supp. 1971).
[51]La. Rev. Stat. Ann., sec. 37: 1301 (1964).
[52]N.Y. Pub. Health Law, sec. 206A (McKinney 1971). Moreover, the New York statutes provide that hospitals must *not* deny or withhold staff membership or diminish privileges of a physician, a dentist, or a *podiatrist* (emphasis supplied) without stating the reasons therefor. The law provides an appeal mechanism to the public health council of the state. N.Y. Public Health Law Section 2801-b (McKinney Supp. 1973). *Fritz v. Huntington Hospital,* 39 N.Y. 2d 339, 384 N.Y.S. 2d 92, 348 N.E. 2d 547 (1976): (A private hospital may not reject applications of two osteopathic physicians solely on the basis that they had not completed an American Medical Association approved training program, since the statute requires that reasons for rejection must be related to standards of patient care or welfare, objectives of the hospital, or character and competency of physician); *Fried v. Straussman,* 393 N.Y.S. 2d 334, 361 N.E. 2d 984, (1977): (If reasons for rejection meet statutory criteria, neither the public health council nor the courts may review the evidence upon which the hospital acted). Moreover, a New York trial court has ruled that a private hospital must at least consider fairly the application of a physician's assistant for privileges to practice, applying relevant criteria of the individual's credentials, training, and experience and granting the applicant procedural due process. The decision was based upon statutory language of the New York Hospital Code setting forth the rules of licensure of hospitals. *Reynolds v. Medical and Dental Staff of Andrus Pavilion of St. John's Riverside Hospital,* 382 N.Y.S. 2d 618, 86 Misc. 2d 418 (Sup. Ct. 1976).
[53]See for example: *Edson v. Griffin,* 21 Conn. Sup. 55, 144 A. 2d 341 (1958); *West Coast Hospital Ass'n v. Hoare,* 64 So. 2d 293 (Fla. 1953); *Levin v. Sinai Hospital,* 186 Md. 174, 46 A. 2d 298 (1946); *Moore v. Andalusia Hospital, Inc.,* 284 Ala. 259, 224 So. 2d 617 (1969): (*Moore* held that the appointment of medical staff to a private hospital is solely in the discretion of the governing body, and a refusal to appoint is not subject to judicial review); *Van Campen v. Olean General Hospital,* 210 App. Div. 204, 205 N.Y.S. 554 (1924).

ment, or a current member of the medical staff who is not to be
reappointed or is subject to discipline, has not been entitled to a
hearing or other procedural safeguards unless the bylaws of the
hospital or medical staff affirmatively provided for such safeguards.[54]
A Wisconsin case decided in 1923 even went so far as apparently
to rule that a staff physician could be dismissed without being afforded
a hearing provided for in the medical staff bylaws, since the staff
bylaws were not binding on the hospital corporation.[55]

Receipt of federal funds through the Hill-Burton or other programs, or receipt of tax revenues from state or local governments,
or a hospital's tax-free status, do not ipso facto change the private
status of a voluntary hospital, and accordingly do not bring into
play the rules pertaining to a government hospital.[56] The recent
cases of *Shulman v. Washington Hospital Center*[57] and *Foote v. Community
Hospital of Beloit*[58] reaffirm the traditional approach, granting to
the voluntary hospital's governing board a nearly absolute discretion
in denying staff privileges, provided only that voluntarily adopted
bylaw requirements relative to procedural safeguards be followed.
In the *Foote* case the Kansas court indicated that it was not necessary
for the hospital to grant a hearing to an applicant for a staff position.
It was proper to give a summary judgment for the hospital which
denied the doctor privileges.[59] In other words, the decision of the

[54] *Joseph v. Passaic Hospital Ass'n*, 26 N.J. 557, 141 A. 2d 18 (1958); *Berberian v.
Lancaster Osteopathic Hospital Ass'n*, 395 Pa. 257, 149 A. 2d 456 (1959).
[55] *State ex rel. Wolf v. LaCrosse Lutheran Hospital Ass'n*, 181 Wis. 33, 193 N.W. 994
(1923). See also: *Natale v. Sisters of Mercy of Council Bluffs*, 243 Iowa 582, 52 N.W.
2d 701 (1952). (Medical staff bylaws providing for a statement of charges against
a physician subject to discipline and a hearing were not binding on the hospital
board, and the board could dismiss the doctor without statement of charges and
hearing.) Cf.: *St. John's Hospital Medical Staff, et al. v. St. John Regional Medical Center,
et al.*, 245 N.W. 2d 472 (S.D. 1976). (Medical staff bylaws adopted and approved
by the hospital's governing body reciting that they are equally binding on the governing
body and medical staff are a "contract" and may not be amended without adherence
to a provision requiring a two-thirds vote of medical staff, citing *Berberian* and *Joseph*,
supra n. 54). See also: *Gashgai v. Maine Medical Association*, 350 A. 2d 571 (Me.
1976). (Bylaws of a medical association were contractual and enforceable by court
in a currently pending disciplinary matter.)
[56] *Shulman v. Washington Hospital Center*, 222 F. Supp. 59 (D.D.C. 1963), 319 F. Supp.
252 (D.D.C. 1970); *West Coast Hosp. v. Hoare*, *supra* n. 53; *Halberstadt v. Kissane*,
51 Misc. 2d 634, 273 N.Y.S. 2d 601 (Sup. Ct. 1966), *aff'd*, 31 A.D. 2d 568, 294
N.Y.S. 2d 841 (1968); *Bricker v. Sceva Speare Memorial Hospital*, 111 N.H. 276, 281
A. 2d 589 (1971), *cert. denied*, 404 U.S. 995 (1971).
[57] *Shulman v. Washington Hosp. Center*, *supra* n. 56.
[58] *Foote v. Community Hosp.*, 195 Kan. 385, 405 P. 2d 423 (1965).
[59] *Id.* A sequel to this case is *Kansas State Board of Healing Arts v. Foote*, 200 Kan.
447, 436 P. 2d 828 (1968), where the Supreme Court of Kansas upheld the Board
of Healing Arts decision in revoking Dr. Foote's license to practice on the grounds
of "extreme incompetency," even though the statute authorizing revocation for
"unprofessional conduct" did not specifically itemize incompetency as embraced within

hospital's governing board is final and not subject to judicial review.[60]

Citing *Shulman, Sams,*[61] and earlier cases, the Illinois Appellate Court has also followed this same traditional approach.[62] The hospital rejected an application from an osteopathic physician because his two physician references were unable or unwilling to comment upon his professional capabilities, and because the applicant lacked an undergraduate degree. The court upheld the rejection, stating, "We refuse to substitute our judgment for that of the hospital authorities regarding the acceptance of the plaintiff for staff membership in a private hospital."[63] Significantly the court observed: "[T]his doctrine is all the more fitting by virtue of the current Illinois law imposing potential liability on a hospital for the imprudent or careless selection of its staff members without limitation to the amount of its liability insurance."[64] There was no problem of unlawful monopoly, the court said, because there were other hospitals in the locality available to the plaintiff.

The traditional judicial attitude of granting the private hospital an almost unlimited discretion, substantively and procedurally, in granting, withholding, and terminating medical staff appointments is tempered, however, by the common law doctrine that interference with a physician's right to practice, committed maliciously, constitutes a cause of action.[65] There is never a privilege to act with malice. Accordingly, where it was established that certain doctors were motivated by their own financial interests in preventing the plaintiff from obtaining staff privileges in the single hospital in the county, an action could be brought against the hospital, the doctors, and the individuals on the governing body.[66]

---

unprofessional conduct. However, under a similar statute the Attorney General of Michigan rendered an opinion contrary to the *Foote* case. *Opinion of the Michigan Attorney General*, no. 4423 (1967). This opinion would appear to support the author's assertion earlier in this text that medical licensing laws are often not adequate to cope with the problem of the quality of medical care rendered within hospitals. However, the Michigan Medical Practice Act has subsequently been revised to strengthen the authority of the licensing board.

[60] See also *Sams v. Ohio Valley General Hosp. Ass'n*, 149 W. Va. 229, 140 S.E. 2d 457 (1965), where the doctor was apparently denied staff privileges as a consequence of his participation in a closed panel group practice, although such was never formally stated as a reason for his exclusion. This state court decision upheld the hospital's denial of privileges to Dr. Sams.

[61] *Id.*

[62] *Mauer v. Highland Park Hosp. Foundation*, 90 Ill. App. 2d 409, 232 N.E. 2d 776 (1967).

[63] *Id.* at 415, 232 N.E. 2d at 779.

[64] *Id.*, citing *Darling v. Charleston Community Memorial Hosp.*, 33 Ill. 2d 326, 211 N.E. 2d 253 (1965), *cert. denied*, 383 U.S. 946 (1966).

[65] *Raymond v. Cregar*, 38 N.J. 472, 185 A. 2d 856 (1962).

[66] *Cowan v. Gibson*, 392 S.W. 2d 307 (Mo. 1965). See also: *Burkhart v. Community Medical Center*, 432 S.W. 2d 433 (Ky. 1968); *Nashville Memorial Hospital, Inc. v. Brinkley*,

State common law pertaining to unlawful restraints of trade can be used as a legal theory or vehicle to attack a voluntary hospital's arbitrary denial of medical staff privileges. The action can be brought against individual members of the board of trustees or the medical staff as well as the hospital corporation, when a trustee or corporation intentionally and without good faith prevents admission to hospital practice on some other basis than the plaintiff's professional qualifications or standards of patient care.[67] In such an action the major problem consists of balancing the interests of the physician in practicing his profession and of the hospital in regulating or preventing his practice. Certainly public policy must play a large role in the court's approach.

In *Blank v. Palo Alto–Stanford Hospital Center*[68] the court held that an exclusive privilege contract with a group of radiologists for the operation of a hospital's radiology department did not violate the California restraint-of-trade concepts when it was established that the contract was entered into to assure high quality care—thus being in the best interests of both the public and the hospital's medical staff. In general however, state statutory enactments regarding restraint of trade cannot be used as a basis for a private cause of action. Such a case would fall outside the purpose of these statutes, either because medical practice does not constitute a "trade" or "commerce" under statutory definitions, or because the doctor cannot show injury to the public.[69]

Federal antitrust statutes, although held applicable to the professions in several recent important decisions, have not yet been used successfully in controversies involving medical staff privileges. One reason for this conclusion is that these statutory laws apply to prohibit

---

534 S.W. 2d 318 (Tenn, 1976): (Allegations of conspiracy without justification or excuse to injure another in the practice of a profession constitute a cause of action. Moreover, express allegations of malice are not necessary, as malice is inferred from allegations that damage was done intentionally without legal justification). *Cf.: Campbell v. St. Mary's Hospital*, 252 N.W. 2d 581 (Minn. 1977). (Unsubstantiated broad allegations of malice do not create a cause of action when staff privileges were revoked).
[67] *Willis v. Santa Ana Community Hosp. Ass'n*, 58 Cal. App. 2d 806, 376 P. 2d 568, 26 Cal. Rptr. 640 (1962).
[68] 234 Cal. App. 2d 377, 44 Cal. Rptr. 572 (1965). See also: *Rush v. City of St. Petersburg*, 205 So. 2d 11 (Fla. 1967): (The court rejected the plaintiff's argument that an exclusive privilege contract with a medical specialist constituted illegal corporate practice of medicine); *Letsch v. Northern San Diego County Hosp. Dist.*, 246 Cal. App. 2d 673, 55 Cal. Rptr. 118 (1966).
[69] *Moles v. White*, 336 So. 2d 427 (Fla. Ct. App. 1976). (An exclusive contract for provision of open heart surgery does not violate a state antitrust statute, since operation of a hospital and practice of medicine are not within the applicability of the statute.)

monopolies or restraints of trade only when interstate commerce is substantially affected.[70]

In the recent case of *Wolf v. Jane Phillips Episcopal–Memorial Medical Center*[71] an osteopathic physician alleged that denial of a staff appointment constituted a per se violation of the Sherman Antitrust Act, which renders illegal every contract, combination, and conspiracy in restraint of trade in interstate commerce.[72] This notable legislation provides a private cause of action for treble damages to victims of a violation. Plaintiff physician claimed that both hospitals in his community were controlled by the defendant and that he had sustained a loss of gross income of $1 million. He sought treble damages and a injunction. The court, however, ruled that plaintiff's cause of action could not succeed. Even if the practice of medicine was subject to antitrust statutes and not exempt as a "learned profession," the Sherman Act was inapplicable because the denial of staff privileges does not substantially affect interstate commerce.[73]

Much more significant than common law concepts of malicious interference with a physician's right of practice, or state law notions of unlawful restraints of trade which circumscribe only to a very limited degree the power of a private hospital to appoint and reappoint medical staff, is the distinct departure in 1963 from the historical and traditional judicial law under which the private hospital had nearly unlimited discretion. This occurred in New Jersey in the landmark case of *Griesman v. Newcomb Hospital.* Without benefit of state statute—or constitutional law doctrine, to be discussed shortly—the court held that a hospital could not arbitrarily refuse to consider the application of an osteopathic physician.[74] The basis of the decision was simply public policy: a private hospital is vested with a public interest and possesses a "fiduciary relationship" to both the patient and the medical community, especially when the hospital is the sole institution in the locality.[75]

---

[70] *Riggal v. Washington County Medical Soc'y*, 249 F. 2d 266 (8th Cir. 1957), *cert. denied*, 355 U.S. 954 (1957).
[71] 513 F. 2d 684 (10th Cir. 1975).
[72] 15 U.S.C. sec. 1.
[73] *Goldfarb v. Virginia State Bar*, 421 U.S. 773, 44 L. Ed. 2d 572, 95 S.Ct. 2004 (1975). (Under federal antitrust statutes there is no exemption for the learned professions). Further, in factual situations other than medical staff appointment controversies, the operation of a hospital may substantially affect interstate commerce, thus conferring jurisdiction in complaints alleging violation of federal antitrust statutes. *Hospital Building Company v. Trustees of Rex Hospital*, 425 U.S. 738, 48 L. Ed. 2d 338, 96 S. Ct. 1848 (1976).
[74] 40 N.J. 389, 192 A. 2d 817 (1963).
[75] *Id.* at 403-4, 192 A. 2d at 825.

Griesman could eventually take its place in history as the basis for a new philosophy with respect to medical staff privileges in a private, nonprofit hospital. The court invalidated bylaw requirements that all staff physicians be graduates of a medical school approved by the American Medical Association and members of the county medical society.[76] Specifically, the court held that the voluntary hospital must at least consider the application of an osteopathic physician. In reaching this conclusion, the case relied heavily upon *Falcone v. Middlesex County Medical Society*, which had determined that the defendant's denial of medical society membership to a licensed osteopathic physician was in violation of the state's public policy.[77] Accordingly the New Jersey court indicated its willingness to inquire into the reasonableness of a rule pertaining to staff privileges, and to strike down the rule if the court found it too arbitrary and not necessarily directly related to standards of patient care.

Following *Griesman*, New Jersey held that a voluntary hospital could not refuse an applicant without giving him the opportunity to have a hearing and learn the reasons for his rejection.[78] The hearing need not be in the nature of a courtroom trial, but the applicant has the right to appear in person if he wishes and present evidence and witnesses in his behalf. An appeal procedure should be provided. This, of course, does not mean that all applicants must be admitted to hospital privileges. It was proper to defer the application of an osteopathic physician whose academic record was shown to be only fair, who had no postgraduate training, and who had privileges elsewhere.[79] In other words, these New Jersey cases have established that all applications must be fully considered and evaluated and that all applicants are entitled to fair consideration in accordance with due process of law.[80]

---

[76] *Id.* at 394, 192 A. 2d at 819.

[77] 34 N.J. 582, 170 A. 2d 791 (1961). See a similar decision in *Blende v. Maricopa County Medical Society*, 96 Ariz. 240, 393 P. 2d 926 (1964). The court ruled that a local medical society cannot arbitrarily deny membership if there is a relationship between society membership and hospital staff privileges. But later litigation established that there was no definite, formal relationship between society membership and hospital staff privileges, and therefore the society could not be required to admit the doctor to membership. *Maricopa County Medical Soc'y v. Blende*, 5 Ariz. App. 454, 427 P. 2d 946 (1967).

[78] *Sussman v. Overlook Hosp. Ass'n*, 95 N.J. Super. 418, 231 A. 2d 389 (1967).

[79] *Schneir v. Englewood Hosp. Ass'n*, 91 N.J. Super. 527, 221 A. 2d 559 (1966).

[80] See also: *Davis v. Morristown Memorial Hospital*, 106 N.J. Super. 33, 254 A. 2d 125 (1969): (Documented evidence of lack of beds in the obstetrical department is sufficient reason to deny a physician's appointment to staff); *Guerrero v. Burlington County Memorial Hospital*, 70 N.J. 344, 360 A. 2d 334 (1976): (A private hospital may deny appointments to the staff of a satellite medical/surgical facility to two

Courts other than those of New Jersey are speaking in terms both of substantive and procedural due process and of unreasonable and discriminatory action when they consider the range of discretion allowed a private hospital in appointment and reappointment of staff physicians.[81] The implication is that the court will intervene on behalf of the doctor if it finds the hospital's action to be unreasonable, arbitrary, or procedurally inconsistent with fairness and objectivity. Essentially then, the position of the voluntary hospital is being equated in New Jersey and other jurisdictions with that of the governmental institution.

California has followed the lead of New Jersey by holding that private as well as public hospitals must provide due process to physicians who are denied staff appointments or who are disciplined, even if hospital bylaws do not require such procedures. In *Ascherman v. San Francisco Medical Society, et al.* the physician had privileges at Franklin Hospital, Hahneman Hospital, and St. Joseph's Hospital.[82] All three institutions denied him annual reappointment to their respective staffs without granting an opportunity for a hearing and without giving him a statement of the reasons for denial. The hospitals maintained that their bylaws required a hearing only if the doctor were disciplined during the term of annual appointment, and that they did not require a hearing when annual reappointment was withheld. Thereupon Dr. Ascherman applied for appointment at

---

eminently qualified surgeons when denial was based upon documented evidence of limited bed capacity, the fact that current staff was providing adequate surgical coverage, and that the needs of the community would not be served by adding to the surgical staff). Cf.: *Walsky v. Pascack Valley Hospital*, 367 A. 2d 1204 (N.J. Super. Ct. 1976). (A moratorium on additions to medical staff, which was adopted in 1969 when hospital utilization was approximately 96 per cent, and renewed annually but sometimes violated in individual cases, and which did not accomplish its intended purpose of reducing utilization, is arbitrary and capricious, violating the constitutional rights of physician applicants and the public policy of the state.)

[81] *Woodard v. Porter Hosp.*, 125 Vt. 419, 217 A. 2d 37 (1966); *Hagan v. Osteopathic General Hosp.*, 102 R.I. 717, 232 A. 2d 596 (1967): (The court held for the hospital in a privilege controversy, stressing that due process of law had been observed and that there were adequate reasons for rejection of the applicant); *Davidson v. Youngstown Hospital Ass'n*, 19 Ohio App. 2d 246, 250 N.E. 2d 892 (1969); *Bricker v. Sceva Speare Memorial Hospital*, 111 N.H. 276, 281 A. 2d 589 (1971), *cert. denied*, 404 U.S. 995, (1971); *Hawkins v. Kinsie*, 540 P. 2d 345 (Colo. App. 1975): (An osteopathic physician stated a claim for damages by alleging that the decision of a private hospital not to renew his privileges was arbitrary, capricious, and unreasonable); *Park Hospital District, et al. v. District Court of the Eighth Judicial District in the County of Larimer*, 555 P. 2d 984 (Colo. 1976); *McElhinney v. William Booth Memorial Hospital*, 544 S.W. 2d 216 (Ky. 1977): (Whether a hospital is public or private, the court will review its bylaws and require sufficiently definite standards prescribing physicians' conduct to justify revocation of staff privileges.) Cf.: *Moles v. White*, 336 So. 2d 427 (Fla. Dist. Ct. App. 1976): (Allegations that the private hospital serves a public purpose did not make it a public institution requiring due process).

[82] 39 Cal. App. 3d 623, 114 Cal. Rptr. 681 (1974).

French Hospital, but this application was rejected, again without a hearing and without stated reasons for the action.

The San Francisco Medical Society had also removed the physician's name from its referral service, apparently because of certain philosophical or political differences which arose between Dr. Ascherman and others in the early 1960s. At that time Dr. Ascherman was an advocate for a federally financed medical care program, eventually legislated by Congress as Medicare. When he challenged the American Society for Internal Medicine as a "lobbying group" for those opposing Medicare and questioned the bona fides of that organization, Dr. Ascherman suddenly found himself excluded from the staffs of four hospitals and without professional referrals. He brought suit against the medical society, the hospitals, the malpractice insurance carrier insuring members of the medical society (which had canceled his insurance), and various individuals who participated in these decisions, asking not only for an injunction which would restore his privileges but for compensatory and punitive damages. The trial court judge directed a verdict as a matter of law in favor of all defendants on all of plaintiff's claims.

The California Court of Appeal disagreed and reversed in part the judgment of the trial court. The opinion rejects the traditional, historical rule that a court will not review the nearly unlimited discretion granted to a private hospital in excluding or disciplining staff physicians. In essence it held that a private institution affects the public interest and possesses a fiduciary duty, thus requiring that minimal due process be afforded staff physicians with respect to both initial appointments and renewal of appointments. Minimal due process includes at least an opportunity for a hearing, preceded by appropriate notice, a written statement of charges or reasons for denial of appointment or reappointment, a right in the physician to call witnesses on his behalf, a right of cross-examination of hospital witnesses, a right that the decision of the hearing body be supported by substantial evidence produced at the hearing, and a right to have a written decision of the hearing body along with the basis of the decision.[83] The physician is not necessarily entitled to have his counsel present at the hearing, but if hospital counsel is present then the doctor is likewise entitled to be represented by his attorney. Most significantly, as in the New Jersey cases, this judicial decision was based simply upon public policy and was not grounded upon rights guaranteed by the Fourteenth Amendment to the U.S. Constitution.

---

[83] 39 Cal. App. 3d 623, 648; 114 Cal. Rptr. 681, 697 (1974).

Accordingly the California Court of Appeal reversed the trial judgment in favor of the San Francisco Medical Society and the several hospitals, requiring them to afford due process to Dr. Ascherman.

Also of major significance in *Ascherman* was the court's ruling that the individual physicians participating in the hearing and peer review process are immune from personal liability in damages so long as they acted in good faith and without malice. Such immunity is provided for by California statute, and the court held the statute to be constitutional.[84] As to whether or not the individual defendants in this particular litigation had acted in good faith without malice, a new trial before a jury was required on the factual issues.

In California, as in some other jurisdictions, a professional society must provide both substantive and procedural fairness when determining eligibility for membership or when disciplining a member.[85] It is noteworthy that this 1974 California case was decided by the California Supreme Court following the California Court of Appeal decision in *Ascherman*. Hence the highest court of the state has essentially affirmed the principles of public policy articulated earlier in 1974 by the court of appeal. This is certainly the trend of judicial opinion: a private organization is no longer privileged to act unreasonably or arbitrarily, since in practical effect it exercises considerable power over a physician's ability to practice, to serve his patients, and to earn a living.

Actually this requirement of granting an aggrieved physician the rights of due process can be of real value to the hospital and the medical staff in their effort to establish and maintain professionally accepted standards of practice. If a hearing is conducted as mandated by *Ascherman* and if the physician persists in pursuing the controversy in the courts, subsequent judicial review of the matter will be limited to determining whether there was sufficient evidence to support the hearing committee's decision. The court will not accept or rule on any new evidence presented on behalf of the rejected or disciplined physician. Hence, as long as rules or standards invoked by the hospital to deny an appointment or discipline a doctor bear a reasonable or rational relation to the standards of patient care or objectives of the hospital, and as long as there is sufficient evidence to justify the decision adverse to the physician, the court will not interfere.

Subsequent to the decision of *Ascherman v. San Francisco Medical*

---

[84] Cal. Civil Code sec. 43.7, 39 Cal. App. 3d 623, 663, 114 Cal. Rptr. 681, 707 (1974).
[85] *Pinsker v. Pacific Coast Society of Orthodontists, et al.*, 12 Cal. 3d 541, 526 P. 2d 253, 116 Cal. Rptr. 245 (1974).

Society the same physician filed suit against St. Francis Memorial Hospital, challenging a medical staff bylaw which required that applicants be supported by three letters of recommendation from active members of the medical staff. The bylaw was struck down as unreasonable, since it would allow active members of the staff to exclude applicants arbitrarily or for discriminatory reasons.[86] This does not mean of course that a hospital cannot require applicants to submit letters of recommendation, but it does require the hospital to grant each applicant a fair hearing and to evaluate letters of recommendation objectively without requiring the letters to be from a particular source.

The fourth development—or source of law—which requires the private hospital to act reasonably and fairly in medical staff appointments is the application of the Fourteenth Amendment and federal civil rights legislation to the physician-hospital relationship. The starting point is to recognize that the Fourteenth Amendment provides that no state shall deny any person equal protection of law or due process of law. Moreover 42 United States Code, Section 1983 authorizes a civil action for deprivation of civil rights when the alleged deprivation is caused by a person "acting under color of state law." Accordingly a physician is entitled to equal protection and due process only when the hospital is engaged in "state action" or when it acts under "color of law." Without question, governmental hospitals are engaged in state action and must therefore grant the physician these constitutional rights, but the situation is not nearly so clear with respect to the private institution.[87]

Initially the legal issue of "state action" is jurisdictional, meaning simply that the court must determine if it has the jurisdiction to review whether or not the hospital extended equal protection and due process to the doctor. Many decisions have now accumulated in both federal and state courts with respect to this issue with varying and inconsistent results.

Although neither regulation by government nor the receipt of governmental funds or such governmental benefits as tax exemptions converts a private hospital per se into a public or governmental institution, an authoritative line of decisions holds that such factors do subject the voluntary hospital to the Fourteenth Amendment.

---

[86] *Ascherman v. St. Francis Memorial Hospital,* 45 Cal. App. 3d 507, 119 Cal. Rptr. 507 (1975).
[87] A governmental hospital must extend equal protection and due process: *Foster v. Mobile County Hospital Board,* 398 F. 2d 227 (5th Cir. 1968); *Sosa v. Board of Managers of Val Verde Hospital,* 437 F. 2d 173 (5th Cir. 1971).

Several of these cases have involved alleged racial discrimination, but the application of constitutional mandates to the private hospital is not restricted to this form of discriminatory conduct.[88]

A leading case held that the receipt by the hospital of substantial amounts of Hill-Burton funds from the federal government entitled the plaintiff physicians to equal protection.[89] The court went on to rule that the private hospital could not exclude the applicants simply on the grounds that their medical office was located outside the county where the hospital was located. Such a rule for medical staff membership had no rational basis and was unreasonable and arbitrary.

Likewise the Supreme Court of Hawaii held in *Silver v. Castle Memorial Hospital* that it would take jurisdiction and require due process even in the absence of allegations of racial discrimination when the defendants had "received more than nominal governmental funding."[90] "State action" was present *in Schlein v. Milford Hospital,* when the Connecticut hospital licensing law required a showing of "demonstrable need" for hospitals in a given area, especially when the defendant was the only hospital in the area.[91] The hospital's denial of staff privileges thus had the effect of constituting a "de facto" geographical restriction on the physician's license to practice medicine anywhere in the state, and the court refused to grant the hospital's motion to dismiss the action. The *Schlein* decision acknowledged the more restrictive view of "state action" articulated by another federal district court in *Barrett v. United Hospital* but distinguished *Barrett* on the basis that it had not considered the significance of the state's involvement in licensing both hospitals and doctors.[92]

---

[88] A leading decision applying the Fourteenth Amendment to a private hospital when there were allegations of racial discrimination is *Simkins v. Moses H. Cone Memorial Hospital,* 323 F. 2d 959 (4th Cir. 1963), *cert. denied,* 376 U.S. 938 (1964). Another is *Eaton v. Grubbs,* 329 F. 2d 710 (4th Cir. 1964). In Eaton a local government unit had appointed members of the original governing board of a private hospital, local taxes were appropriated to the hospital's use, and the deed to the hospital's land provided for title to revert to the county if hospital use should cease.

[89] *Sams v. Ohio Valley General Hospital Ass'n,* 413 F. 2d 826 (4th Cir. 1969).

[90] 53 Hawaii 475, 497 P. 2d 564 (1972), *cert. denied,* 405 U.S. 1048 (1972). Another case finding "state action" to be present when governmental funding of the hospital was present is *Citta v. Delaware Valley Hospital,* 313 F. Supp. 301 (E.D. Pa. 1970).

[91] *Schlein v. Milford Hospital,* 383 F. Supp. 1263 (Conn. 1974). Subsequent litigation, however, determined that the physician had been accorded sufficient due process. An opportunity to appear before the hospital's credentials committee to refute adverse reports, a written statement of reasons for denial of privileges, a hearing before an ad hoc committee of the medical staff, and the right of appeal to the hospital's executive committee established that the hospital had not acted arbitrarily. *Schlein v. Milford Hospital,* 423 F. Supp. 541 (Conn. 1976).

[92] *Barrett v. United Hospital,* 376 F. Supp. 791 (S.D.N.Y. 1974), *aff'd,* 506 F. 2d 1395 (2d Cir. 1974).

In *Barrett* a private hospital revoked the physician's privileges following his plea of guilty in a criminal assault proceeding. His license to practice medicine was also revoked. Subsequently, after his license was restored, the hospital board upon recommendation of medical staff denied reestablishment of hospital privileges. Dr. Barrett then brought suit alleging violation of his civil and constitutional rights. The court granted the defendant's motion for summary judgment, dismissing the plaintiff's complaint and ruling that the hospital was not engaged in "state action" or "acting under color of state law."

In arriving at this conclusion the court rejected the view that receipt of governmental funds, even in substantial amounts, brings into play the Fourteenth Amendment or the civil rights statutes, in the absence of allegations of racial discrimination or when the hospital was not placed in the role of conducting a "public function." Receipt by the hospital of other governmental benefits, such as tax-exempt status, the existence of various state regulatory laws pertaining to private hospitals, and the fact that United Hospital was the only general hospital in the community did not alter this conclusion. Relying in part upon analogous case precedent within its circuit as well as upon decisions in other federal circuits, the district court articulated a "three-pronged test" for the presence of "state action." The plaintiff must show that the state's involvement with the private hospital is significant, that the state is involved with the activity that caused the injury, and that the state aided, encouraged, or connoted approval of the activity.

The second of these requirements—involvement of the state in causing the injury—is the "nexus" requirement. Governmental funding and regulation do not satisfy the "nexus" requirement, since these activities of government do not cause the plaintiff's injury. Nor does government thereby aid, encourage, or approve of the complained of activity. The "public function" exception to the three-pronged test for the presence of state action is confined to situations where private organizations perform a function traditionally performed by the state: for example, ownership and operation of a company town or of a public park. A private hospital is not "governmental in nature"; even if it is performing a public function with respect to patient care, it is not so acting in the appointment of medical staff or the hiring and firing of other staff personnel. Accordingly, since the hospital was not engaged in "state action" or "acting under color-of-law" the court did not extend constitutional protections to the physician.[93]

Where the hospital's facilities are owned by a county government, however, and leased to a private corporation, and where some governmental officials are members of the board of the corporation, all in addition to the receipt of governmental funds, "state action" is present.[94]

The Oklahoma Supreme Court recently adopted the three-pronged test of *Barrett* and held that it would not review the termination of privileges of a radiologist who had allegedly been a disruptive force on the medical staff of a private hospital. Even though the hospital had received substantial sums of money from both the federal and local government, there was not "state action" justifying judicial intervention.[95]

The hesitation of the courts to intervene in disputes about medical staff appointments and privileges, either on the basis that a private hospital is subject only to a requirement that it adhere to voluntarily adopted bylaws, or on the basis that the hospital is not subject to "state action" and thus need not afford constitutional law protections to the physician, is commendable in one sense. Judicial tribunals are not competent to make managerial decisions more properly vested in the governing board of the institution. Nevertheless, in the light of conflicting judicial opinion in both federal and state courts with respect to both the common law of public policy and the applicability of constitutional law to the hospital-physician relationship, all hospitals should develop policies and procedures that ensure substantive and procedural due process. Such policies will minimize the prospects of lawsuits by physicians challenging the hospital's decisions regarding medical staff appointments and the delineation of privileges.

Moreover, in addition to local case law which requires the private

---

[93]Illustrative of cases reaching the same conclusion with respect to "state action" are: *Mulvihill v. Julia L. Butterfield Memorial Hospital,* 329 F. Supp. 1020 (S.D.N.Y. 1971); *Berrios v. Memorial Hospital, Inc.,* 403 F. Supp. 1222 (E.D. Tenn. 1975); *Ward v. St. Anthony Hospital,* 476 F. 2d 671 (10th Cir. 1973); *Ascherman v. Presbyterian Hospital of Pacific Medical Center, Inc.,* 507 F. 2d 1103 (9th Cir. 1974); *Monyek v. Parkway General Hospital,* 273 So. 2d 430 (Fla. App. 1973): (A proprietary hospital receiving governmental funds); *Sokol v. University Hospital, Inc.,* 402 F. Supp. 1029 (Mass. 1975); *Gotsis v. Lorain Community Hospital,* 46 Ohio App. 2d 8 (1974); *Briscoe v. Bock,* 540 F. 2d 392 (8th Cir. 1976); *Ford v. Harris County Medical Society,* 535 F. 2d 321 (5th Cir. 1976).
[94]*O'Neill v. Grayson County War Memorial Hospital,* 472 F. 2d 1140 (6th Cir. 1973).
[95]*Ponca City Hospital, Inc. v. Murphree,* 545 P. 2d 738 (Okla. 1976).

hospital to act reasonably and not arbitrarily and to afford procedural fairness, both the "Conditions for Participation—Hospitals" contained in the Medicare regulations and the Standards of the Joint Commission on Accreditation of Hospitals dictate essentially the same conclusions. The "Conditions" require the hospital's governing body to appoint physicians and define privileges on the basis of written, defined criteria. Criteria for selection are: individual character, competence, training, experience, and judgment.[96] All qualified candidates are to be considered by the credentials committee of the medical staff, which then makes recommendations to the board of trustees. The interpretation of the Standards of the Joint Commission require delineation of privileges commensurate with an individual's training, experience, competence, judgment, character, and current capability.[97] Further, the Joint Commission's *Guidelines for the Formulation of Medical Staff By-laws, Rules and Regulations*, published in 1971, carefully provide for procedural due process.

The sole, overall guideline for policy with respect to medical staff appointments and the delineation of privileges should be simply the quality of professional care rendered in the light of the hospital's objectives and capabilities. Any rule or criterion for medical staff appointment that relates objectively to standards of patient care, the objectives and purposes of the hospital, or the clinical and ethical behavior of the individual physician will be upheld as reasonable and not arbitrary, and thus consistent with substantive equal protection and due process. A host of cases support hospitals' efforts to upgrade and maintain programs to improve quality. To illustrate, a hospital may require physicians to sign and abide by reasonable medical staff bylaws,[98] to serve on a rotating basis in the emergency room,[99] and to be responsible for timely completion of medical records.[100] It may require applicants for a staff appointment to supply references,[101] and it may require consultation in surgical or medical cases as defined

---

[96] 20 C.F.R. sec. 405.1021, 405.1023 (1973).

[97] *Accreditation Manual for Hospitals,* Joint Commission on Accreditation of Hospitals, Chicago (1976), 108. See also the revised and expanded interpretation of new standards in the *Second Supplement to Manual* (1977), 103–9.

[98] *Yeargin v. Hamilton Memorial Hospital,* 225 Ga. 661, 171 S.E. 2d 136 (1969), *cert. denied,* 397 U.S. 963 (1970)

[99] *Yeargin v. Hamilton Memorial Hospital,* 229 Ga. 870, 195 S.E. 2d 8 (1972).

[100] *Board of Trustees of the Memorial Hospital of Sheridan County v. Pratt,* 72 Wyo. 120, 262 P. 2d 682 (1953); *Peterson v. Tucson General Hospital, Inc.,* 559 P. 2d 186 (Ariz. Ct. App. 1976).

[101] *Rao v. Board of County Commissioners,* 80 Wash. 2d 695, 497 P. 2d 591 (1972).

by medical staff.[102] Physicians may be required by a hospital to carry malpractice insurance coverage.[103] Further, surgical or specialty privileges can be restricted; for example, major surgery in a given specialty may be limited to those who are board certified or board eligible or have been admitted to fellowship in the American College of Physicians and Surgeons, or to those with a minimum of ten years' experience in the specialty, as approved by the medical staff executive committee.[104] Such restrictions on the conduct of major surgery may be adopted by the board of trustees upon recommendation of medical staff and even be applied to physicians who had previously been performing major surgery. It is not unreasonable, arbitrary, or capricious to exclude a physician from further practice of a specialty when he is unable to meet professionally approved criteria.

Both public and private hospitals act reasonably in refusing to appoint, or to suspend the appointment of, physicians and in disciplining physicians for documented professional incompetence.[105] Even when the physician is legally entitled to due process, summary suspension for clinical incompetence will be upheld as long as the physician is afforded a hearing within a reasonable time after suspension.[106] After a right to a hearing, dismissal from staff as a result of "intolerable personal behavior" in violation of adequately defined standards of conduct is proper.[107] An application for appointment may be rejected if the physician fails to document his

---

[102] *Fahey v. Holy Family Hospital,* 32 Ill. App. 3d 537, 336 N.E. 2d 309 (1975). (A rule requiring that any physician not a member of the department of obstetrics and gynecology must obtain consultation before performing major surgery in this specialty is reasonable and may be enforced against a physician who had been performing such surgery without consultation.)

[103] *Pollock v. Methodist Hospital,* 392 F. Supp. 393 (E.D. La. 1975). Accord: *Homes v. Hoemako Hospital,* 573 P. 2d 477 (Ariz. 1977); see also: *Jones v. State Board of Medicine,* 555 P. 2d 399 (Idaho 1976). (Statutory requirement that both physicians and hospitals obtain malpractice insurance as condition of licensure is constitutional.)

[104] *Khan v. Suburban Community Hospital,* 45 Ohio St. 2d 39, 340 N.E. 2d 398 (1976). *Cf.:* Armstrong v. Board of Directors of Fayette County General Hospital, 553 S.W. 2d 77 (Tenn. 1977). (A public hospital may not require board certification or eligibility for major surgical privileges.)

[105] Illustrative cases are: *Koelling v. Skiff Memorial Hospital,* 259 Iowa 1185, 146 N.W. 2d 284 (1966); *Mizell v. North Broward Hospital District,* 175 So. 2d 583 (Fla. App. 1965); *Sosa v. Board of Managers of Val Verde Hospital,* 437 F. 2d 173 (5th Cir. 1971); *Moore v. Board of Trustees of Carson-Tahoe Hospital,* 88 Nev. 207, 495 P. 2d 605 (1972), *cert. denied,* 409 U.S. 879 (1972). *Klinge v. Lutheran Charities Association of St. Louis,* 383 F. Supp. 287 (Mo. 1974), *modified,* 523 F. 2d 56 (8th Cir. 1975).

[106] *Citta v. Delaware Valley Hospital,* 313 F. Supp. 301 (E.D. Pa. 1970).

[107] *Anderson v. Caro Community Hospital,* 10 Mich. App. 348, 159 N.W. 2d 347 (1968).

"ability to work with others" when such a requirement is specified in the bylaws.[108]

A private hospital may limit the use of its laboratory facilities to members of its medical staff and physicians licensed by the state board of medical examiners, thus excluding the patients of chiropractors. Since such a policy was recommended by a state agency, the board of medical examiners, the adoption of the policy by the hospital was "state action." However, such a policy of discrimination against chiropractors was reasonable and constitutionally permissible, since state licensing laws distinguish between the several professions practicing different systems of treating disease; moreover, the action of the hospital was additionally based upon protecting its status of accreditation by the Joint Commission on Accreditation of Hospitals.[109]

It is therefore readily apparent that courts will uphold the efforts of hospital boards which are following documented recommendations of relevant committees of medical staff in programs to improve quality of care, at least when the procedures in enforcing the programs are fundamentally fair. As recently stated by the Supreme Court of Ohio, "It is the board, not the court, which is charged with the responsibility of providing a staff of competent physicians. The board has chosen to rely upon the advice of medical staff, and the court may not surrogate for the staff in discharging their responsibility."[110]

The responsibility of the governing board to select a competent medical staff includes the authority to enter into an exclusive contract with a given physician or group of physicians for specialty services. Hospitals frequently enter into exclusive contractual arrangements for staffing the radiology and pathology departments, for example. Such contracts have been upheld, even for a governmental hospital, as long as adequate reasons relating to standards of patient care and efficient hospital operation exist and can be satisfactorily documented.[111] In *Adler v. Montefiore Hospital Association of Western Pennsylvania* a private hospital employed Dr. Edward Curtiss as

[108] *Huffaker v. Bailey*, 540 P. 2d 1398 (Oregon 1975).
[109] *Aasum v. Good Samaritan Hospital*, 395 F. Supp. 363 (Oregon 1975), *modified* and *aff'd*, 542 F. 2d 792 (9th Cir. 1976). (A private tax-exempt hospital is not engaged in state action even though three of seven board members were appointed by public authority, the hospital received federal funds, and policy with respect to chiropractors' use of laboratory facilities was recommended by the Board of Medical Examiners.)
[110] *Khan v. Suburban Community Hospital*, 45 Ohio St. 2d 39, 43-44, 340 N.E. 2d 398, 402 (1976).
[111] *Rush v. City of St. Petersburg*, 205 So. 2d 11 (Fla. App. 1967); *Benell v. City of Virginia*, 258 Minn. 559, 104 M.W. 2d 633 (1960); *Blank v. Palo Alto-Stanford Hospital Center*, 234 Cal. App. 2d 377, 44 Cal. Rptr. 572 (1965) (radiology).

full-time salaried director of the cardiology laboratory and granted him the exclusive privilege of performing cardiac catheterizations, thereby excluding other qualified cardiologists from performing this specialized procedure. In the subsequent lawsuit by Dr. Adler challenging this arrangement it was stipulated by the parties that the hospital was "at least a quasi-public institution" and that the doctrine of "state action" would apply. Nevertheless the exclusive arrangement was upheld as reasonable and related to the hospital's objectives, especially since it was a teaching institution.[112] Catheterization, the court held, was a laboratory procedure like radiology—as distinct from surgery, for example—and thus there had been no denial of plaintiff's right to admit his private patients to the hospital or treat them; nor was there denial of a corresponding right in the patient to select his own physician. The exclusive contract was a part of the general advancement of medical specialization designed to protect both the patient's safety and the hospital's operation, as evidenced by the following factors established by expert witness testimony: the procedure of catheterization requires a team, and a single physician can best train and supervise the team; the physician can best maintain his competence if he performs more than just a few catheterizations over a period of time; failure of equipment can be minimized by having only one physician responsible for its use and maintenance; scheduling problems for patients can be reduced or minimized; a full-time physician is better able to teach students; it is in the best interests of patient care that the physician performing the procedure be on the hospital premises at all times in the event of complications; and finally, the hospital board can better monitor the quality of care when one person is in charge of the laboratory. Accordingly there was no violation of Dr. Adler's rights to substantive due process and equal protection, since he must yield to reasonable rules intended to benefit the hospital's patients and their physicians, the university and its students, and the public.

Consistent with *Adler* was the action of the Arizona Court of Appeals which upheld an exclusive contract with two internists to provide nuclear medicine services.[113] The reasons given for approving the arrangement were the same as in *Adler*, namely, improved patient care and efficient hospital operation. The legal issues in the Arizona litigation were, however, different from those resolved in the Penn-

---

[112] *Adler v. Montefiore Hospital Association of Western Pennsylvania*, 453 Pa. 60, 311 A. 2d 634 (1973), *cert. denied*, 414 U.S. 1131 (1974).
[113] *Dattilo v. Tucson General Hospital*, 23 Ariz. App. 392, 533 P.2d 700 (1975).

sylvania decision. Dr. Dattilo alleged that the contract was an unreasonable restraint of trade in violation of both the common law and
federal or state antitrust statutes, and that it thus entitled him to
damages as the victim of the illegal monopoly. Ruling against this
contention the court applied the "rule of reason" and a "balancing
test." The rule of reason, applicable to both the federal antitrust
legislation (the Sherman Act) and similar state statutes, means simply
that only *unreasonable* restraints are unlawful. Although the common
law does provide a right of action where an individual's right to
pursue a lawful business or occupation is intentionally interfered
with,[114] justification for the contract is determined "by balancing,
in the light of all the circumstances, the relative importance to society
and the parties of protecting the activities interfered with on one
hand and permitting the interference on the other." [115] In the light
of improved standards of patient care and efficient operation of
the department of nuclear medicine the contract was justified.

In three other recent cases, courts have refused to intervene in
decisions of hospital authorities to confer exclusive privileges on
designated physicians. All concerned arrangements for exclusive
rights with respect to medical diagnosis and care and treatment of
patients, in contradistinction to services characterized in some of
the cases previously discussed as "laboratory procedures." Hence
these cases have the effect of restricting medical staff privileges of
other qualified and competent staff physicians. In *Dell v. St. Joseph
Mercy Hospital of Detroit, Inc.,* a contract between the hospital and
certain private cardiologists designated the latter as possessing the
exclusive right to make "official interpretations of electrocardiograms
for the official hospital records." Although Dr. Dell, a fully qualified
internist whose competence was not questioned, was not actually
prohibited from interpreting the electrocardiograms of his private
patients, the exclusive arrangement had the effect of prohibiting
his interpretation from becoming a part of the "official records."
Since both the hospital and the possessors of the exclusive right
billed the patient or the patient's insurance carrier for the "official"
interpretation, the plaintiff physician was in actuality unable to collect
for his services in connection with any diagnosis that he might make

---

[114] *Willis v. Santa Anna Community Hospital Ass'n,* 58 Cal. 2d 806, 376 P. 2d 568,
26 Cal. Rptr. 640 (1962). See *supra* n. 65–72.
[115] 533 P. 2d at 703, 704. See also: *Harron v. United Hospital Center, Inc., Clarksburg,
W. Va.,* 522 F. 2d 1133 (4th Cir. 1975), *cert. denied,* 96 S. Ct. 1116 (1976). (An
exclusive radiology contract does not violate the federal Sherman Antitrust Act or
the civil rights statutes, 42 U.S.C. sec. 1981, 1983, and 1985.

for his patient following an electrocardiogram. His suit alleged
violations of constitutional and civil rights. The federal district court
dismissed the action, commenting that it was "unable to comprehend
in what manner plaintiff's constitutional rights have been violated."[116]
In *Sokol v. University Hospital, Inc.*, the plaintiff, a cardiac surgeon,
challenged the hospital's restriction of cardiac surgery to a single
surgeon on two grounds: he alleged, first, that the contract violated
antitrust statutes; and, secondly, that his civil rights were impaired.
Again the court dismissed the suit, saying that no claim was stated
under the federal Sherman Antitrust Act. Further, it was held, the
private university hospital was not engaged in "state action," and
hence the court would not review the allegations of deprivation of
civil rights.[117]

Similarly, the Florida District Court of Appeal has reached the
same results. A professional service corporation and a heart surgeon
alleged that an exclusive contract for open-heart surgery violated
state antitrust statutes, deprived the plaintiffs of their right to
constitutional equal protection and due process of law, and finally,
was contrary to general state common law or public policy, which
should require private hospitals serving a public purpose to evaluate
fairly an applicant's training, experience, and current competence
when making a decision on an application for appointment and
delineation of privileges. In actuality, the hospital's chief executive
officer had summarily rejected the surgeon's application without
referral to the credentials committee or to the medical staff for
recommendation. This decision was upheld and the suit was properly
dismissed. The court held that state antitrust legislation was not
applicable to the practice of medicine or the operation of a hospital
in the absence of clear legislative intention to the contrary, since
the statutes pertain only to "trade" or "commerce." Moreover, since
a private hospital is not engaged in state action, constitutional
protections do not apply; finally, a mere allegation that the hospital
serves a public purpose does not mandate that the physician be
provided due process.[118]

A private hospital having an affiliation agreement with a university
medical school which restricts the medical staff of the hospital to
those physicians who also hold a university faculty appointment acts
"reasonably," since the rule is necessary for successful operation of

---

[116] *Dell v. St. Joseph Mercy Hospital of Detroit, Inc.*, Civil no. 4070668 (E.D. Mich. 1974)
(*unreported opinion*).
[117] 402 F. Supp. 1029 (Mass. 1975).
[118] *Moles v. White*, 336 So. 2d 427 (Fla. Ct. App. 1976).

a teaching institution.[119] Rejected by the appellate court was an argument by plaintiff that the arrangement constituted an abdication of the responsibility of the hospital's governing body to appoint medical staff, or constituted at least an unauthorized delegation of responsibility to the university medical school. In response to un-contradicted expert testimony that without this type of affiliation agreement the hospital would lose its status as a teaching institution, the court held that in actuality the ultimate power of staff appoint-ments continued to rest with the hospital's board of trustees.

Hospital administrators can expect further challenges to exclusive contracts or closed staffs. Attorney James E. Ludlam has pointed out that the litigation often concerns the matter of *how* the contract was entered into as well as *what* was done. Accordingly he cautions that the procedure of making and implementing the decision deserves major attention. Specifically recommended are the following guide-lines. The governing body of the hospital should first decide on the desirability of a closed staff, preferably without considering the individual or individuals who are to receive the contract. This decision must be accompanied by fully documented written recommendations from the medical staff stating the reasons for the decision. Qualifi-cations of the persons to receive the contract should be determined and specified in writing; a joint board–medical staff search committee should be created, with authority to recommend the individual to receive the contract; the contract itself should be carefully drafted and contain a full description of the mutual rights and responsibilities of the parties; and the economic arrangements, standards of per-formance, and the right of termination should be carefully delineated. If a physician should challenge the contract he should be given the opportunity for a hearing, although the issue at the hearing should be confined to the initial decision to enter into the exclusive contract and should avoid questions relative to the professional qualifications of any individual who was awarded the contract or who challenges the award.[120]

Procedure in making and implementing decisions is fully as impor-tant as substance in deterring lawsuits or providing a successful defense to a suit. Procedural due process has been referred to throughout this chapter and discussed in some depth in the context

---

[119] *Dillard v. Rowland,* 520 S.W. 2d 81 (Mo. App. 1974).
[120] Ludlam, "Legal Pitfalls in Exclusive Physician-Hospital Agreements," *The Hospital Medical Staff,* December 1975, 6–10.

of staff appointments in the governmental hospital.[121] An excellent case further illustrating the importance of procedural fairness is *Klinge v. Lutheran Charities Association of St. Louis.*[122]

In 1972 Dr. Klinge's surgical practice was placed under certain restrictions following a review of his cases by a record review committee. Approximately two years later all privileges were revoked upon further accumulation of evidence that the physician simply could not practice surgery. This documented evidence, obtained fairly and objectively by the medical staff review committees, assured that the physician had been afforded substantive due process. Procedurally the physician was given a hearing before a panel of staff physicians; he was also provided with a written statement of fifteen specific charges against him, given access to approximately ninety-five hospital documents supporting the alleged professional inadequacies, furnished with a copy of the hearing panel's findings sustaining ten of the charges, and finally given an opportunity to appear before the full board of trustees prior to ultimate termination of privileges. The hospital prepared a transcript of the hearing.

The chairman of the panel was an experienced attorney acting in a nonadversary capacity. This fact does not deprive the physician of due process; nor does the fact that the hearing panel was made up of staff physicians violate due process, because fundamental fairness under all the facts and circumstances does not necessarily require a hearing panel of physicians totally divorced from or unaware of the case. To be noted also from *Klinge* is that the expense of the hearing is to be borne by the hospital.

Due process does not require that the physician be permitted legal counsel at the hearing.[123] If the hospital attorney is present, however, then the physician should likewise be permitted his lawyer. Moreover, if the doctor simply requests that his attorney be allowed to represent him at the hearing, some experienced hospital attorneys recommend that the request be granted.

Some hospitals' medical staff bylaws provide that applications for appointment and pending disciplinary matters be referred to the

---

[121] See especially the federal district court's opinion in *Sosa v. Board of Managers of Val Verde Hosp.*, *supra* n. 28.

[122] 523 F. 2d 56 (8th Cir. 1975).

[123] *Ascherman v. San Francisco Medical Society, et al.*, 39 Cal. App. 3d 623, 114 Cal. Rptr. 681 (1974). But see: *Garrow v. Elizabeth General Hospital and Dispensary*, 155 N.J. Super. 78, 382 A. 2d 393 (1977). (A private hospital must permit a physician to be represented by counsel at a hearing upon application for appointment.)

entire staff for consideration and a vote. Such provisions are inadvisable and invite legal attack, although whether or not a particular provision is invalid will depend upon the facts and circumstances of each case. In one reported case, a requirement that applicants receive an affirmative vote from 75 per cent of the entire staff in a secret ballot was held to be constitutionally invalid as applied to physicians of a minority race.[124] In contrast, in a pending disciplinary matter, the doctor was not denied due process when he declined the opportunity of a hearing before the entire medical staff, at least in the absence of any indication that the procedural details to be followed would violate the rules of fairness.[125]

A medical staff numbering well over a hundred physicians, however, such as the one in *Suckle*, certainly cannot be fully informed regarding all of the facts and evidence in a medical staff appointment or privilege controversy. The entire staff is not capable of making professional recommendations to the hospital board with respect to particular individuals seeking privileges; and to utilize the staff as a hearing panel—ignoring a sound medical staff committee structure—is to risk the loss of a lawsuit on grounds that due process has been denied.

An issue of current interest and importance is whether or not physicians holding administrative or medico-administrative positions are entitled to procedural due process when removed from their position. First of all, of course, any applicable bylaw provisions providing for notice and hearing must be adhered to; secondly, if the administrator-physician has a specific contract with the hospital the terms of the contract must be honored. As a practical matter, neither a bylaw nor a contractual provision is likely to provide the administrative person with the procedural details of due process—for example, furnishing the reasons for removal in writing, the opportunity at a hearing to introduce evidence in his behalf and rebut adverse evidence, and the opportunity of an appeal.

Traditionally, for many sound reasons, the appointment and removal of persons serving the hospital in an administrative capacity has been viewed as a right of management unencumbered by the requirements of due process. At this writing no court has yet imposed the doctrine of "state action" on a private hospital to require due process in the selection and retention of administrative personnel.

---

[124] *Cypress v. Newport News and Nonsectarian Hospital Ass'n,* 375 F. 2d 648 (4th Cir. 1967).
[125] *Suckle v. Madison General Hospital,* 499 F. 2d 1364 (7th Cir. 1974).

Hence, where all terms of a contract were followed, it was proper to remove a physician from his administrative position as chairman of the surgery department.[126]

The best guide would seem to be this: only when their clinical, medical competence is in question are physicians entitled to due process hearings. The obvious difficulty with this guideline, of course, is that it is not always possible or practical to separate administrative and medical competence. Hence in doubtful cases it would be sound policy for hospital management to grant due process, thus surrendering some managerial "prerogatives" in the interests of preventive law and in furthering better understanding with the medical community.

The granting of procedural due process may seem to some physicians—and hospital board members—to be unduly complicated, time consuming, traumatic, and monetarily expensive. Accordingly some may contend that the implementation of a hearing and appeals procedure is unnecessary or even unwise in the absence of a local case requiring a private hospital to handle medical staff privilege controversies in this fashion. However, failure to recognize and to implement both substantive and procedural due process causes substantial risks. The most evident risk is that failure to be objective and fair invites lawsuits against the hospital by the physician. The emphasis should be on seeing that the implementation of programs to assure quality and of decisions concerning medical staff privileges is kept within the hospital and out of the courts. This is best accomplished by recognizing the doctor's right to due process.

---

[126] *Martin v. Catholic Medical Center of Brooklyn and Queens, Inc.*, 35 N.Y. 2d 901, 324 N.E. 2d 362, 364 N.Y.S. 2d 893 (1974).

Table of Cases

467

Index